Insomnia

Editor

JACK D. EDINGER

SLEEP MEDICINE CLINICS

www.sleep.theclinics.com

Consulting Editor
TEOFILO LEE-CHIONG Jr

September 2013 • Volume 8 • Number 3

ELSEVIER

1600 John F. Kennedy Boulevard • Suite 1800 • Philadelphia, Pennsylvania, 19103-2899

http://www.theclinics.com

SLEEP MEDICINE CLINICS Volume 8, Number 3
September 2013, ISSN 1556-407X, ISBN-13: 978-0-323-18872-2

Editor: Katie Saunders
Developmental Editor: Donald E. Mumford

Sleep Medicine Clinics (ISSN 1556-407X) is published quarterly by Elsevier Inc., 360 Park Avenue South, New York, NY 10010-1710. Months of issue are March, June, September and December. Business and Editorial Offices: 1600 John F. Kennedy Blvd., Ste. 1800, Philadelphia, PA 19103-2899. Customer Service Office: 3251 Riverport Lane, Maryland Heights, MO 63043. Periodicals postage paid at New York, NY and additional mailing offices. Subscription prices are $184.00 per year (US individuals), $91.00 (US residents), $383.00 (US institutions), $226.00 (Canadian and foreign individuals), $127.00 (Canadian and foreign residents) and $422.00 (Canadian and foreign institutions). Foreign air speed delivery is included in all *Clinics* subscription prices. All prices are subject to change without notice. **POSTMASTER:** Send change of address to *Sleep Medicine Clinics*, Elsevier Health Sciences Division, Subscription Customer Service, 3251 Riverport Lane, Maryland Heights, MO 63043. Customer Service: **Tel: 1-800-654-2452 (U.S. and Canada); 314-447-8871 (outside U.S. and Canada). Fax: 314-447-8029. E-mail: journalscustomerservice-usa@elsevier.com (for print support); journalsonlinesupport-usa@elsevier.com (for online support)**.

Reprints. For copies of 100 or more of articles in this publication, please contact the Commercial Reprints Department, Elsevier Inc., 360 Park Avenue South, New York, NY 10010-1710. Tel.: 212-633-3874; Fax: 212-633-3820; E-mail: reprints@elsevier.com.

Printed and bound by CPI Group (UK) Ltd, Croydon, CR0 4YY

Transferred to digital print 2013

PROGRAM OBJECTIVE

The goal of *Sleep Clinics of North America* is to keep practicing physicians up to date with current clinical practice by providing timely articles reviewing the state of the art in patient care.

TARGET AUDIENCE

All practicing physicians and other healthcare professionals.

LEARNING OBJECTIVES

Upon completion of this activity, participants will be able to:

1. Review the role of genes in the insomnia phenotype.
2. Discuss the use of internet and mobile media for delivery of cognitive-behavioralinsomnia therapy
3. Recognize lessons learned from the National Dissemination of Cognitive Behavioral Therapy for Insomnia in the Veterans Health Administration and the impact of training on therapists' self-efficacy and attitudes.

ACCREDITATION

The Elsevier Office of Continuing Medical Education (EOCME) is accredited by the Accreditation Council for Continuing Medical Education (ACCME) to provide continuing medical education for physicians.

The EOCME designates thisenduringmaterial for a maximum of 15 *AMA PRA Category 1 Credit*(s) ™. Physicians should claim only the credit commensurate with the extent of their participation in the activity.

All other health care professionals requesting continuing education credit for this enduring material will be issued a certificate of participation.

DISCLOSURE OF CONFLICTS OF INTEREST

The EOCME assesses conflict of interest with its instructors, faculty, planners, and other individuals who are in a position to control the content of CME activities. All relevant conflicts of interest that are identified are thoroughly vetted by EOCME for fair balance, scientific objectivity, and patient care recommendations. EOCME is committed to providing its learners with CME activities that promote improvements or quality in healthcare and not a specific proprietary business or a commercial interest.

The planning committee, staff, authors and editors listed below have identified no financial relationships or relationships to products or devices they or their spouse/life partner have with commercial interest related to the content of this CME activity:

Wendy Batdorf, PhD; Enda Byrne, PhD; Nicole Congleton; Megan R.Crawford, PhD; Julio Fernandez-Mendoza, PhD; Philip R.Gehrman, PhD, CBSM;Julia Gimeno, BA; Katie Hartner; Allison G.Harvey, PhD; Brynne Hunter; Denise C.Jarrin, PhD; Katherine A. Kaplan, PhD; Bradley E.Karlin, PhD; Sandy Lavery; Nicole Lovato, PhD; Rachel Manber, PhD; Brian McKinstry, MD; Jill McNair; Mahalakshmi Narayanan; Jared Minkel, PhD; Charles M. Morin, PhD; Jason Ong, PhD; Cory Pfeiffenberger, PhD; Dieter Riemann, PhD; Josée Savard, PhD; Marie-Helene Savard, PhD; Allison T. Siebern, PhD, CBSM; Adriane M. Soehner, MA; Kai Spiegelhalder, MD, PhD; C. Barr Taylor, MD; Mickey Trockel, MD; Alexandros N. Vgontzas, MD.

The planning committee, staff, authors and editors listed below have identified financial relationships or relationships to products or devices they or their spouse/life partner have with commercial interest related to the content of this CME activity:

Jack Edinger, PhD has a research grant from Philips-Respironics, Inc., and has royalties/patents from Springer Press and Oxford University Press.

Colin A. Espie, PhD, FBPsS has stock ownership and royalties/patents with Sleepio Ltd/UK; is a consultant/advisor and is on speakers bureau for Novartis; and is on speakers bureau for Boots UK and UCB Pharma.

Peter Hames, MA(Oxon) is employed by and has stock ownership and royalties/patents with Sleepio Ltd/UK.

Andrew D. Krystal, MD is a consultant/advisor for Teva Pharmaceutical Industries, Transcept Pharmaceuticals Inc., Phillips, Somaxon Pharmaceuticals; has research grants with Teva Pharmaceutical Industries, Sunovion Pharmaceuticals Inc., Transcept Pharmaceuticals Inc., Phillips, Astellas Pharma, Abbott Laboratories, and Somaxon Pharmaceuticals.

Leon Lack, PhD is a consultant for and has stock ownership and a research grant with Re-time Pty. Ltd., a wholly owned subsidiary of Flinders University.

Teofilo L. Lee-Chiong Jr, MD is a consultant/advisor for CareCore National and Elsevier; has stock ownership in Philips Respironics; has royalties/patents in Elsevier, Wiley, Lippencott, Oxford University and CreateSpace.

Charles M. Morin, PhD is a consultant/advisor for Merck, Valeant and Novartis; is on speakers bureau for Valeant; and has research grant from Novartis.

UNAPPROVED/OFF-LABEL USE DISCLOSURE

The EOCME requires CME faculty to disclose to the participants:

1. When products or procedures being discussed are off-label, unlabelled, experimental, and/or investigational (not US Food and Drug Administration (FDA) approved); and

2. Any limitations on the information presented, such as data that are preliminary or that represent ongoing research, interim analyses, and/or unsupported opinions. Faculty may discuss information about pharmaceutical agents that is outside of FDA-approved labelling. This information is intended solely for CME and is not intended to promote off-label use of these medications. If you have any questions, contact the medical affairs department of the manufacturer for the most recent prescribing information.

TO ENROLL
To enroll in the Sleep Medicines Clinic Continuing Medical Education program, call customer service at 1-800-654-2452 or sign up online at http://www.theclinics.com/home/cme. The CME program is available to subscribers for an additional annual fee of USD $126.

METHOD OF PARTICIPATION
In order to claim credit, participants must complete the following:
1. Complete enrolment as indicated above.
2. Read the activity.
3. Complete the CME Test and Evaluation. Participants must achieve a score of 70% on the test. All CME Tests and Evaluations must be completed online.

CME INQUIRIES/SPECIAL NEEDS
For all CME inquiries or special needs, please contact elsevierCME@elsevier.com.

SLEEP MEDICINE CLINICS

Contributors

CONSULTING EDITOR

TEOFILO LEE-CHIONG Jr, MD
Professor of Medicine, Division of Pulmonary,
Critical Care and Sleep Medicine, Department
of Medicine, National Jewish Health, University
of Colorado, Denver, Colorado; Chief Medical
Liaison, Philips Respironics, Pennsylvania

EDITOR

JACK D. EDINGER, PhD
Professor, Department of Medicine, National
Jewish Health, Denver, Colorado; Adjunct
Professor, Duke University Medical Center,
Durham, North Carolina

AUTHORS

WENDY BATDORF, PhD
Mental Health Services, U.S. Department of
Veterans Affairs Central Office, Washington,
DC; EBP Training Program Coordinator (ACT,
CBT-D, CBT-I), Department of Veterans Affairs,
Urbandale, Iowa

ENDA M. BYRNE, PhD
Queensland Brain Institute, University of
Queensland, St Lucia, Queensland, Australia

MEGAN R. CRAWFORD, PhD
Postdoctoral Fellow, Department of Behavioral
Science, Rush University Medical Center,
Chicago, Illinois

COLIN A. ESPIE, PhD, FBPsS
Professor of Behavioural Sleep Medicine,
Nuffield Department of Clinical Neurosciences,
Sleep and Circadian Neuroscience Institute,
John Radcliffe Hospital, University of Oxford,
Oxford, United Kingdom

JULIO FERNANDEZ-MENDOZA, PhD
Postdoctoral Scholar, Department of
Psychiatry, Sleep Research & Treatment
Center, Pennsylvania State University College
of Medicine, Hershey, Pennsylvania

PHILIP R. GEHRMAN, PhD, CBSM
Department of Psychiatry, Perelman School of
Medicine, University of Pennsylvania,
Philadelphia, Pennsylvania

JULIA GIMENO, BA
Social Science Research Assistant, Psychiatry
& Behavioral Sciences, Stanford University,
Stanford, California

PETER HAMES, MA(Oxon)
CEO, Sleepio Ltd, London, United Kingdom

ALLISON G. HARVEY, PhD
Professor, Department of Psychology,
University of California, Berkeley, California

DENISE C. JARRIN, PhD
Centre de recherche Université Laval
Robert-Giffard, School of Psychology,
Québec, Canada

KATHERINE A. KAPLAN, MA
Graduate Student, Department of Psychology,
University of California, Berkeley, Berkeley,
California

BRADLEY E. KARLIN, PhD
National Mental Health Director, Psychotherapy and Psychogeriatrics, Mental Health Services, U. S. Department of Veterans Affairs Central Office, Washington, DC; Adjunct Associate Professor, Department of Mental Health, Bloomberg School of Public Health, Johns Hopkins University, Baltimore, Maryland

ANDREW D. KRYSTAL, MD, MS
Professor of Psychiatry and Behavioral Sciences, Duke University School of Medicine, Durham, North Carolina

LEON LACK, PhD
Faculty of Social and Behavioural Sciences, School of Psychology, Flinders University, Bedford Park, Adelaide, South Australia, Australia

NICOLE LOVATO, PhD
Faculty of Social and Behavioural Sciences, Research Associate, School of Psychology, Flinders University, Bedford Park, Adelaide, South Australia, Australia

RACHEL MANBER, PhD
Professor, Psychiatry & Behavioral Sciences and the Stanford Center for Sleep Sciences and Medicine, Stanford University, Stanford, California

BRIAN MCKINSTRY, MD
Professor of Primary Care E-Health, Centre for Population Health Sciences, University of Edinburgh, Edinburgh, United Kingdom

JARED MINKEL, PhD
Medical Instructor, Department of Psychiatry and Behavioral Sciences, Duke University School of Medicine, Durham, NC; Department of Psychiatry, University of North Carolina School of Medicine, NC

CHARLES M. MORIN, PhD
Centre de recherche Université Laval Robert-Giffard, School of Psychology, Québec, Canada

JASON C. ONG, PhD
Assistant Professor, Department of Behavioral Science, Rush University Medical Center, Chicago, Illinois

CORY PFEIFFENBERGER, PhD
Translational Research Laboratories, Center for Sleep and Circadian Neurobiology, Perelman School of Medicine, University of Pennsylvania, Philadelphia, Pennsylvania

DIETER RIEMANN, PhD
Department of Psychiatry and Psychotherapy, University of Freiburg Medical Center, Freiburg, Germany

JOSÉE SAVARD, PhD
Professor, School of Psychology, Laval University; Centre de recherche du CHU de Québec, Laval University Cancer Research Center, Québec, Québec, Canada

MARIE-HÉLÈNE SAVARD, PhD
Research Professional, Centre de recherche du CHU de Québec, Laval University Cancer Research Center, Québec, Québec, Canada

ALLISON T. SIEBERN, PhD
Clinical Assistant Professor, Psychiatry & Behavioral Sciences and the Stanford Center for Sleep Sciences and Medicine, Stanford University, Redwood City, California

ADRIANE M. SOEHNER, MA
Graduate Student, Department of Psychology, University of California, Berkeley, Berkeley, California

KAI SPIEGELHALDER, MD, PhD
Department of Psychiatry and Psychotherapy, University of Freiburg Medical Center; Freiburg Institute of Advanced Studies (FRIAS), University of Freiburg, Freiburg, Germany

C. BARR TAYLOR, MD
Emeritus (Active) Professor, Psychiatry & Behavioral Sciences, Stanford University, Stanford, California

MICKEY TROCKEL, MD, PhD
Clinical Assistant Professor, Psychiatry & Behavioral Sciences, Stanford University, Stanford, California

ALEXANDROS N. VGONTZAS, MD
Professor, Department of Psychiatry, Sleep Research & Treatment Center, Pennsylvania State University College of Medicine, Hershey, Pennsylvania

Contents

This article summarizes recent epidemiologic evidence on insomnia, including its prevalence, incidence, and risk factors, as well as its course and consequences. Insomnia is a significant public health problem. It is a highly prevalent condition, both as a symptom and a syndrome, and is often a persistent condition over time. Its persistence is associated with increased risk for mental, physical, and occupational health problems. Chronic insomnia also carries heavy economic burden. These findings have direct implications for community-based prevention and intervention programs and for future research.

In this article, the evidence for hyperarousal in insomnia is reviewed, with an emphasis on neurobiological studies. Indicators of physiologic hyperarousal include electroencephalography-derived polysomnographic, autonomic, and neuroendocrine variables and outcome parameters of neuroimaging studies. Most studies documented an increased physiologic arousal in patients with insomnia, but it is not known whether physiologic hyperarousal is a cause or consequence of insomnia, what is the genetic basis of hyperarousal and what is the impact of early-life stressors and other life events, and what is the neurobiological basis of hyperarousal and how can it be modified in the most efficient manner.

We review evidence that insomnia with objective short sleep duration is associated with physiologic hyperarousal; higher risk for hypertension, diabetes, neurocognitive impairment, and mortality; and with a persistent course. We propose that objective measures of sleep be included in the diagnosis of insomnia and its subtypes, objective measures of sleep obtained in the home environment of the patient would become part of the routine assessment and diagnosis of insomnia in a clinician's office setting, and insomnia with short sleep duration may respond better to biologic treatments, whereas insomnia with normal sleep duration may respond primarily to psychological therapies.

With the development of genetic model systems for sleep, it seems logical to use them to screen human insomnia genetic studies for bona fide hits and to further characterize the mechanisms behind insomnia. This must be an important component of future research on the genetics of insomnia. Understanding of the role of genes in the insomnia phenotype is limited. There are several molecular genetic tools available that were not in existence even a few years ago. The time is ripe for research on the genetics of insomnia that may finally shed light on the mechanisms of this common sleep disorder.

the syndrome level. This review summarizes available prevalence estimates and empirical evidence on the evolution of insomnia complaints throughout the cancer care trajectory. Potential etiologic factors (predisposing, precipitating, and perpetuating factors) are discussed. Available empirical findings on the efficacy of nonpharmacologic treatments for sleep difficulties in patients with cancer, in particular cognitive-behavioral therapy (CBT), are presented. Several areas for future research are proposed, including strategies to improve accessibility to CBT for insomnia in clinical settings.

Emerging evidence suggests that comorbid insomnia has a negative impact on the treatment of obstructive sleep apnea (OSA), particularly with adherence to positive airway pressure therapy. Furthermore, the two conditions together are associated with greater morbidity of psychiatric, medical, and other sleep disorders. In discussing the clinical implications of such evidence, sleep clinicians should conduct comprehensive evaluations for both OSA and insomnia. Moreover, patient management should include considerations to treating both OSA and insomnia. Future research should include studies aimed at understanding the pathophysiology of the comorbid condition, improving diagnostic tools and evaluating the effectiveness of treatment combinations.

Cognitive behavioral therapy for insomnia (CBT-I) is a highly effective and well-established treatment, but patient access is limited because few clinicians are trained to deliver the therapy. The Veterans Health Administration (VHA) is nationally disseminating CBT-I as part of its efforts to make evidence-based psychotherapies widely available to Veterans. As part of this dissemination effort, the VHA has implemented a national, competency-based CBT-I training program. This article describes the training methods and the impact of training on therapists' use of CBT-I and on their self-efficacy to deliver and attitudes toward CBT-I.

Cognitive behavioral therapy (CBT) is an effective treatment of insomnia disorder. CBT has traditionally been delivered by a therapist in a clinic; however, the ubiquitous nature of the Internet and increasing penetration of mobile devices offers new possibilities. Moreover, there are limitations to face-to-face therapy, particularly in relation to between-session home implementation. This article, therefore, presents the opportunity afforded by technological development, not only to meet the need and demand for CBT but also to improve insomnia care both at the level of the individual patient and at population level.

Foreword
Insomnia

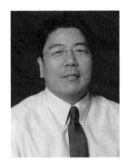

Teofilo Lee-Chiong Jr, MD
Consulting Editor

I have often wondered how individuals managed their insomnias before our current era of hypnotic medications and cognitive behavioral therapy.

Undoubtedly, ancient civilizations did not possess any technology that would have permitted the development of jet lag—not even their fastest sailing ships (or balloons as some archeological evidence seems to suggest were being used then) could have reached speeds fast enough to traverse multiple time zones within a single day. Were there other means of rapid travel invented by humans eons ago that, regrettably, have been forgotten in the mists of unrecorded history? Even if there were, these would have been very limited.

Shift work was very limited in past ages as well. Surely, the security of the townspeople required night watchmen to guide their towers, ports, or borders. The Great Wall protected the Chinese nation for centuries not so much by the expanse of its mortared walls but by a system of watchtowers—with watchmen on duty 24 hours each day—situated strategically above the horizon that enabled an almost instantaneous relay of lighted torches alarming the populace of invading armies. There may also have been messengers that had to travel nonstop to deliver urgent messages, either on foot or on horseback, regarding royal edicts or enemy troop movements to distant townships or army camps. Finally, there were stargazers who tracked the movements of heavenly bodies across the evening sky in order to record the passing of the seasons as well as to discern from patterns unfolding in the firmaments that reveal once heretofore hidden predictions of future events. Mastery over the night was as essential to civilization then as now; hence, ancient societies needed shift workers as much as we do today.

But what of the lone individual who stayed awake all night amidst a family or tribe asleep within the same cave, hut, or open night sky? What became of him? Did he ruminate about past anxieties or plan for forthcoming activities? Were delayed sleep phasers left behind when the rest of the pack arose with the sun and moved on? Similarly, was advanced sleep phase ever a problem then if everyone else fell asleep early as night enveloped them? Which did he fear more—the night itself or the imagined dangers possibly lurking within its darkness? Was the campfire a friend or foe to his sleep—in short, did light afford better sleep that was unencumbered by fears of unsuspected attacks or did he, instead, distracted by the illuminescence, turn away from it to slumber in the shadows of the evening?

Did man create alcohol not so much as to celebrate his victories or forget defeats but to somehow ease his seemingly endless sleeplessness? Did he experiment with different plants, fruits, and flowers, boiling some and drying others, in order to extract soporific essences from them—and if he did (and we are almost certain he did so), how many failed attempts, adverse effects, and, even, fatal ingestions, did ancient botanists endure as they sought the cure for man's sleep

Sleep Med Clin 8 (2013) xiii–xiv
http://dx.doi.org/10.1016/j.jsmc.2013.08.002

disturbances? Did man trephine, bleed, paste, paint, stab, or immerse his body to cease the insomniac's turmoil? Or did he appeal to his gods or simply leave it to fate?

I have often wondered how future generations would think of the ways we manage insomnia today—would they find our therapies abhorrent or will they be amused by our failures? Will future sleep clinicians and researchers find the ultimate cure for insomnia that would, finally and for all times, render all insomnia specialists irrelevant and end our profession and careers? I have often wondered about these things, and others, during my own sleepless nights.

Teofilo Lee-Chiong Jr, MD
Professor of Medicine
National Jewish Health
Denver, Colorado 80123, USA

Professor of Medicine
University of Colorado Denver
Aurora, Colorado 80044, USA

Chief Medical Liaison
Philips Respironics
Monroeville, Pennsylvania 15146, USA

E-mail address:
Lee-ChiongT@NJC.ORG

Preface
Insomnia

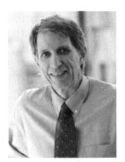

Jack D. Edinger, PhD
Editor

It is often said that a little knowledge is a dangerous thing. Well, maybe lacking knowledge is not always dangerous, but the naiveté accompanying this state can often lead you to underestimate the challenges you actually face. As I look back 31 years when I entered the field of sleep medicine and began to focus my clinical and research efforts on insomnia patients, I recall thinking what a simple and straightforward group of patients they comprised. In fact, I often tell the story that I became intrigued with this patient group after I successfully treated my first insomnia patient following one reading of a chapter written by Richard Bootzin describing stimulus control therapy. I specifically recall how relatively gratifying it was to implement such an easy-to-administer intervention and have the patient show marked improvement in just a few weeks. This experience was so unlike the more haphazard outcomes I observed with other forms of psychological interventions I had tried to that early point in my career. This one experience led me to spend the last 31 years specializing in insomnia treatment and focusing the majority of my research toward the understanding and management this disorder. During my professional voyage over this time period, I have become nothing but truly convinced how naïve my initial view of this patient group really was.

Perhaps it is not until one bloodies his or her professional nose that the realization comes as to how complex a chosen field of study actual is. Probably some of my more humbling professional experiences have come in my work focused on the diagnostic classification of insomnia. On the one hand I can say I have been fortunate to have had opportunities to lead the insomnia classification workgroups for both the second and the third editions of the International Classification of Sleep Disorders (ICSD-2 and ICSD-3). On the other hand I have to admit that such experiences have been eye-opening and in many ways unsettling. In our work on the ICSD-2, we tried to improve the diagnostic criteria sets for the original ICSD insomnia diagnoses and provide more operation definitions for insomnia subtyping. While we were quite proud of our work, we subsequently learned through a large collaborative study that the reliability and validity of many of the insomnia subtypes we carefully tried to define were dismally poor.[1] Moreover, by rubbing shoulders with my fellow nosologists, I have learned that what we know about the pathophysiology and subtyping of insomnia pales in comparison to what is known about other types of sleep disorders. And about that first patient I treated 31 years ago…. Well, I ran into him about 6 years ago in one of my clinics and found that not only had his insomnia returned over the years, but he also developed significant comorbid depression and anxiety problems as well. Moreover he had forgotten that I had ever seen him in the past—a humbling experience indeed.

It is just that humble and hopefully more enlightened spirit that led me to accept this invitation to serve as guest editor for this sleep insomnia issue of *Sleep Medicine Clinics*. After all, it wouldn't hurt to learn a bit more about this topic field and continue to chip away at the nascent naiveté that seduced me into my career while I was still

Sleep Med Clin 8 (2013) xv–xvi
http://dx.doi.org/10.1016/j.jsmc.2013.07.011

professionally wet behind the ears. Of course much has been learned about insomnia over the past 30+ years but what has been learned has also informed us about how much more there is to learn. In forging this issue, I thought it best to offer readers a bit of a journey through insomnia as a sort of past, present, and future tour of this topic area. Thus, the articles included in this issue provide the reader a fairly thorough historic review of selected areas of insomnia research and also pose new and exciting directions for us to pursue.

This issue is divided into two major sections. Section 1, entitled, "Understanding the Nature, Impact, and Etiology of Insomnia," includes a selection of articles describing the prevalence, morbidity, and potentially important factors related to the pathophysiology and etiology of insomnia disorders. The initial article by Morin and Jarrin provides the reader an up-to-date overview of what is known about the epidemiology of insomnia. The subsequent article by Spiegelhalder and Dieter Riemann provides a review of what is known about the potential role of hyperarousal in insomnia, whereas the article by Vgontzas and Fernandez-Mendoza poses an interesting hypothesis about the role of psychophysiological hyperarousal in the development of a particularly serve insomnia subtype. Finally, the article by Gehrman, Pfeiffenberger, and Byrne provides a cutting-edge update about genetic research on insomnia and where such research may take us.

Section 2, entitled, "Challenges and Methods in Insomnia Management," provides a collection of articles focused on insomnia treatment methods and the challenges posed in managing the range of patient types who present clinically. The initial article by Minkel and Krystal provides an exhaustive review of what is known about the pharmacological management of insomnia patients and highlights areas for future development in this area. The subsequent article by Lovato and Lack discusses the use of bright light therapy in the management of insomnia sufferers with sleep onset and sleep maintenance complaints. The subsequent four articles have been written by groups who are on the frontier of learning how best to management various forms of comorbid insomnia. Specifically, these articles focus on the management of insomnia occurring comorbid to serious psychiatric illnesses (Soehner, Kaplan, and Harvey), chronic pain (Finan, Buenaver, Coryell, and Smith), cancer (Savard and Savard), and sleep apnea (Ong and Crawford). In the final two articles, the authors describe two rather distinctive approaches to address the challenge of too few providers for too many patients. Specifically, these articles describe methods for disseminating cognitive behavioral insomnia therapy (CBT). The article by Manber, Trockel, Batdorf, Siebern, Taylor, Gimeno, and Karlin describes the largest provider-training program ever devised for the dissemination of CBT within a health care system. Finally, the article by Espie, Hames, and McKinstry provides a very entertaining and provocative description of an animated online intervention program for CBT delivery.

For the novice, this issue should provide an updated overview of where we have been and where we hope to go in our understanding and management of insomnia. In contrast, it is hoped that this issue will provide the more seasoned expert new research ideas that help move the field forward. And, for both, it is hoped that this issue will eliminate any naiveté that leads to underestimating the challenges a true mastery of this topic area poses.

Jack D. Edinger, PhD
Department of Medicine
National Jewish Health
Denver, CO, USA

Duke University Medical Center
Durham, NC, USA

E-mail address:
EdingerJ@NJHealth.org

REFERENCE

1. Edinger JD, Wyatt JK, Stepanski EJ, et al. Testing the reliability and validity of DSM-IV-TR and ICSD-2 insomnia diagnoses: results of a multi-method/multi-trait analysis. Arch Gen Psychiatry 2011;68(10): 992–1002.

Section 1: Understanding the Nature, Impact and Etiology of Insomnia

Epidemiology of Insomnia
Prevalence, Course, Risk Factors, and Public Health Burden

Charles M. Morin, PhD*, Denise C. Jarrin, PhD

KEYWORDS

• Insomnia • Sleep disorders • Epidemiology • Prevalence • Incidence • Risk factors

KEY POINTS

- The epidemiology of insomnia has received increased attention in the last decade and investigators have moved from a purely cross-sectional approach to a more prospective and longitudinal approach.
- Progress on the epidemiology of insomnia has been hampered by important methodological shortcomings including, but not limited to, the lack of a consistent case definition and standardized assessment procedures across studies.
- Additional prospective and longitudinal studies are needed to identify early precursors of insomnia and factors moderating its trajectories over time.
- A better understanding of how insomnia evolves over time and what factors trigger an episode or perpetuate it over time is critical for developing effective prevention and treatment programs.

INTRODUCTION

Insomnia is a significant public health problem, which affects large segments of the population at one point or another in life. The burden of chronic insomnia is also widespread both for the individual, in terms of reduced quality of life, and for society at large, in terms of work absenteeism, disability, and health care costs. Although significant advances have been made in therapeutics, there is more limited knowledge on its epidemiology, risk factors, long-term course, and prognosis. A better understanding of these critical issues would be informative to develop more effective therapies. This article summarizes the evidence on the epidemiology of insomnia, including its natural history, prevalence, incidence, and risk factors, as well as its long-term consequences and public health burden. In addition, some directions for future population-based research and for developing effective prevention programs are outlined.

NATURE OF INSOMNIA AND UPDATED DIAGNOSTIC CRITERIA

Insomnia is characterized by a spectrum of complaints reflecting dissatisfaction with the quality, duration, or continuity of sleep. The predominant nocturnal symptoms include difficulties falling asleep at bedtime, waking up in the middle of the night and having difficulty going back to sleep, or waking up too early in the morning with an inability to return to sleep.[1,2] These difficulties are not mutually exclusive, as a person may experience mixed problems initiating and maintaining sleep. In

Disclosure: Preparation of this article was supported by the Canadian Institutes of Health Research (MOP42504) and by the National Institutes of Health (MH078188 and MH60413).
Centre de Recherche, Institut Universitaire en Santé Mentale de Québec, Université Laval Robert-Giffard, School of Psychology, Québec, Canada
* Corresponding author. Université Laval, School of Psychology, Pavillon Félix-Antoine Savard, 2325, rue des Bibliothèques, Québec, QC G1V 0A6, Canada.
E-mail address: cmorin@psy.ulaval.ca

Sleep Med Clin 8 (2013) 281–297
http://dx.doi.org/10.1016/j.jsmc.2013.05.002

addition to nighttime sleep difficulties, daytime symptoms represent an integral component of insomnia. These symptoms include fatigue or decreased energy, cognitive impairments involving attention, concentration and memory, and mood disturbances (eg, irritability, dysphoria).[3–5] These latter symptoms contribute to significant role impairments[6] and are often the primary concern prompting patients to seek treatment.[7]

Several important changes have been made to the diagnostic criteria of insomnia in the *Diagnostic and Statistical Manual of Mental Disorders, Fifth Edition* DSM-5[2] and in the *International Classification of Sleep Disorders, Third Edition* (ICSD-III).[8] For example, the symptom of nonrestorative sleep has been eliminated from the insomnia definition, mainly because this complaint is ill defined and not specific to insomnia. In the DSM-5,[2] the duration threshold for chronic insomnia has also been increased from 1 to 3 months, a change based on evidence that 3 months is a critical period, after which insomnia is more likely to persist[9] and its morbidity becomes more noticeable.[10] Likewise, a minimal frequency of 3 nights per week has been added to further operationalize the definition of clinical insomnia. More importantly, the DSM-V[2] no longer makes a distinction between primary insomnia and insomnia secondary to a psychiatric, medical, or another sleep disorder. This change was predicated on the evidence that when insomnia is comorbid with another disorder (eg, major depression), it is often difficult, if not impossible, to determine which disorder is the cause and which is the consequence. Historically, clinicians generally have assumed that insomnia was symptomatic of a more important disorder and that treating the underlying disorder (eg, depression, pain) would also improve sleep; as such, insomnia was often overlooked and undertreated. There is now solid evidence that insomnia is a prevalent residual symptom, even after successful treatment of depression[11] and its persistence increases the risk of relapse of depression.[12] Furthermore, although insomnia has long been conceptualized as a symptom of another disorder, there is strong evidence showing that chronic insomnia is also a precursor or a risk factor for new-onset psychiatric disorders.[13] By moving away from the need to make a causal attribution between insomnia and coexisting disorders, it is hoped that clinicians will pay more attention to insomnia as a disorder on its own. Recent treatment studies have shown that when insomnia is comorbid with another psychiatric or medical disorder, treatment outcome is better when attending to both insomnia and the comorbid condition than when attending to the comorbid condition alone.[14,15]

PREVALENCE AND CORRELATES OF INSOMNIA
Prevalence

At least 50 epidemiologic studies on insomnia were published between the first population-based surveys by Karacan and colleagues[16] and Bixler and colleagues[17] in the 1970s and a landmark review paper in 2002 by Ohayon[18] and, since then, at least another 20 studies have been published. Prevalence estimates of insomnia vary widely across studies, partly because of differences in case definitions, assessment procedures, sample characteristics, and length of assessment intervals. With regard to the last point, most studies used point estimates (ie, past month), although some have relied on longer intervals (ie, past year or even lifetime). Depending on the specific definitions used (ie, insomnia symptoms vs disorder, sleep dissatisfaction), prevalence rates have varied from as low as 5% to as high as 50%.[18] In general, population-based data indicate that about one-third of adults (30%–36%) report at least one nocturnal insomnia symptom (ie, difficulty initiating or maintaining sleep, nonrestorative sleep), but this rate decreases to between 10% and 15% when daytime consequences (eg, fatigue) are added to the case definition. Rates of sleep dissatisfaction, without regard to specific sleep diagnosis, also vary widely (10%–25%) in the adult population. When using more stringent and operational DSM[2] or ICSD[19] diagnostic criteria, prevalence rates tend to cluster between 6% and 10%.[6,7,20–22] These highly variable estimates underscore the need to rely on operational definitions and standardized assessment procedures to derive accurate and comparable prevalence rates across studies.

Although the most common single symptom of insomnia is difficulty maintaining sleep, mixed difficulties in sleep onset and maintenance are more prevalent than any single complaint.[6,7,20,22] Among subtypes of sleep maintenance problems, both middle-of-the-night and early morning awakenings are equally prevalent, although the latter are more common among older adults.[22,23] Nonrestorative sleep is also a prevalent complaint, but less frequently as a single complaint; it is typically reported in association with other insomnia symptoms and also in association with several other sleep disorders. Its nonspecificity has led to its exclusion from the insomnia definition in both DSM-5[2] and ICSD-III.[8]

Insomnia is also highly prevalent in primary care medicine, usually the first entry point to access professional care for insomnia, with about 40% of patients reporting significant sleep disturbances.[24]

Patients with more severe and more chronic insomnia, more comorbid medical or psychiatric disorders, and those who are better educated are more likely to seek treatment of insomnia.[25]

Correlates of Insomnia

Insomnia is consistently more prevalent among women, middle-aged and older adults, shift workers, and patients with coexisting medical and psychiatric disorders. With regard to gender, a meta-analysis[26] revealed a risk ratio of 1.41 for women versus men. Although insomnia has a greater overall prevalence in middle-aged and older adults, the nature of insomnia interacts with age, such that sleep maintenance difficulties are more common among middle-aged and older adults, whereas sleep initiation difficulties are more frequent among younger adults.[6,18,22]

Strong associations (odds ratios = 4.0–6.0) have been reported between insomnia and poor mental and physical health, psychological distress, anxiety and depressive symptoms, as well as with somatic symptoms and poor self-rated physical health.[6,7,20,27,28] Insomnia has also been associated with lower socioeconomic status and with living alone (eg, single, separated, or widowed). Hormonal replacement therapy was found in one study to be a protective factor against insomnia in older adults.[23]

Prevalence Across Ethnicities and Cultures

In a nation-wide sleep survey in the United States, insomnia in adults was diagnosed in 10% of Whites, 7% of Hispanics, 4% of Asians, and 3% of African Americans.[29] Likewise, insomnia prevalence rates in European American, African American, and Mexican American adolescents were 5.3%, 5.2%, and 3.5%, respectively.[30] Comparative studies between immigrants and nonimmigrants have provided mixed results, with some research indicating immigrants report fewer,[31,32] more,[33] or similar numbers[34] of sleep complaints or insomnia symptoms compared with their nonimmigrant counterparts. These discrepancies may be attributed to the differences in sleep attitudes and beliefs reported across diverse ethnicities and cultures, including what individuals believe to be the causes and the consequences of sleep problems,[34] as well as the priority placed on obtaining adequate sleep within cultures.[32]

Although there are few direct cross-cultural comparisons of insomnia, a worldwide study found that the highest prevalence rates of insomnia were in Brazil (79.8%), followed by South Africa (45.3%), Eastern Europe (32%), Asia (28.3%), and Western Europe (23.2%).[35] In another cross-country survey, the highest prevalence rates of insomnia symptoms were reported in Western Europe (37.2%), followed by the United States (27%), and Japan (6.6%).[36] Prevalence rates of restless sleep (as opposed to insomnia) across 23 countries in Europe were less than 10% in Mediterranean and Nordic countries, ranged from 11% to 22% in Western European countries, and from 25% to 37% in Eastern European countries among working-aged adults.[37] Likewise, the highest prevalence rates of sleep problems were found in the United States (56%), followed by Western Europe (31%) and Japan (23%).[38] Cross-cultural studies in pediatric samples suggest that toddlers and children from Asian cultures (eg, Hong Kong, India, Singapore) tend to go to bed at later times, wake up at earlier times, report shorter sleep durations, and are perceived by parents to show more sleep problems compared with children from White cultures (eg, Canada, United Kingdom, New Zealand).[39,40]

People from different cultures experience, perceive, and understand health problems differently, possibly as a result of religious beliefs, stigma, reasoning fallacy, differences in symptom presentation, processing, and expressing experiences.[41,42] These cultural differences can affect whether insomnia is perceived as normal (part of everyday life) or abnormal. For example, waking up in the middle of the night is sometimes seen as a gift for some religions, because it provides an additional opportunity to pray. Further qualitative research would be helpful to better understand cross-cultural and ethnic differences in the phenomenologic experience and expression of insomnia, because this may help develop more targeted prevention and intervention strategies.

INCIDENCE AND RISK FACTORS
Incidence

There are few longitudinal incidence studies (**Table 1**) compared with the large number of cross-sectional prevalence studies. Nonetheless, incidence rates vary extensively across studies, depending on the case definition (eg, symptoms vs syndrome) and the interval used to track new onset. For instance, four population-based studies using the same 12-month interval between baseline and follow-up assessments revealed incidence rates of 2.8% in Sweden,[21] 6.0% in the United States,[27] 7.4% in Canada,[43] and 15% in the United Kingdom,[44] with the variability being partly accounted for by different case definitions across studies. For example, a Canadian study[43] found an incidence rate of 30.7% for insomnia symptoms compared with 7.4% for an insomnia

Table 1
Summary of prevalence, incidence, and persistence rates of insomnia in population-based longitudinal, prospective studies

Author	Sample (Number, Age [y])	Follow-up Interval	Case Definition	Prevalence (%)	Incidence (%)	Persistence (%)
Ellis et al,[46] 2012	General population (1095, 32.72)	1 mo 3 mo	Acute insomnia: previous/ongoing problems with initiating/maintaining sleep, early awakenings, feeling unrefreshed upon waking (3 d–3 mo) DSM-5 & prolonged sleep onset, wake after sleep onset, low quality of life First onset: acute insomnia, no past sleep problem, no comorbidity Recurrent episode: first onset with previous sleep problem	Acute insomnia: 7.9 First onset: 33.7 Recurrent: 48.8	Acute insomnia: 1 mo: 4.37 3 mo: 9.15 DSM-5: 1 mo: 3.4 3 mo: 7.8 First onset: 1 mo: 61.1 3 mo: 4.4	—
LeBlanc et al,[43] 2009	General population (464 [good sleepers], ≥18)	6 mo 1 y	Symptoms: initial, maintenance, or late insomnia (≥3 nights/wk) or use of sleep-promoting medication Syndrome: dissatisfied with sleep, initial, maintenance, or late insomnia (≥3 nights/wk) for at least a month & daytime impairment or use of prescribed medication (≥3 nights/wk)	—	Overall symptoms (no previous insomnia): 30.7 (28.8) 6 mo: 14.4 (5.77) 1 y: 13.5 (6.82) Overall syndrome: 7.3 (3.9) 6 mo: 2.37 (1.57) 1 y: 4.52 (2.09)	—
Ford & Kramer,[27] 1989	Community sample (7954, 18–≥65)	1 y	Diagnostic interview (DSM-III) Report difficulty initiating/maintaining sleep, or early awakening (≥2 wk) in past 6 mo	10.2	6	31

Study	Sample	Duration	Definition			
Roberts et al,[47] 1999	General population (2380, 50–102)	1 y	Report difficulty initiating/maintaining sleep in past 2 wk	23.4	9	13
Fok et al,[54] 2010	Community sample (656, ≥65)	1 y	Report trouble sleeping in past month	44.7	21.4	66.3
Jansson & Linton,[120] 2006	General population (1530, 20–60)	1 y	Report difficulty initiating/maintaining sleep, early awakening & daytime problems (≥3 nights/wk) in past 3 mo	10	6	—
Morphy et al,[44] 2007	General population (2363, 18–98)	1 y	Symptoms: report difficulty initiating/maintaining sleep, nocturnal awakenings (on most nights) in past month Syndrome: symptoms & waking up tired	Overall: 36.8 Symptoms: 30.4 Syndrome: 13.2	Overall: 14.6 Symptoms: 13.3 Syndrome: 6.8	Overall: 69.2 Symptoms: 67.9 Syndrome: 54.8
Jansson-Frojmark et al,[21] 2008	General population (1746, 20–60)	1 y	Report difficulty initiating/maintaining sleep, early awakening & daytime problems (≥3 nights/wk) in past 3 mo	6.8–9.7	2.8	44.4
Jansson-Frojmark & Lindblom,[121] 2008	General population (1498, 20–60)	1 y	Report sleep problem & difficulty initiating/maintaining sleep (3 nights/wk) in past 3 mo	15	—	14
Skapinakis et al,[122] 2012	Adults (2406, 16–74)	1.5 y	Report difficulty initiating/maintaining sleep in past month	57.7	15.8	—
Kim et al,[55] 2009	Community sample (909, ≥65)	2 y	Report difficulty initiating/maintaining sleep Symptoms: 1–2 nights/wk over month Syndrome: ≥3 nights/wk over month	Overall: 27 Symptoms: 32 Syndrome: 21	Overall: 23 Symptoms: 37 Syndrome: 20	Overall: 40 Symptoms: 38 Syndrome: 41
Komada et al,[123] 2012	General population (1434, ≥20)	2 y	Pittsburgh Sleep Quality Index cutoff score ≥5.5	30.7	12.9	18.7

(continued on next page)

Table 1
(continued)

Author	Sample (Number, Age [y])	Follow-up Interval	Case Definition	Prevalence (%)	Incidence (%)	Persistence (%)
Morin et al,[53] 2009	Population-based (388, M = 44.8 [13.9])	3 y	Symptoms: initial, maintenance, or late insomnia (>3 nights/wk) or use of sleep-promoting medication Syndrome: dissatisfied with sleep, initial, maintenance, or late insomnia (≥3 nights/wk) for at least a month & daytime impairment or use of prescribed medication (≥3 nights/wk)	—	—	Symptoms: 1 y: 23.4 2 y: 8.4 3 y: 37.2 ≥1 y: 69.0 Syndrome: 1 y: 11.3 2 y: 9.0 3 y: 66.1 ≥1 y: 86.4
Breslau et al,[45] 1996	HMO group (1007, 21–30)	3.5 y	Report difficulty initiating/ maintaining sleep, early morning awakening (2 wk) Lifetime history of insomnia	Insomnia (no comorbidity): 16.6 Lifetime history: 24.6	Overall: 13.3 Lifetime history: 45 No lifetime: 8.7	—
Morgan & Clark,[56] 1997	Elderly adults (1042, ≥65)	4 y	Report sleep problem "often or all the time" in past week	—	3.1 (weighted)	36.1
Zhang et al,[28] 2012	Adults (2316, 46.3)	5.2 y	Report difficulty initiating/ maintaining sleep, early morning awakening, daytime symptoms Symptoms: 3/wk over 1 y Syndrome: symptoms & daytime symptoms	Symptoms: 7.1 Syndrome: 4.8	Overall: 5.9 Symptoms: 3.6 Syndrome: 2.3	Overall: 36.5 Symptoms: 29.5 Syndrome: 47.0
Fernandez-Mendoza et al,[124] 2012	Random general population (1395, ≥20)	7.5 y	Poor sleep: moderate/severe difficulty initiating/ maintaining sleep, early final awakening, daytime symptoms Insomnia: insomnia complaint lasting >1y	Poor sleep: 32.3	Poor sleep: 18.4 Poor sleep to insomnia: 16.8	38.4

Study	Population	Follow-up	Definition			
Vgontzas et al,[125] 2012	Random general population (1395, ≥20)	7.5 y	Insomnia compliant lasting >1y	11.9	—	43.6
Singareddy et al,[126] 2012	Random general population (1395, ≥20)	7.5 y	Chronic insomnia: "Do you feel you have insomnia with a duration of at least 1 y?"	10.6	9.3 (weighted)	—
Silversen et al,[69] 2012	Population-based (24,715, 19–80)	11 y	DSM-IV, onset, terminal, later insomnia & daytime symptoms in past month	5.1	6.5	19.2
Buysse et al,[66] 2008	Population sample (278 [all 6 interviews], baseline age 20)	20 y	Based on symptom, duration & frequency of episodes in past year 1 mo: sleep difficulties for ≥1 mo & daytime impairments 2–3 wk: at least once over past year Recurrent brief: <2 wk recurring at least monthly over past year Occasional brief: <2 wk duration occurring less than monthly	Cumulative weighted 1 mo: 19.8 2–3 wk: 9.7 Recurrent brief: 20.6 Occasional brief: 17.5	—	At any future interview: 1 mo: 39 2–3 wk: 31 Recurrent brief: 40 Occasional brief: 30

Note: Summary of results are presented from shortest to longest follow-up intervals.

syndrome. Another important variable explaining some of the variability is whether investigators make a distinction between incident cases of first episode (ie, no previous history of insomnia) and cases of recurrence (ie, with past insomnia episodes). For example, the 7.4% incidence rates in the LeBlanc and colleagues[43] study decreased almost by half (3.9%) when only individuals without previous lifetime episode of insomnia were included in the case definition. A similar finding had also been reported (13.1% vs 8.7%) in a sample of young adults.[45]

Another variable that affects incidence rates is whether the reported rate includes all cumulative cases emerging between baseline and follow-up assessments (cumulative incidence) or only new cases present at the second assessment (point estimate). Because insomnia is a condition that often fluctuates over time, it is plausible that a new case might emerge after baseline assessment but remit by the follow-up assessment point. A recent study[46] examined the distribution of three subtypes of acute insomnia as a function of duration and found a significant difference between the 1-month (4.4%) and 3-month (9.2%) incidence rates; in addition, recurrent acute insomnia (3.8%) was more common than first episode of acute insomnia (2.6%) and comorbid acute insomnia (1.4%).

A related issue that may explain some of the variability in incidence rates is the time frame used to assess insomnia. In the LeBlanc and colleagues[43] study, assessment of insomnia at each time point was based on the previous month only, rather than the entire 6-month and 12-month intervals, which may have yielded more conservative rates because it did not capture those cases that developed insomnia and subsequently remitted within the follow-up intervals. Because insomnia is often waxing and waning, it is plausible that the incidence rates have been underestimated in some of these studies.

Risk Factors

Although several insomnia correlates have been identified reliably across studies, the data about risk factors predisposing to insomnia are more tentative. Nonetheless, the most commonly hypothesized factors predisposing to insomnia include demographic factors, such as female gender and older age, and a personal or familial history of insomnia. Women are at greater risk for insomnia, and perhaps more so during menopause, because of hormonal changes. The risk of insomnia also increases with aging, but this may be the result of increased health problems with aging rather than age per se.[47] The risk of insomnia

is also higher among first-degree family members of individuals with insomnia than in the general population,[48,49] although it remains unclear whether this link is inherited through a genetic predisposition, learned by observations of parental models, or simply a by-product of another (eg, psychiatric) disorder. A past personal history of insomnia has also been identified as an important risk for future episodes of insomnia.[43]

Psychological and a biological predisposition are two additional factors that have been linked to greater risk to develop insomnia. The psychological vulnerability to insomnia is typically characterized by an anxiety-prone personality, with increased scores on measures of anxiety and depressive symptoms, worries, perfectionism, introversion, and lower abilities to cope with day-to-day stressful situations.[43] On the other hand, the biological vulnerability is characterized by indices of hyperarousability and increased hypothalamic-pituitary-adrenal axis activity.[50] Although this latter hypothesis has been around for some time,[51,52] it still remains unclear whether hyperarousal is a state that characterizes an individual's response to sleep difficulties or their apprehension, or a more enduring trait that predisposes some individuals to develop insomnia under stressful circumstances.

COURSE OF INSOMNIA: PERSISTENCE, REMISSION, RELAPSE

The course of insomnia is of significant interest to both epidemiologists and clinicians. The extent to which insomnia is a transient, recurrent, or persistent condition has important implications in terms of whether and when to initiate treatment and long-term prognosis and morbidity.

Several longitudinal studies have documented the course of insomnia over various time intervals (see **Table 1**), but most of those have used only 2 assessment points. The evidence is clear that insomnia is often a persistent problem over time, with persistence rates varying as a function of the intervals between assessments. For example, data derived from some of the same longitudinal studies assessing incidence have produced persistence rates over a 1-year period of 31% in the United States,[27] 44.4% (syndrome like) in Sweden,[21] 69% (symptoms) in the United Kingdom,[44] and 74% (symptoms and syndromes combined) in Canada.[53] Studies conducted with cohorts of older adults have produced persistence rates of 66.3%[54] for 1-year, 40% for a 2-year period,[55] and 36.1% for a 4-year period.[56] In a cohort of 4467 older adults involved in the Cardiovascular Health Study,[57] rates of persistent insomnia over a 1-year to 4-year period were

15.4% for trouble falling asleep and 22.7% for frequent awakenings, compared with 13.4% for excessive daytime sleepiness.

Factors associated with persistence of insomnia are often the same as those associated with its incidence (ie, female gender, older age, and presence of medical or mental health problems),[54] with depression and mental health problems presenting stronger associations than physical health problems. Insomnia can also be a persistent condition, independent of mental disorders.

As part of our ongoing longitudinal study,[53] we are following 4000 adults annually throughout Canada, and at each assessment these individuals are classified as good sleepers, individuals with insomnia symptoms, or individuals with an insomnia syndrome (disorder). Sleep status is based on information derived from standard assessment instruments (Insomnia Severity Index, Pittsburgh Sleep Quality Index) and is defined by an algorithm using a combination of insomnia diagnostic criteria (DSM and ICD) and the use of sleep-promoting medication.[43,53] For instance, individuals with an insomnia syndrome must report dissatisfaction with sleep, symptoms of initial, middle, or late insomnia at least 3 nights per week for a month, and significant distress or daytime impairments. Also included in this group are those taking prescribed sleep-promoting medication 3 nights or more per week for at least 1 month. Individuals classified with insomnia symptoms report some of these same symptoms but do not fulfill all diagnostic criteria for an insomnia syndrome. Individuals using prescribed medications fewer than 3 nights per week or over-the-counter medications for sleep at least 1 night per week are also classified in this group. Good sleepers do not report any sleep complaint and do not use medications to promote sleep.

Preliminary data from a subsample of 388 participants completing the first 3 annual follow-ups showed that 46% of individuals with insomnia (symptoms or syndrome) at baseline continued to report insomnia (symptoms or syndrome) at the 3-year follow-up, and for the remaining 54% who went into remission at some point in time, half of them eventually relapsed.[53] Different insomnia trajectories were observed across severity levels, with individuals presenting an insomnia syndrome at baseline showing a more persistent course over time, whereas individuals with subsyndromal insomnia had a more fluctuating trajectory, with a greater likelihood of remission status at a subsequent follow-up.

This study has also shown that insomnia status may change considerably even within a 12-month period. For example, an individual with insomnia at baseline may become a good sleeper 6 months later and again have insomnia 12 months later. This fluctuation over time underscores the need to adopt a more microscopic approach in longitudinal studies of insomnia. To examine this issue, we conducted monthly evaluations over a 12-month period with a subgroup of 100 individuals.[9] At baseline, 42 participants were classified as good sleepers, 34 met criteria for insomnia symptoms and 24 for an insomnia syndrome. There were significant fluctuations of insomnia over time, with 66% of the participants changing sleep status at least once over the 12 monthly assessments. Changes in sleep status were significantly more frequent among individuals with insomnia symptoms at baseline (M = 3.55) than among those initially classified as good sleepers (M = 2.14).

Among the subgroup with insomnia symptoms at baseline, 85.3% reported improved sleep (ie, became good sleepers) at least once over the 12 monthly assessments compared with 29.4% whose sleep worsened (ie, met criteria for an insomnia syndrome) during the same period. Among individuals classified as good sleepers at baseline, risks of developing insomnia symptoms and syndrome at least once over the subsequent months were respectively 14.4% and 3.2%. An interval of 6 months was found most reliable to estimate incidence rates, whereas an interval of 3 months proved the most reliable to estimate persistence rate. These results suggest significant sleep variability over a 12-month period and highlight the importance of conducting repeated assessment at a shorter than the typical yearly interval in order to reliably capture the natural course of insomnia over time.

CONSEQUENCES AND BURDEN OF INSOMNIA

Insomnia is associated with significant short-term and long-term consequences. Although the essential features of insomnia are nocturnal complaints, daytime impairments and distress over daytime functioning are also defining criteria of insomnia,[1,2] and this component has been identified as a research priority by insomnia expert panels.[58,59]

Short-Term Consequences of Insomnia

Short-term, daily consequences include physical discomfort upon awakening, fatigue, tiredness, unpleasant body sensations (eg, heavy eyes), hypersensitivity to noise and light, and low energy/motivation throughout the day.[60] Insomnia is associated with mood disturbances (eg, irritability), heightened emotional reactiveness,[60,61] negative interactions with children[62] and partners,[63] reduced optimism and self-esteem,[64] as well as overall poor quality of life (eg, vitality).[61]

In a recent qualitative study, participants with insomnia symptoms reported feeling segregated and misunderstood by others (eg, friends, physicians), described daily life as an effort or struggle, and raised concerns over the cumulative and long-term impact of insomnia on physical and mental health, occupational and vocational functioning, as well as on social domains.[60] Although subjective complaints are not always corroborated with objective measurements, a recent meta-analysis[5] found subtle and selective, yet reliable deficits in studies using objective cognitive functioning measures. For instance, individuals with insomnia show deficits in cognitive performance, most notably in attention, concentration, and memory-related tasks; all of which can produce pervasive consequences in every aspect of daily life. Not surprisingly, daytime complaints are recognized as a primary determinant of help-seeking behaviors among individuals with insomnia.[7]

Long-Term Consequences of Insomnia

Psychological health

In addition to the strong association between insomnia and poor mental health derived from cross-sectional studies, prospective studies indicate that persistent insomnia is also a risk factor for worsening of mental health and the development of several psychiatric disorders.[28,45,65] Persistent insomnia is associated with 2 times higher likelihood of future anxiety[44] and 4 times greater likelihood of future depression in adults,[45,66] adolescents,[67] and children.[68] A meta-analysis summarizing the findings of 21 longitudinal studies found that participants with insomnia had a 2-fold greater risk for developing depression than participants without sleep complaints.[13] One putative mechanism hypothesized that the link between persistent insomnia and depression is the alteration of the arousal system and its subsequent impact on affective and cognitive systems.[65]

The relationship between insomnia and depression can be bidirectional, such that insomnia may be the cause or the result of depression and vice versa, and this relationship may change over time. In a prospective population-based study,[69] non-depressed participants with insomnia at baseline had a 6 times greater risk of developing depression at follow-up compared with counterparts without insomnia. Likewise, depressed participants without insomnia at baseline also had 6 times more risk of developing insomnia 11 years later compared with nondepressed participants. In addition, insomnia and sleep disturbances are

associated with increased risk for suicide intentions, attempts, and successes in both clinical[70] and nonclinical samples.[71] In a longitudinal study conducted with 75,000 adults from Norway over a 20-year follow-up period, the age-adjusted and sex-adjusted hazard ratios for suicide were 1.9, 2.7, and 4.3 for reporting sleeping problems sometimes, often, or almost every night, respectively, compared with participants who reported no sleeping problems. Associations were stronger in younger (<50 years) participants, but even after adjusting for mental disorder and alcohol use at baseline, participants with the worst sleep patterns remained at a 2-fold increased risk of suicide.[72]

Physical health

In addition to its association with mental health problems, insomnia is linked with poor physical health as well. Evidence from cross-sectional studies indicates that various medical conditions (eg, hypertension, diabetes) are more common among individuals with insomnia relative to those without insomnia.[73] Individuals with chronic insomnia also show poorer immune functioning (eg, lower natural killer cell activity) compared with good sleepers.[74] Further, insomnia symptoms are linked with alterations in appetite-regulating hormones[75] and notably, the subsequent development of metabolic syndrome.[76] A recent longitudinal study showed that individuals with insomnia had a 40% to 60% increased risk of developing headaches such as migraines and tension-type headaches, respectively, over 11 years after adjusting for age, sex, and sleep medication.[77]

Chronic insomnia is associated with increased nocturnal systolic blood pressure and reduced day-to-night decrease of blood pressure.[78] Chronic insomnia is also considered a significant risk factor in the development of mild to moderate hypertension.[79,80] Yet, the insomnia-hypertension relationship remains equivocal; Phillips and colleagues[81] found that insomnia complaints (eg, difficulty initiating sleep) did not predict hypertension 6 years later and reduced the risk in an older cohort of non–African American men (average age of 73 years).

Additional evidence suggests that insomnia is a risk factor for future cardiac events, including acute myocardial infarction[82] and coronary heart disease,[83] even among individuals free of cardiovascular disease.[80] Individuals reporting multiple insomnia symptoms (ie, difficulties initiating/maintaining sleep, early morning awakening) at baseline showed increased incident rates of coronary heart disease compared with those with only one or without any symptoms at baseline.[84] In particular, frequent reports of difficulty initiating and maintaining sleep, as well as nonrestorative sleep, were associated with increased hazard ratios of 1.45, 1.30, and 1.27, respectively, for acute myocardial infarction.[82] Further, insomnia symptoms are significantly associated with cardiovascular and all-cause mortality up to 17 years after insomnia symptoms are detected.[85] This effect is most conspicuous among men with objectively determined short sleep duration.[86] A meta-analysis[87] found that those endorsing insomnia symptoms have a 45% increased risk of cardiovascular morbidity and mortality. However, other studies with shorter follow-up assessments (eg, 6 years) and additional covariates (eg, sleep duration, depression)[88,89] did not identify insomnia as a significant risk factor for future cardiovascular disease or all-cause mortality.[90]

Difficulties initiating or maintaining sleep are associated with 57% to 84% increased risk, respectively, for incident diabetes[91] up to 22 years later.[85] This finding is especially more pronounced among individuals with frequent reports of sleep disturbances[92]; however, this finding was not found in a study of older women[93] or in a more recent study of middle-aged Chinese adults.[28]

Occupational health

Insomnia is often associated with role impairments, particularly in the work environment. Workers with insomnia syndrome report reduced productivity, are absent 8.1 hours more per 3-month period,[94] and have a greater tendency to show up to work late than those without insomnia.[95] Insomnia is associated with a reduced likelihood of future professional advancements (eg, promotion, salary increase)[96–98] and an increased risk of permanent work disability, even after controlling for baseline exposure to disability, sick leave, sleep duration, and other possible confounders.[97,98] Compared with good sleepers, those with sleep disturbances report more intentions of switching occupations, have reduced job satisfaction, fewer adaptive coping skills, rely more on emotion-oriented coping strategies than problem-solving strategies, and report lower feelings of mastery.[99] Insomnia is thus recognized as a significant barrier in the achievement of career and life goals.

Insomnia is closely linked with greater cognitive failures in everyday activities,[5] and thus, is also associated with an increased proneness for occupational mishaps, accidents, or errors.[100] Daley and colleagues[101] found that patients with insomnia syndrome were almost twice more likely to have experienced personal and work-related accidents than were good sleepers. Among the elderly, insomnia (and not hypnotic use) was shown to predict falls over a 5-month to 7-month observation period, with the highest risk noted among residents who remained untreated or remained unresponsive to treatment at follow-up.[102] Drivers reporting insomnia symptoms, poor sleep quality, prolonged wakefulness, or sleepiness also have an increased risk of being involved in nocturnal[103] and diurnal automobile accidents.[104]

Economic Burden of Insomnia

Insomnia carries significant economic burden for the health care system. One study[105] projected that the costs for medical expenditures (ie, claims for inpatients/outpatients, pharmacy, emergency room services) were $934 more for young to middle-aged adults with insomnia (18–64 years) and $1143 more for older adults with insomnia (>65 years) compared with well-matched individuals without insomnia. Insomnia severity and frequency also show a dose-response effect with direct costs, such that annual health care costs among members of a health plan in the United States are estimated to be $1323 for those with moderate to severe insomnia, $907 for subthreshold insomnia, and $757 for good sleepers.[106] In a similar study,[107] participants with frequent complaints of insomnia symptoms reported higher annual medical costs ($2552) than did those with less frequent insomnia symptoms ($1510). In a population-based sample, Daley and colleagues[94] reported the annual per person insomnia-related direct costs were $293 for individuals with an insomnia syndrome, $160 for those with insomnia symptoms, and $45 for good sleepers. Cost-benefit analyses for insomnia treatment estimated lower monthly health care costs and increased quality-adjusted life year among remitted patients compared with their nonremitted counterparts.[108,109]

The indirect costs of insomnia can also add to the economic burden of society. Using an administrative database, annual mean incremental costs for sick leave, short-term and long-term disability, and workers' compensation was $567 more for employees with insomnia compared with employees without insomnia.[110] The estimated expenditures of employed health plan members because of absenteeism[105] and presenteeism (ie, attending work while ill, leading to low work performance) were significantly more among employees with insomnia than employees without insomnia.[111] Costs for reduced productivity were highest for employed health plan members with moderate to severe insomnia, followed by those with insomnia symptoms, and those without insomnia.[106] Similar reports were documented in a population-based sample for overall indirect costs, with the highest cost per person for those with an insomnia syndrome estimated to be at $4717 annually, followed by those with insomnia symptoms at $1271 and good sleepers at $376.[94] The annual indirect costs for resources lost were nearly 10 times higher than the direct costs specific to treating insomnia.[94] Although insomnia carries a significant economic burden, it is difficult from the available evidence to separate expenses that are caused specifically by insomnia from those expenses driven by common co-occurring conditions such as depression and pain.

COMMUNITY/PUBLIC HEALTH EDUCATION AND PREVENTION OF INSOMNIA

Despite the considerable health, social, and economic burden of insomnia, it is often underrecognized and untreated in both pediatric[112] and adult populations. Although there is solid evidence showing the efficacy of insomnia therapies[113] and strong incentives for prevention strategies, methods for preventing insomnia remain underdeveloped.[114,115] As such, it is imperative to find appropriate strategies for the prevention of insomnia.

Although some risk factors are unmodifiable, (eg, age, sex, genetics), others are modifiable (eg, maladaptive sleep practices). Unmodifiable risk factors can be used to identify at-risk individuals, whereas education and behavioral interventions that are practical and easily sustainable[116] can be used to alter modifiable risk factors. For example, given the greater likelihood of insomnia within a family,[48,49] prevention approaches can be particularly helpful to alter lifestyle behaviors (eg, maintain a regular sleep schedule, reduced intake of stimulants) and sleeping environment (eg, reduced noise level), all of which may have a significant impact on the general population, but particularly among vulnerable populations.

From a public health perspective, an important step in insomnia prevention involves increasing awareness on the importance of adequate sleep and the debilitating effects of insomnia.[114,115] Some individuals hold misconceptions or lack knowledge about healthy sleep patterns and sleep disorders (eg, causes, consequences, treatment) which, in turn, can contribute to poor sleep practices. Public health education campaigns can prove beneficial to increase awareness about the importance of sleep and about behavioral practices to prevent sleep problems. Although it is

recognized that health care professionals should routinely evaluate sleep and provide some sleep education as part of patient care, many professionals rate their own sleep knowledge as fair or poor.[117] Furthermore, during consultations, health care professionals do not typically initiate inquiries about their patient's sleep, unless the patient, a family member, or patient's caretaker presents sleep-related concerns.[112,117] Thus, an important step is increasing education and training on sleep for health care professionals.[114]

Sleep counseling may lead to changes in patients' attitudes, knowledge, and behaviors toward sleep. Borrowing successful strategies from other prevention programs may also lead to changes. For instance, providing accurate information about the importance of sleep and differences in sleep needs as a function of different age groups may bring people to make sleep more of a priority in their life. Likewise, making simple and specific behavioral recommendations (eg, reduce time spent awake in bed and get up at the same time every morning), can be effective to alleviate insomnia before it reaches clinical threshold. Although the relation between sleep knowledge and sleep practices is mixed, sleep education remains an essential step in promoting healthy sleep. In fact, general education interventions targeted at children[118] and parents[119] have yielded promising results.

Given the heavy burden that insomnia places on the individual and society, implementing prevention strategies at the community level is important. Recently, Kraus and Rabin[115] proposed launching a public-wide awareness campaign entitled *Sleep America*, with specific aims to (1) promote insomnia education using various mediums (eg, Web-based initiatives), (2) increase accessibility of insomnia treatments (eg, behavioral sleep medicine), and (3) monitor and potentially refute misleading claims about non–evidence-based insomnia treatments. Future research is needed to evaluate the cost-effectiveness of prevention strategies that focus on modifiable risk factors, emphasize knowledge translation on sleep education, and can be delivered at the individual and societal level. This research should be implemented, particularly, among at-risk populations for an effective campaign that improves public health.

KEY POINTS AND SUGGESTIONS FOR FUTURE EPIDEMIOLOGIC STUDIES

The epidemiology of insomnia has received increased attention in the last decade, and investigators have moved from a purely cross-sectional approach of estimating prevalence of insomnia and its correlates to a more prospective and longitudinal approach aimed at documenting its natural history, risk factors, and long-term consequences. There is now substantial evidence that insomnia is a highly prevalent and persistent condition, both as a symptom and as a syndrome. Its persistence is associated with increased risk for mental (eg, major depression), physical (eg, hypertension), and occupational health problems (eg, disability). At least half a dozen studies have documented the economic burden of insomnia, with the main finding being that insomnia is a costly health problem. Notably, treating insomnia (eg, professional consultations, medications, sleep-promoting aids) is far less costly compared with the loss of human resources (eg, absenteeism) due to insomnia.

Recent findings concerning the epidemiology of insomnia have direct implications for clinical studies, including: (1) the need for large, population-based studies aimed at evaluating whether insomnia can be prevented in cohorts of at-risk individuals; (2) clinical studies that evaluate whether the morbidity associated with chronic insomnia can be reversed; and (3) prospective health economic evaluations (ie, cost-benefit, cost-usefulness, cost-effectiveness) of different therapeutic approaches and treatment delivery models (eg, individual vs group vs self-help therapies). Such studies might have the greatest impact on decision makers and the allocation of health care resources for insomnia.

Progress on the epidemiology of insomnia has been hampered by important methodological shortcomings, including, but not limited to, inconsistent case definitions and standardized assessment procedures across studies. These methodological problems have contributed to producing extensive variability in estimates of prevalence, incidence, and persistence rates of insomnia. It will be essential in future studies to rely on standard case definition and assessment procedures in order to derive more reliable estimates of insomnia. Given the recent efforts to harmonize insomnia diagnostic criteria between the DSM and ICSD nosology, it may be easier for investigators to follow this recommendation. Studies attempting to quantify the economic burden of insomnia have also produced variable and imprecise cost estimates because investigators have not separated the costs driven specifically by insomnia from those costs attributable to frequently comorbid psychiatric or medical disorders.

Although there is extensive evidence about the prevalence and incidence of insomnia, there is less information about its natural history and long-term course and prognosis. Also, little is known about moderating and mediating variables that modulate the course of insomnia (ie, remission, relapse). Additional prospective and longitudinal studies are especially important to identify early precursors and precipitating factors of insomnia. It is important to monitor these factors at regular intervals in relation to onset, remission, and relapse. Although there is evidence that insomnia is a condition that may wax and wane, it is difficult to predict whether an acute insomnia episode will be transient or develop a more chronic course. Previous studies have not examined course modifiers (eg, treatment initiation). Additional research is needed to achieve more precise identification of moderating and mediating factors likely to be associated with natural course changes. Information about life events, health status, treatment and products used to alleviate sleep problems would help to characterize more precisely the natural history of insomnia and potential course modifiers. A better understanding of how insomnia evolves over time and what factors trigger an episode or perpetuate it over time is critical for developing effective prevention and treatment programs.

REFERENCES

1. American Academy of Sleep Medicine. International classification of sleep disorders: diagnostic and coding manual. 2nd edition. Westchester (IL): American Academy of Sleep Medicine; 2005.
2. American Psychiatric Association. Diagnostic and statistical manual of mental disorders (DSM5). Washington, DC: American Psychiatric Association; 2013.
3. Buysse DJ, Thompson W, Scott J, et al. Daytime symptoms in primary insomnia: a prospective analysis using ecological momentary assessment. Sleep Med 2007;8:198–208.
4. Edinger JD, Bonnet MH, Bootzin RR, et al. Derivation of research diagnostic criteria for insomnia: report of an American Academy of Sleep Medicine work group. Sleep 2004;27:1567–96.
5. Fortier-Brochu E, Beaulieu-Bonneau S, Ivers H, et al. Insomnia and daytime cognitive performance: a meta-analysis. Sleep Med Rev 2012;16:83–94.
6. Roth T, Jaeger S, Jin R, et al. Sleep problems, comorbid mental disorders, and role functioning in the national comorbidity survey replication. Biol Psychiatry 2006;60:1364–71.
7. Morin CM, LeBlanc M, Daley M, et al. Epidemiology of insomnia: prevalence, self-help treatments, consultations, and determinants of help-seeking behaviors. Sleep Med 2006;7:123–30.
8. Edinger J, Morin CM. Insomnia disorder: A unified approach. Paper presented at SLEEP 2013.

Proceedings of the 27th APSS, 2013 June 1–5; Baltimore, MD, USA.

9. Morin CM, LeBlanc M, Ivers H, et al. Monthly fluctuations of insomnia symptoms in a population-based sample. Under review.

10. Ohayon MM, Riemann D, Morin C, et al. Hierarchy of insomnia criteria based on daytime consequences. Sleep Med 2012;13:2–7.

11. Nierenberg AA, Keefe BR, Leslie VC, et al. Residual symptoms in depressed patients who respond acutely to fluoxetine. J Clin Psychiatry 1999;60:221–5.

12. Perlis ML, Giles DE, Buysse DJ, et al. Self-reported sleep disturbance as a prodromal symptom in recurrent depression. J Affect Disord 1997;42:209–12.

13. Baglioni C, Battagliese G, Feige B, et al. Insomnia as a predictor of depression: a meta analytic evaluation of longitudinal epidemiological studies. J Affect Disord 2011;135:10–9.

14. Fava M, McCall WV, Krystal A, et al. Eszopiclone co-administered with fluoxetine in patients with insomnia coexisting with major depressive disorder. Biol Psychiatry 2006;59:1052–60.

15. Manber R, Edinger JD, Gress JL, et al. Cognitive behavioral therapy for insomnia enhances depression outcome in patients with comorbid major depressive disorder and insomnia. Sleep 2008;31:489–95.

16. Karacan I, Thornby JI, Anch M, et al. Prevalence of sleep disturbance in a primarily urban Florida County. Soc Sci Med 1976;10:239–44.

17. Bixler ED, Kales A, Soldatos CR, et al. Prevalence of sleep disorders in the Los Angeles metropolitan area. Am J Psychiatry 1979;136:1257–62.

18. Ohayon MM. Epidemiology of insomnia: what we know and what we still need to learn. Sleep Med Rev 2002;6:97–111.

19. American Academy of Sleep Medicine. International Classification of Sleep Disorders: Diagnostic and Coding Manual. 2nd ed. Westchester, IL: American Academy of Sleep Medicine; 2005.

20. Morin CM, LeBlanc M, Bélanger L, et al. Epidemiology of insomnia in the adult Canadian population. Can J Psychiatry 2011;56:540–8.

21. Jansson-Frojmark M, Linton SJ. The course of insomnia over one year: a longitudinal study in the general population in Sweden. Sleep 2008;31:881–6.

22. Ohayon MM, Reynolds CF 3rd. Epidemiological and clinical relevance of insomnia diagnosis algorithms according to the DSM-IV and the International Classification of Sleep Disorders (ICSD). Sleep Med 2009;10:952–60.

23. Jaussent I, Dauvilliers Y, Ancelin ML, et al. Insomnia symptoms in older adults: associated factors and gender differences. Am J Geriatr Psychiatry 2011;19:88–97.

24. Simon GE, VonKorff M. Prevalence, burden, and treatment of insomnia in primary care. Am J Psychiatry 1997;154:1417–23.

25. Aikens JE, Rouse ME. Help-seeking for insomnia among adult patients in primary care. J Am Board Fam Pract 2005;18:257–61.

26. Zhang B, Wing YK. Sex differences in insomnia: a meta-analysis. Sleep 2006;29:85–93.

27. Ford DE, Kamerow DB. Epidemiologic study of sleep disturbances and psychiatric disorders. An opportunity for prevention? J Am Med Assoc 1989;262:1479–84.

28. Zhang J, Lam SP, Li SX, et al. Long-term outcomes and predictors of chronic insomnia: a prospective study in Hong Kong Chinese adults. Sleep Med 2012;13:455–62.

29. National Sleep Foundation (NSF) (n.d.). Sleep in America Poll. Retrieved from February 4, 2013. http://www.sleepfoundation.org/category/article-type/sleepamerica-polls.

30. Roberts RE, Roberts CR, Chan W. Ethnic differences in symptoms of insomnia among adolescents. Sleep 2006;29:359–65.

31. Paine SJ, Gander PH, Harris R, et al. Who reports insomnia? Relationships with age, sex, ethnicity, and socioeconomic deprivation. Sleep 2004;27:1163–9.

32. Seicean S, Neuhauser D, Strohl K, et al. An exploration of differences in sleep characteristics between Mexico-born US immigrants and other Americans to address the Hispanic paradox. Sleep 2011;34:1021–31.

33. Jean-Louis G, Magai CM, Cohen CI, et al. Ethnic differences in self-reported sleep problems in older adults. Sleep 2001;24:926–33.

34. Clever MN, Bruck D. Comparisons of the sleep quality, daytime sleepiness, and sleep cognitions of Caucasian Australians and Zimbabwean and Ghanaian black immigrants. S Afr J Psychol 2013;43:81–93.

35. Soldatos C, Allaert F, Ohta T, et al. How do individuals sleep around the world? Results from a single-day survey in ten countries. Sleep Med 2005;6:5–13.

36. Leger D, Poursain B. An international survey of insomnia: under-recognition and under-treatment of a polysymptomatic condition. Curr Med Res Opin 2005;21:1785–92.

37. Dregan A, Armstrong D. Cross-country variation in sleep disturbance among working and older age groups: an analysis based on the European Social Survey. Int Psychogeriatr 2011;23:1413–20.

38. Leger D, Poursain B, Neubauer D, et al. An international survey of sleeping problems in the general population. Curr Med Res Opin 2008;24:307–17.

39. Liu X, Liu L, Owens JA, et al. Sleep patterns and sleep problems among schoolchildren in the United States and China. Pediatrics 2005;115:241–9.

40. Mindell J, Sadeh A, Wiegand B, et al. Cross-cultural differences in infant and toddler sleep. Sleep Med 2010;11:274–80.
41. Ban L, Kashima Y, Haslam N. Does understanding behaviour make it seem normal? Perceptions of abnormality among Euro-Australians and Chinese-Singaporeans. J Cross Cult Psychol 2012; 43:286–98.
42. Sayar K, Kirmayer LJ, Taillefer SS. Predictors of somatic symptoms in depressive disorder. Gen Hosp Psychiatry 2003;25:108–14.
43. LeBlanc M, Mérette C, Savard J, et al. Incidence and risk factors of insomnia in a population-based sample. Sleep 2009;32:1027–37.
44. Morphy H, Dunn KM, Lewis M, et al. Epidemiology of insomnia: a longitudinal study in a UK population. Sleep 2007;30:274–80.
45. Breslau N, Roth T, Rosenthal L, et al. Sleep disturbance and psychiatric disorders: a longitudinal epidemiological study of young adults. Biol Psychiatry 1996;39:411–8.
46. Ellis JG, Perlis ML, Neale LF, et al. The natural history of insomnia: focus on prevalence and incidence of acute insomnia. J Psychiatr Res 2012; 46:1278–85.
47. Roberts RE, Shema SJ, Kaplan GA. Prospective data on sleep complaints and associated risk factors in an older cohort. Psychosom Med 1999;61: 188–96.
48. Dauvilliers Y, Morin CM, Cervena K, et al. Family studies in insomnia. J Psychosom Res 2005;58: 271–8.
49. Beaulieu-Bonneau S, LeBlanc M, Merette C, et al. Family history of insomnia in a population-based sample. Sleep 2007;30:1739–45.
50. Vgontzas AN, Bixler EO, Lin HM, et al. Chronic insomnia is associated with nyctohemeral activation of the hypothalamic-pituitary-adrenal axis: clinical implications. J Clin Endocrinol Metab 2001;86: 3787–94.
51. Riemann D, Spiegelhadler R, Feige B, et al. The hyperarousal model of insomnia: a review of the concept and its evidence. Sleep Med Rev 2010; 14:19–31.
52. Bonnet MH, Arand DL. Hyperarousal and insomnia: state of the science. Sleep Med Rev 2010;14:9–15.
53. Morin CM, Bélanger L, LeBlanc M, et al. The Natural History of Insomnia: a population-based 3-year longitudinal study. Arch Intern Med 2009;169: 447–53.
54. Fok M, Stewart R, Besset A, et al. Incidence and persistence of sleep complaints in a community older population. Int J Geriatr Psychiatry 2010;25: 37–45.
55. Kim JM, Stewart R, Kim SW, et al. Insomnia, depression, and physical disorders in late life: a 2-year longitudinal community study in Koreans. Sleep 2009;32:1221–8.
56. Morgan K, Clarke D. Longitudinal trends in late-life insomnia: implications for prescribing. Age Ageing 1997;26:179–84.
57. Quan SF, Katz R, Olson J, et al. Factors associated with incidence and persistence of symptoms of disturbed sleep in an elderly cohort: the cardiovascular health study. Am J Med Sci 2005; 329:163–72.
58. Buysse DJ, Ancoli-Israel S, Edinger JD, et al. Recommendations for a standard research assessment of insomnia. Sleep 2006;29:1155–73.
59. National Institutes of Health. National Institutes of Health State of the Science conference statement: manifestations and management of chronic insomnia in adults, June 13–15, 2005. Sleep 2005;28:1049–57.
60. Kyle SD, Espie CA, Morgan K. "… Not just a minor thing, it is something major, which stops you from functioning daily": quality of life and daytime functioning in insomnia. Behav Sleep Med 2010;8: 123–40.
61. LeBlanc M, Beaulieu-Bonneau S, Mérette C, et al. Psychological and health-related quality of life factors associated with insomnia in a population-based sample. J Psychosom Res 2007;63:157–66.
62. Novak M, Mucsi I, Shapiro CM, et al. Increased utilization of health services by insomniacs–an epidemiological perspective. J Psychosom Res 2004;56: 527–36.
63. Hasler PB, Troxel WM. Couples' nighttime sleep efficiency and concordance: evidence for bidirectional associations with daytime relationship functioning. Psychosom Med 2010;72:794–801.
64. Lemola S, Räikkönen K, Gomez V, et al. Optimism and self-esteem are related to sleep. Results from a large community-based sample. Int J Behav Med 2012. http://dx.doi.org/10.1007/s12529-012-9272-z.
65. Baglioni C, Riemann D. Is chronic insomnia a precursor to major depression? Epidemiological and biological findings. Curr Psychiatry Rep 2012;14: 511–8.
66. Buysse DJ, Angst J, Gamma A, et al. Prevalence, course, and comorbidity of insomnia and depression in young adults. Sleep 2008;31:473–80.
67. Roberts RE, Duong HT. Depression and insomnia among adolescents: a prospective perspective. J Affect Disord 2012;148:66–71.
68. Gregory AM, Rijsdijk FV, Lau JY, et al. The direction of longitudinal associations between sleep problems and depression symptoms: a study of twins aged 8 and 10 years. Sleep 2009;32: 189–99.
69. Sivertsen B, Salo P, Mykletun A. The bidirectional association between depression and

insomnia: the HUNT study. Psychosom Med 2012;74:758–65.

70. Krakow B, Ribeiro JD, Ulibarri VA, et al. Sleep disturbances and suicidal ideation in sleep medical center patients. J Affect Disord 2011;131:422–7.

71. Carli V, Roy A, Bevilacqua L, et al. Insomnia and suicidal behaviour in prisoners. Psychiatry Res 2011;185:141–4.

72. Bjørngaard JH, Bjerkeset O, Romundstad P, et al. Sleeping problems and suicide in 75,000 Norwegian adults: a 20 year follow-up of the HUNT I Study. Sleep 2011;34:1155–9.

73. Pearson NJ, Johnson L, Nahin RL. Insomnia, trouble sleeping, and complementary and alternative medicine: analysis of the 2002 National Health Interview Survey Data. Arch Intern Med 2006;166: 1775–82.

74. Savard J, Laroche L, Simard S, et al. Chronic insomnia and immune functioning. Psychosom Med 2003;65:211–21.

75. Motivala SJ, Tomiyama AJ, Ziegler M, et al. Nocturnal levels of ghrelin and leptin and sleep in chronic insomnia. Psychoneuroendocrinology 2009;34:540–5.

76. Troxel WM, Buysse DJ, Matthews KA, et al. Sleep symptoms predict the development of the metabolic syndrome. Sleep 2010;33:1633–40.

77. Odegård SS, Sand T, Engstrøm M, et al. The long-term effect of insomnia on primary headaches. A prospective population-based cohort study (HUNT-2 and HUNT-3). Headache 2011;51:570–80.

78. Lanfranchi PA, Pennestri MH, Fradette L, et al. Nighttime blood pressure in normotensive subjects with chronic insomnia: implications for cardiovascular risk. Sleep 2009;32:760–6.

79. Suka M, Yoshida K, Sugimori H. Persistent insomnia is a predictor of hypertension in Japanese male workers. J Occup Health 2003;45: 344–50.

80. Phillips B, Mannino DM. Do insomnia complaints cause hypertension or cardiovascular disease? J Clin Sleep Med 2007;3:489–94.

81. Phillips B, Bůžková P, Enright P. Insomnia did not predict incident hypertension in older adults in the cardiovascular health study. Sleep 2009;32: 65–72.

82. Laugsand LE, Vatten LJ, Platou C, et al. Insomnia and the risk of acute myocardial infarction. Circulation 2011;124:2073–81.

83. Chandola T, Ferrie JE, Perski A, et al. The effect of short sleep duration on coronary heart disease risk is greatest among those with sleep disturbance: a prospective study from the Whitehall II cohort. Sleep 2010;33:739–44.

84. Loponen M, Hublin C, Kalimo R, et al. Joint effect of self-reported sleep problems and three components of the metabolic syndrome on risk of

coronary heart disease. J Psychosom Res 2010; 68:149–58.

85. Nilsson PM, Roost M, Engstrom G, et al. Incidence of diabetes in middle-aged men is related to sleep disturbances. Diabetes Care 2004;27: 2464–9.

86. Vgontzas AN, Liao D, Pejovic S, et al. Insomnia with short sleep duration and mortality: the Penn State Cohort. Sleep 2010;33:1159–64.

87. Sofi F, Cesari F, Casini A, et al. Insomnia and risk of cardiovascular disease: a meta-analysis. Eur J Prev Cardiol 2012. http://dx.doi.org/10.1177/2047487312460020.

88. Kripke DF, Garfinkel L, Wingard DL, et al. Mortality associated with sleep duration and insomnia. Arch Gen Psychiatry 2002;59:131–6.

89. Phillips BA, Mannino DM. Does insomnia kill? Sleep 2005;28:965–71.

90. Schwartz SW, Cornoni-Huntley J, Cole SR, et al. Are sleep complaints an independent risk factor for myocardial infarction? Ann Epidemiol 1998;8: 384–92.

91. Cappuccio FP, D'Elia L, Strazzullo P, et al. Quantity and quality of sleep and incidence of type 2 diabetes: a systematic review and meta-analysis. Diabetes Care 2010;33:414–20.

92. Kawakami N, Takatsuka N, Shimizu H. Sleep disturbance and onset of type 2 diabetes. Diabetes Care 2004;27:282–3.

93. Bjorkelund C, Bondyr-Carlsson D, Lapidus L, et al. Sleep disturbances in midlife unrelated to 32-year diabetes incidence: the prospective population study of women in Gothenburg. Diabetes Care 2005;28:2739–44.

94. Daley M, Morin CM, LeBlanc M, et al. The economic burden of insomnia: direct and indirect costs for individuals with insomnia syndrome, insomnia symptoms, and good sleepers. Sleep 2009;32: 55–64.

95. David B, Morgan K. Workplace performance, but not punctuality, is consistently impaired among people with insomnia. Proceedings of the 19th Congress of the European Sleep Research Society, Glasgow 2008. J Sleep Res 2008;17:193.

96. Johnson LC, Spinweber C. Quality of sleep and performance in the navy: a longitudinal study of good and poor sleepers. In: Guilleminault C, Lugaresi E, editors. Sleep/wake disorders. New York: Raven Press; 1983. pp.13–28.

97. Sivertsen B, Overland S, Pallesen S, et al. Insomnia and long sleep duration are risk factors for later work disability. The Hordaland health study. J Sleep Res 2009;18:122–8.

98. Sivertsen B, Overland S, Neckelmann D, et al. The long-term effect of insomnia on work disability: the HUNT-2 historical cohort study. Am J Epidemiol 2006;163:1018–24.

99. Morin CM, Rodrigues S, Ivers H. Role of stress, arousal, and coping skills in primary insomnia. Psychosom Med 2003;65:259–67.

100. Shahly V, Berglund PA, Coulouvrat C, et al. The associations of insomnia with costly workplace accidents and errors: results from the America Insomnia Survey. Arch Gen Psychiatry 2012;69: 1054–63.

101. Daley M, Morin CM, LeBlanc M, et al. Insomnia and its relationship to health-care utilization, work absenteeism, productivity and accidents. Sleep Med 2009;10:427–38.

102. Avidan AY, Fries BE, James ML, et al. Insomnia and hypnotic use, recorded in the minimum data set, as predictors of falls and hip fractures in Michigan nursing homes. J Am Geriatr Soc 2005;53: 955–62.

103. Philip P, Sagaspe P, Lagarde E, et al. Sleep disorders and accidental risk in a large group of regular registered highway drivers. Sleep Med 2010;11: 973–9.

104. Lucidi F, Mallia L, Violani C, et al. The contributions of sleep-related risk factors to diurnal car accidents. Accid Anal Prev 2013;51:135–40.

105. Ozminkowski RJ, Wang S, Walsh JK. The direct and indirect costs of untreated insomnia in adults in the United States. Sleep 2007;30:263–73.

106. Sarsour K, Kalsekar A, Swindle R, et al. The association between insomnia severity and healthcare and productivity costs in a health plan sample. Sleep 2011;34:443–50.

107. Foley KA, Sarsour K, Kalsekar A, et al. Subtypes of sleep disturbance: associations among symptoms, comorbidities, treatment, and medical costs. Behav Sleep Med 2010;8:90–104.

108. Botteman M. Health economics of insomnia therapy: implications for policy. Sleep Med 2009;10: S22–5.

109. Morgan K, Dixon S, Mathers N, et al. Psychological treatment for insomnia in the regulation of long-term hypnotic drug use. Health Technol Assess 2004;8:1–68.

110. Kleinman NL, Brook RA, Doan JF, et al. Health benefit costs and absenteeism due to insomnia from the employer's perspective: a retrospective, case-control, database study. J Clin Psychiatry 2009;70:1098–104.

111. Kessler RC, Berglund PA, Coulouvrat C, et al. Insomnia and the performance of US workers: results from the America Insomnia Survey. Sleep 2011;34:1161–71.

112. Owens JA. The practice of pediatric sleep medicine: results of a community survey. Pediatrics 2001;108:E51.

113. Morin CM, Benca R. Chronic insomnia. Lancet 2012;379:1129–41.

114. Institute of Medicine of the National Academies (IMNA). Sleep disorders and sleep deprivation. Washington, DC: The National Academies Press; 2006.

115. Kraus SS, Rabin LA. Sleep America: managing the crisis of adult chronic insomnia and associated conditions. J Affect Disord 2012;138:192–212.

116. Pawson R, Owen L, Wong G. Legislating for health: locating the evidence. J Public Health Policy 2010; 31:164–77.

117. Rosen RC, Zozula R, Jahn EG, et al. Low rates of recognition of sleep disorders in primary care: comparison of a community-based versus clinical academic setting. Sleep Med 2001;2:47–55.

118. Sousa IC, Araújo JF, Azevedo CV. The effect of a sleep hygiene education program on the sleep-wake cycle of Brazilian adolescent students. Sleep Biol Rhythms 2007;5:251–8.

119. Jones CH, Owens JA, Pham B. Can a brief educational intervention improve parents' knowledge of healthy children's sleep? A pilot test. Health Educ J 2012. http://dx.doi.org/10.1177/0017896912452073.

120. Jansson M, Linton SJ. Psychosocial work stressors in the development and maintenance of insomnia: a prospective study. J Occup Health Psychol 2006;11:241–8.

121. Jansson-Fröjmark M, Lindblom K. A bidirectional relationship between anxiety and depression, and insomnia? A prospective study in the general population. J Psychosom Res 2008;64:443–9.

122. Skapinakis P, Rai D, Anagnostopoulos F, et al. Sleep disturbances and depressive symptoms: an investigation of their longitudinal association in a representative sample of the UK general population. Psychol Med 2013;43:329–39.

123. Komada Y, Nomura T, Kusumi M, et al. A two-year follow-up study on the symptoms of sleep disturbances/insomnia and their effects on daytime functioning. Sleep Med 2012;13:1115–21.

124. Fernandez-Mendoza J, Vgontzas AN, Bixler EO, et al. Clinical and polysomnographic predictors of the natural history of poor sleep in the general population. Sleep 2012;35:689–97.

125. Vgontzas AN, Fernandez-Mendoza J, Bixler EO, et al. Persistent insomnia: the role of objective short sleep duration and mental health. Sleep 2012;35: 61–8.

126. Singareddy R, Vgontzas AN, Fernandez-Mendoza J, et al. Risk factors for incident chronic insomnia: a general population prospective study. Sleep Med 2012;3:346–53.

Hyperarousal and Insomnia

Kai Spiegelhalder, MD, PhD[a,b,*], Dieter Riemann, PhD[a]

KEYWORDS

- Insomnia • Hyperarousal • Psychopathology • Brain function

KEY POINTS

- Studies investigating polysomnographically derived variables in patients with insomnia support the assumption that insomnia is characterized by physiologic hyperarousal.
- Most studies investigating autonomic variables and some of the studies investigating neuroendocrine variables are also in line with the hyperarousal assumption.
- No clear-cut picture of the pathophysiology of insomnia has emerged from neuroimaging studies.

INTRODUCTION

Insomnia is characterized by difficulties with initiating or maintaining sleep, or nonrestorative sleep, accompanied by daytime impairment. Primary insomnia (PI) is a largely exclusionary diagnosis of poor sleep, ruling out psychiatric, medical, and additional sleep-related disease. Current etiologic models of PI highlight the role of cognitive, emotional, and physiologic hyperarousal for the development and maintenance of the disorder.[1–9] In this article, the evidence for hyperarousal in insomnia is reviewed, with an emphasis on neurobiologically oriented studies. Most of the studies presented include comparisons between patients with PI and healthy good sleepers. Indicators of physiologic hyperarousal include electroencephalography (EEG)-derived polysomnographic (PSG) variables (standard PSG parameters, spectral analysis, cycling alternating pattern [CAP], event-related potentials [ERPs] during sleep) and autonomic and neuroendocrine variables, as well as outcome parameters of neuroimaging studies.

PSG
Standard PSG Parameters

PSG-derived sleep continuity is disturbed in insomnia, with a prolonged sleep onset latency, an increased wake time after sleep onset, and a reduced sleep efficiency,[10–12] all of which have been interpreted as consequences of the postulated hyperarousal in this patient group. However, decades of PSG studies in insomnia have revealed that the absolute values of the differences from healthy good sleepers are not large (eg, 20–40 minutes with respect to total sleep time) and that objectively determined sleep parameters are less disturbed than expected from subjective patients' reports. Furthermore, there is a remarkable night-to-night variability in patients with insomnia, suggesting large fluctuations also in arousal levels.[13] With respect to sleep architecture, some large investigations and a meta-analysis described a reduction of slow-wave sleep and rapid eye movement sleep in patients with insomnia.[14,15] Both phenomena have been interpreted as supporting the hyperarousal assumption[16,17]; however, it is not clear why other sleep stages are less affected by increased arousal levels. In the Multiple Sleep Latency Test, patients with insomnia show prolonged sleep latencies compared with healthy good sleepers[18–23] supporting the concept of 24-hour hyperarousal.

Spectral Analysis

A considerable body of evidence indicates that EEG spectral power in the β range is increased

---

[a] Department of Psychiatry and Psychotherapy, University of Freiburg Medical Center, Hauptstrasse 5, Freiburg 79104, Germany; [b] Freiburg Institute of Advanced Studies (FRIAS), University of Freiburg, Albertstrasse 19, Freiburg 79104, Germany
* Corresponding author. Department of Psychiatry and Psychotherapy, University of Freiburg Medical Center, Freiburg, Germany.
E-mail address: kai.spiegelhalder@uniklinik-freiburg.de

Sleep Med Clin 8 (2013) 299–307
http://dx.doi.org/10.1016/j.jsmc.2013.04.008
1556-407X/13/$ – see front matter © 2013 Elsevier Inc. All rights reserved.

in patients with insomnia during sleep[24–33] (**Fig. 1**; for a conflicting result, see Ref.[34]). Furthermore, there is preliminary evidence that cognitive-behavioral therapy for insomnia, the first-line treatment of PI, reduces β activity in patients with insomnia.[35,36] Given that β activity has been shown to be associated with sensorimotor and cognitive processes,[37] the finding of increased β power in insomnia suggests that nocturnal hyperarousal is an important part of the disorder.[7] However, up to now, there have been no longitudinal studies investigating whether increased β power is a cause or consequence of insomnia. In addition, future studies are needed to further investigate the effect of insomnia treatment, including psychotherapy and pharmacologic treatment, on EEG spectral power in sleep-disordered patients. There is a strong inter-subject variability in absolute EEG spectral parameters,[38,39] thus requiring large sample sizes in case-control designs.

CAP

CAP is a periodic EEG activity during non–rapid eye movement (NREM) sleep that is characterized by transient electrocortical events that are distinct from background EEG activity and recur at up to 1-minute intervals.[40,41] CAP is assumed to be an arousal phenomenon and, consequently, it has been hypothesized that the CAP rate is increased in patients with insomnia. Terzano and colleagues[42] compared 47 patients with PI and 25 good sleeper controls and found an increased CAP rate in the PI group. Despite the comparatively large sample size of this investigation, the conclusions are limited because all patients received a placebo during the evaluation night and some patients received hypnotic medication in the night before the evaluation night. However, further investigations by the same investigators replicated the finding of an increased CAP rate in different subtypes of insomnia.[43,44] Furthermore, there is evidence that hypnotic treatment decreases CAP rates to normal levels.[42,45,46] CAP rates seem to be a promising indicator of hyperarousal in insomnia.

ERPs During Sleep

ERPs are averaged brain responses to frequently presented stimuli. During wakefulness, different ERP components are assumed to be caused by different stages of cortical processing of the stimulus. The amplitude of early components increases with increasing stimulus intensity, whereas the amplitude of later components is linked to stimulus salience.[47] During sleep, the functional meaning of ERP components is less clear; however, it is assumed that the amplitude of ERP components during sleep onset or in a given sleep stage can be used to determine arousal levels.

Devoto and colleagues[48] investigated 11 patients with PI and 11 healthy good sleepers and found that disturbed sleep was associated with higher P300 amplitudes during wakefulness in

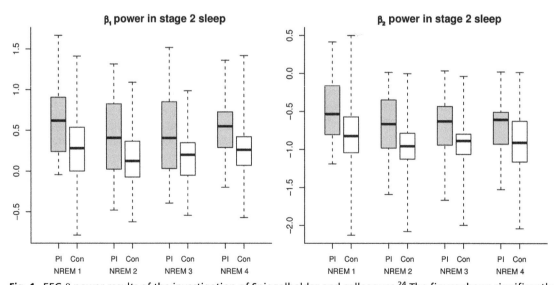

Fig. 1. EEG β power results of the investigation of Spiegelhalder and colleagues.[24] The figure shows significantly increased β₁ and β₂ power across the first 4 cycles of stage 2 sleep in patients with PI compared with healthy good sleepers. Con, healthy controls; NREM, non–rapid eye movement sleep cycle. (*From* Spiegelhalder K, Regen W, Feige B, et al. Increased EEG sigma and beta power during NREM sleep in primary insomnia. Biol Psychol 2012;91:332; with permission.)

patients with insomnia. The same group replicated this result of increased waking P300 amplitudes in an independent sample of 7 patients with PI and 7 healthy good sleepers[49] and interpreted their finding as supporting the assumption of a hyperarousal in patients with PI, because previous studies have linked increased P300 amplitudes to increased arousal levels. However, later studies by other groups did not replicate this finding or reported differing results. Sforza and Haba-Rubio examined ERP amplitudes during evening and morning wakefulness in 15 patients with PI, 45 patients with sleep-related breathing disorder, and 13 healthy good sleepers.[50] No significant differences between patients with PI and healthy good sleepers were found in any of the investigated variables (N100, P200, and P300). Bastien and colleagues[51] also studied ERP amplitudes during evening and morning wakefulness as well as during sleep onset in 15 patients with PI and 16 healthy good sleepers. During wakefulness, patients with PI showed increased N100 amplitudes, an indicator of increased arousal levels. During sleep onset, P200 was increased in the patient group and N350 was reduced. The same group of investigators performed 2 additional studies, which further supported the assumption that the N100 and P200 amplitudes are altered in patients with insomnia.[52,53] Another ERP study targeting the sleep onset period was conducted by Kertesz and Cote[54] in 13 patients with insomnia and 12 healthy good sleepers. In contrast to the findings by Bastien and colleagues, these investigators reported a decreased P200 amplitude in patients with insomnia, which is more consistent with the idea of hyperarousal than an increased P200 amplitude. During sleep, Yang and Lo[55] examined ERPs in 15 patients with PI and 15 healthy good sleepers and found an increased N100 amplitude as well as a decreased P200 amplitude to rare tones and a smaller N350 to standard tones during the first 5 minutes of stage 2 sleep.

The results of ERP studies in insomnia are not consistent; however, most of the findings, especially with respect to increased N100 and decreased P200 amplitudes, suggest increased arousal levels in patients with insomnia.

Summary

Summarizing the results from PSG-derived variables, a large body of evidence supports the hyperarousal perspective. However, most of the studies cited are limited by small sample sizes and some of the findings have not been replicated. The investigation of EEG spectral analysis, CAP, and ERPs may have the potential to provide deeper insights into insomnia psychopathology than EEG sleep staging according to standard criteria.[56,57] More specifically, these techniques may allow us to increase our knowledge about the neurobiological basis of hyperarousal in insomnia.

AUTONOMIC AND NEUROENDOCRINE VARIABLES
Autonomic Variables

Several autonomic variables, including heart rate, heart rate variability, body temperature, whole-body metabolism and galvanic skin response, have been investigated as indicators for hyperarousal in patients with insomnia.

There is some evidence that heart rate is increased in patients with insomnia, both in the presleep period and during nighttime sleep.[58–63] However, these results have been challenged by other studies that failed to find significant between-group differences.[64–69] Although resting heart rate in insomnia was increased in most of these investigations, showing nonsignificant group differences, interindividual variance exceeded the between-group difference. Accordingly, it can be assumed that heart rate is susceptible to many influences, of which insomnia is probably a minor one (**Fig. 2**). Using indices of heart rate variability in 12 patients with PI and 12 healthy good sleepers,

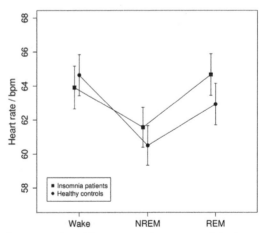

Fig. 2. Results with respect to heart rate of the investigation of Spiegelhalder and colleagues.[69] The figure shows a significant interaction effect GROUP x STAGE on heart rate, indicating that heart rate reduction from wakefulness to sleep is lower in patients with insomnia (*filled rectangles*) compared with healthy good sleepers (*filled circles*). However, no significant main effect GROUP was found in this investigation. Values are mean ± standard errors. (*From* Spiegelhalder K, Fuchs L, Ladwig J, et al. Heart rate and heart rate variability in subjectively reported insomnia. J Sleep Res 2011;20:141; with permission.)

1 study[60] reported that nocturnal sympathetic activity is increased in patients with insomnia, whereas parasympathetic activity is reduced. However, several subsequent studies with larger sample sizes could only partially replicate these findings, with many nonsignificant between-group comparisons.[62,63,67–70]

With respect to body temperature, Lack and colleagues[71] summarized the literature and came to the conclusion that core body temperature seems to be increased in elderly patients with insomnia during the night but not during daytime. However, an association between insomnia and impaired thermoregulation has not been consistently reported. Investigating whole-body metabolism by measuring body oxygen use, Bonnet and Arand found an increased basal metabolic rate in patients with insomnia, providing another possible indicator of physiologic hyperarousal.[20] Concerning galvanic skin response, results are inconsistent. Broman and Hetta[72] found higher electrodermal activity in a daytime study implying a higher arousal level in patients with insomnia. However, during the night, Monroe[64] found an increase in basal skin resistance in patients with insomnia, whereas Freedman and Sattler[65] found no significant between-group differences.

Most studies measuring autonomic variables in insomnia documented an increased physiologic arousal in this patient group. However, most findings were not replicated unequivocally and small sample sizes are a major limitation of this research area. Because of the cross-sectional nature of the investigations, causal inferences cannot be made, and it remains unclear whether increased autonomic activity is causing insomnia or whether insomnia triggers increased autonomic activity.

Neuroendocrine Variables

Cortisol has been frequently investigated as an indicator of the activity of the hypothalamic-pituitary-adrenal axis and as an indicator of hyperarousal in patients with insomnia. Vgontzas and colleagues[73] reported a positive correlation between the amount of nocturnal wake times and urinary cortisol excretion in a sample of young patients with insomnia. The same group of investigators[74] found an increased evening and early-night cortisol secretion in another sample of 11 patients with insomnia compared with 13 healthy good sleepers. Furthermore, Rodenbeck and colleagues[75] replicated this finding in a small sample of 7 middle-aged patients with insomnia. However, there is also conflicting evidence. Riemann and colleagues[76] as well as Varkevisser and colleagues[67] did not find any between-group

differences in cortisol secretion between patients with PI and healthy good sleepers. Furthermore, Backhaus and colleagues[77] investigated 14 patients with PI and 15 healthy good sleepers and reported significantly decreased levels of morning cortisol secretion in the patient group. The investigators of this study speculated that decreased morning cortisol may be caused by increased nocturnal cortisol; however, no data on nocturnal cortisol secretion were provided in this investigation. In light of this mixed evidence, it does not seem reasonable to confidently conclude that cortisol secretion is increased in patients with PI. However, this line of research seems to be important because it provides a potential neurobiological link between insomnia and depression.[78] A major limitation of these studies is, again, that only small samples have been investigated.

Summary

Most studies investigating autonomic variables and some of the studies investigating neuroendocrine variables are in line with the assumption that insomnia is characterized by physiologic hyperarousal. Again, the causal direction of the relationship between hyperarousal and alterations in autonomic and neuroendocrine variables remains unstudied. With respect to this question, chronic sleep loss leads to autonomic and neuroendocrine alterations that are similar to the ones observed in insomnia.[79]

NEUROIMAGING STUDIES IN INSOMNIA

Neuroimaging methods allow a direct investigation of brain structure and function and are therefore assumed to allow a direct measurement of arousal levels in patients with insomnia. Consequently, this is a rapidly growing field of research.

The first functional neuroimaging study in insomnia[80] used single-photon emission computed tomography to investigate regional cerebral blood flow during the first NREM sleep cycle in 5 patients with insomnia and 4 healthy good sleepers. Contrary to expectation, patients with insomnia showed a pattern of hypoperfusion across 8 preselected regions of interest, with the strongest effect in the basal ganglia. After successful treatment of 4 patients with insomnia, regional cerebral blood flow normalized in these patients,[81] which may, at least in part, be explained by statistical regression to the mean.

In a frequently cited positron emission tomography study, 7 patients with PI and 20 good sleeper controls were investigated during wakefulness and NREM sleep.[82] In this study, an increased glucose metabolism was found in patients with insomnia both during sleep and during wakefulness. Furthermore, patients with PI showed a smaller decline of glucose metabolism from wakefulness to sleep in the general arousal system, the emotion-regulating system, and the cognitive system. These results were interpreted as direct evidence for central nervous system hyperarousal and have contributed to the conceptualization of insomnia as a disorder of corticolimbic overactivity that interferes with sleep-promoting brain structures (see Refs.[83,84]). In an extension of this work, Nofzinger and colleagues[85] reported a correlation between increased brain metabolism and wake after sleep onset in a sample of 15 patients with PI.

Functional magnetic resonance (MR) imaging was used in 3 studies to investigate patients with insomnia. In the first one, Altena and colleagues[86] investigated 21 patients with PI and 12 healthy good sleepers with a category fluency task and a letter fluency task. Patients with insomnia showed a hypoactivation of medial and inferior prefrontal cortical areas during this task in the absence of behavioral differences compared with healthy good sleepers. Rescanning after successful cognitive-behavioral therapy was associated with a normalization of these brain activity patterns. In an investigation of working memory performance in 25 patients with PI and 25 healthy good sleepers, Drummond and colleagues[87] reported an abnormal pattern of neural function in the patient group by using an N-back working memory task. However, the investigators of these 2 studies do not claim that their results relate directly to arousal levels in insomnia. Huang and colleagues[88] investigated amygdala resting-state functional connectivity in 10 patients with PI and 10 healthy good sleepers. These investigators reported decreased connectivity between the amygdala and other limbic areas, possibly suggesting a dysfunction of the emotion-regulating system.

Neurochemical alterations in insomnia have been investigated using magnetic resonance spectroscopy measuring cortical γ-aminobutyric acid (GABA), the most important inhibitory neurotransmitter in the central nervous system. The rationale for this approach is the assumption that hyperarousal may be related to a decreased cortical influence of GABA. In line with this theory, 2 studies reported decreased GABA levels in insomnia[89,90]; however, another investigation by a different research group found the opposite effect.[91]

With respect to brain morphometry in insomnia, studies using conventional T2-weighted MR images reported inconsistent results. Although several cross-sectional investigations suggested that hippocampus volumes may be reduced in patients with insomnia,[92–94] other studies did not find this effect.[95–99] In the largest study so far,[96] 28 well-characterized patients with insomnia and 38 good sleeper controls were investigated using automated parcellation and pattern recognition approaches as well as voxel-wise analyses of gray and white matter volumes. In this investigation, no significant between-group differences were observed in any of the investigated brain morphometry variables. Thus, insomnia does not seem to be associated with substantial brain morphometry changes on a macroscopic level. However, all published investigations may have been statistically underpowered. For example, the investigation by Spiegelhalder and colleagues[96] provided a power analysis showing that, for the main analysis, only effect sizes of at least 0.71 could have been detected with a power of 0.80. Smaller brain morphometry changes in insomnia cannot be ruled out with certainty, and either large samples sizes or longitudinal within-subjects investigations seem needed to clarify the relationship between insomnia and brain morphometry. Furthermore, the relationship between brain morphometry and trait arousal levels has not yet been investigated.

Given the heterogeneity of neuroimaging methods applied and the small sample sizes in the cited studies, it is not surprising that no clear-cut picture of the pathophysiology of insomnia emerges. Nevertheless, neuroimaging studies showed that insomnia may be associated with functional and structural brain abnormalities. However, replication studies are urgently needed to determine the robustness of previous findings. With respect to this situation, some of the results may be false-positive because of the flexibility in data collection and analysis inherent in structural and functional neuroimaging studies.[100,101] Although these problems are not restricted to neuroimaging research, they are particularly relevant when small sample sizes are investigated, when liberal statistical thresholds are used, when there is greater flexibility in designs, definitions, outcomes, and analyses, and when a scientific field draws wide attention.[102,103]

SUMMARY

For decades, insomnia has been primarily conceptualized as a psychological disorder. Psychological stress and maladaptive behaviors were regarded as the most important causes that lead to the subjective experience of disturbed sleep. This review emphasizes the role of physiologic hyperarousal in insomnia and, thus, points out that insomnia can be conceptualized as a psychobiological disorder. From our point of view, this psychobiological perspective seems to be more adequate than a pure psychological framework alone. We do not want to devalue the importance of psychological constructs for the etiologic understanding of insomnia and we do not argue for a dominance of the biological over the psychological perspective. Psychological constructs have been shown to be extremely fruitful in this field, especially with respect to the development of cognitive-behavioral treatment of insomnia.

From our point of view, it is a public health priority to develop widely applicable and effective treatment strategies for insomnia, because the disorder is highly prevalent and has severe consequences.[104] These treatment strategies should be based on a deep knowledge of the cause of the disorder, thus requiring longitudinal studies on the interplay between behavior, cognition, emotion, and physiology in insomnia. In our opinion, the most important open questions with respect to the assumption that physiologic hyperarousal is crucially involved in the pathophysiology of insomnia are:

1. Is physiologic hyperarousal a cause or consequence of insomnia?
2. If it is a cause, what causes physiologic hyperarousal? What is the genetic basis of this construct? What is the impact of early-life stressors and other life events?
3. What is the neurobiological basis of hyperarousal? How can it be modified in the most efficient manner without causing severe adverse effects?

REFERENCES

1. Ong JC, Ulmer CS, Manber R. Improving sleep with mindfulness and acceptance: a metacognitive model of insomnia. Behav Res Ther 2012;50: 651–60.
2. Bonnet MH, Arand DL. Hyperarousal and insomnia: state of the science. Sleep Med Rev 2010;14:9–15.
3. Riemann D, Spiegelhalder K, Feige B, et al. The hyperarousal model of insomnia: a review of the concept and its evidence. Sleep Med Rev 2010; 14:19–31.
4. Espie CA, Broomfield NM, MacMahon K, et al. The attention-intention-effort pathway in the development of psychophysiologic insomnia: a theoretical review. Sleep Med Rev 2006;10:215–45.
5. Harvey AG. A cognitive model of insomnia. Behav Res Ther 2002;40:869–93.
6. Lundh LG, Broman JE. Insomnia as an interaction between sleep-interfering and sleep-interpreting processes. J Psychosom Res 2000;49:299–310.
7. Perlis ML, Giles DE, Mendelson WB, et al. Psychophysiological insomnia: the behavioural model and a neurocognitive perspective. J Sleep Res 1997;6: 179–88.
8. Morin CM. Insomnia: psychological assessment and management. New York: Guilford Press; 1993.
9. Spielman AJ, Caruso LS, Glovinsky PB. A behavioral perspective on insomnia treatment. Psychiatr Clin North Am 1987;10:541–53.
10. Benca RM, Obermeyer WH, Thisted RA, et al. Sleep and psychiatric disorders: a meta-analysis. Arch Gen Psychiatry 1992;49:651–68.
11. Reite M, Buysse DJ, Reynolds CF, et al. The use of polysomnography in the evaluation of insomnia. Sleep 1995;18:58–70.
12. Hudson JI, Pope HG, Sullivan LE, et al. Good sleep, bad sleep: a meta-analysis of polysomnographic measures in insomnia, depression and narcolepsy. Biol Psychiatry 1992;32:958–75.
13. Buysse DJ, Cheng Y, Germain A, et al. Night-to-night variability in older adults with and without chronic insomnia. Sleep Med 2010;11:56–64.
14. Baglioni C, Regen W, Teghen A, et al. Sleep changes in the disorder of insomnia: A meta-analysis of polysomnographic studies. Sleep Med Rev, in press.
15. Feige B, Al-Shajlawi A, Nissen C, et al. Does REM sleep contribute to subjective wake time in primary insomnia? A comparison of polysomnographic and subjective sleep in 100 patients. J Sleep Res 2008; 17:180–90.
16. Riemann D, Spiegelhalder K, Nissen C, et al. REM sleep instability–a new pathway for insomnia? Pharmacopsychiatry 2012;45:167–76.
17. Pigeon WR, Perlis ML. Sleep homeostasis in primary insomnia. Sleep Med Rev 2006;10: 247–54.
18. Huang L, Zhou J, Li Z, et al. Sleep perception and the multiple sleep latency test in patients with primary insomnia. J Sleep Res 2012;21:684–92.
19. Roehrs TA, Randall S, Harris E, et al. MSLT in primary insomnia: stability and relation to nocturnal sleep. Sleep 2011;34:1647–52.
20. Bonnet MH, Arand DL. 24-Hour metabolic rate in insomniacs and matched normal sleepers. Sleep 1995;18:581–8.
21. Sugerman JL, Stern JA, Walsh JK. Daytime alertness in subjective and objective insomnia: some preliminary findings. Biol Psychiatry 1985;20: 741–50.
22. Stepanski E, Lamphere J, Badia P, et al. Sleep fragmentation and daytime sleepiness. Sleep 1984;7: 18–26.
23. Seidel WF, Ball S, Cohen S, et al. Daytime alertness in relation to mood, performance, and nocturnal sleep in chronic insomniacs and noncomplaining sleepers. Sleep 1984;7:230–8.

24. Spiegelhalder K, Regen W, Feige B, et al. Increased EEG sigma and beta power during NREM sleep in primary insomnia. Biol Psychol 2012;91:329–33.

25. Buysse DJ, Germain A, Hall ML, et al. EEG spectral analysis in primary insomnia: NREM period effects and sex differences. Sleep 2008;31:1673–82.

26. Marzano C, Ferrara M, Sforza E, et al. Quantitative electroencephalogram (EEG) in insomnia: a new window on pathophysiological mechanisms. Curr Pharm Des 2008;14:3446–55.

27. Staner L, Cornette F, Maurice D, et al. Sleep microstructure around sleep onset differentiates major depressive insomnia from primary insomnia. J Sleep Res 2003;12:319–30.

28. Krystal AD, Edinger JD, Wohlgemuth WK, et al. NREM sleep EEG frequency spectral correlates of sleep complaints in primary insomnia subtypes. Sleep 2002;25:630–40.

29. Perlis ML, Kehr EL, Smith MT, et al. Temporal and stagewise distribution of high frequency EEG activity in patients with primary and secondary insomnia and in good sleeper controls. J Sleep Res 2001;10:93–104.

30. Perlis ML, Smith MT, Andrews PJ, et al. Beta/Gamma EEG activity in patients with primary and secondary insomnia and good sleeper controls. Sleep 2001;24:110–7.

31. Perlis ML, Merica H, Smith MT, et al. Beta EEG activity and insomnia. Sleep Med Rev 2001;5:363–74.

32. Merica H, Blois R, Gaillard JM. Spectral characteristics of sleep EEG in chronic insomnia. Eur J Neurosci 1998;10:1826–34.

33. Freedman RR. EEG power spectra in sleep-onset insomnia. Electroencephalogr Clin Neurophysiol 1986;63:408–13.

34. Bastien CH, LeBlanc M, Carrier J, et al. Sleep EEG power spectra, insomnia, and chronic use of benzodiazepines. Sleep 2003;26:313–7.

35. Cervena K, Dauvilliers Y, Espa F, et al. Effect of cognitive behavioural therapy for insomnia on sleep architecture and sleep EEG power spectra in psychophysiological insomnia. J Sleep Res 2004;13:385–93.

36. Jacobs GD, Benson H, Friedman R. Home-based central nervous system assessment of a multifactor behavioral intervention for chronic sleep-onset insomnia. Behav Ther 1993;24:159–74.

37. Engel AK, Fries P. Beta-band oscillations–signalling the status quo? Curr Opin Neurobiol 2010;20:156–65.

38. de Gennaro L, Marzano C, Fratello F, et al. The electroencephalographic fingerprint of sleep is genetically determined: a twin study. Ann Neurol 2008;64:455–60.

39. Ambrosius U, Lietzenmaier S, Wehrle R, et al. Heritability of sleep electroencephalogram. Biol Psychiatry 2008;64:344–8.

40. Terzano MG, Mancia D, Salati MR, et al. The cyclic alternating pattern as a physiologic component of normal NREM sleep. Sleep 1985;8:137–45.

41. Terzano MG, Parrino L, Sherieri A, et al. Atlas, rules, and recording techniques for the scoring of cyclic alternating pattern (CAP) in human sleep. Sleep Med 2001;2:537–53.

42. Terzano MG, Parrino L, Spaggiari MC, et al. CAP variables and arousals as sleep electroencephalographic markers for primary insomnia. Clin Neurophysiol 2003;114:1715–23.

43. Chouvarda I, Mendez MO, Rosso V, et al. Cyclic alternating patterns in normal sleep and insomnia: structure and content differences. IEEE Trans Neural Syst Rehabil Eng 2012;20:642–52.

44. Parrino L, Milioli G, De Paolis F, et al. Paradoxical insomnia: the role of CAP and arousals in sleep misperception. Sleep Med 2009;10:1139–45.

45. Ozone M, Yagi T, Itoh H, et al. Effects of zolpidem on cyclic alternating pattern, an objective marker of sleep instability, in Japanese patients with psychophysiological insomnia: a randomized crossover comparative study with placebo. Pharmacopsychiatry 2008;41:106–14.

46. Parrino L, Smerieri A, Giglia F, et al. Polysomnographic study of intermittent zolpidem treatment in primary sleep maintenance insomnia. Clin Neuropharmacol 2008;31:40–50.

47. Picton TW, Lins OG, Scherg M. The recording and analysis of event-related potentials. In: Boller F, Grafman J, editors. Handbook of Neuropsychology, 10. Amsterdam: Elsevier; 1995. p. 3–73.

48. Devoto A, Violani C, Lucidi F, et al. P300 amplitude in subjects with primary insomnia is modulated by their sleep quality. J Psychosom Res 2003;54:3–10.

49. Devoto A, Manganelli S, Lucidi F, et al. Quality of sleep and P300 amplitude in primary insomnia: a preliminary study. Sleep 2005;28:859–63.

50. Sforza E, Haba-Rubio J. Event-related potentials in patients with insomnia and sleep-related breathing disorders: evening-to-morning changes. Sleep 2006;29:805–13.

51. Bastien CH, St-Jean G, Morin CM, et al. Chronic psychophysiological insomnia: hyperarousal and/or inhibition deficits? An ERPs investigation. Sleep 2008;31:887–98.

52. Turcotte I, St-Jean G, Bastien CH. Are individuals with paradoxical insomnia more hyperaroused than individuals with psychophysiological insomnia? Event-related potentials measures at the peri-onset of sleep. Int J Psychophysiol 2011;81:177–90.

53. Turcotte I, Bastien CH. Is quality of sleep related to the N1 and P2 ERPs in chronic psychophysiological insomnia sufferers? Int J Psychophysiol 2009;72:314–22.

54. Kertesz RS, Cote KA. Event-related potentials during the transition to sleep for individuals with sleep-onset insomnia. Behav Sleep Med 2011;9:68–85.

55. Yang CM, Lo HS. ERP evidence of enhanced excitatory and reduced inhibitory processes of auditory stimuli during sleep in patients with primary insomnia. Sleep 2007;30:585–92.

56. American Academy of Sleep Medicine, AASM. The AASM manual for the scoring of sleep and associated events: rules, terminology and technical specifications. Westchester (IL): AASM; 2007.

57. Rechtschaffen A, Kales A. A manual of standardized terminology, techniques and scoring system for sleep stages of human subjects. Washington, DC: US Government Printing Office; 1968.

58. Haynes SN, Adams A, Franzen M. The effects of pre-sleep stress on sleep-onset insomnia. J Abnorm Psychol 1981;90:601–6.

59. Stepanski E, Glinn M, Zorick F, et al. Heart rate changes in chronic insomnia. Stress Med 1994; 10:261–6.

60. Bonnet MH, Arand DL. Heart rate variability in insomniacs and matched normal sleepers. Psychosom Med 1998;60:610–5.

61. Nelson J, Harvey AG. An exploration of pre-sleep cognitive activity in insomnia: imagery and verbal thought. Br J Clin Psychol 2003;42:271–88.

62. Yang AC, Tsai SJ, Yang CH, et al. Reduced physiologic complexity is associated with poor sleep in patients with major depression and primary insomnia. J Affect Disord 2011;131:179–85.

63. de Zambotti M, Covassin N, De Min Tona G, et al. Sleep onset and cardiovascular activity in primary insomnia. J Sleep Res 2011;20:318–25.

64. Monroe LJ. Psychological and physiological differences between good and poor sleepers. J Abnorm Psychol 1967;72:255–64.

65. Freedman RR, Sattler HL. Physiological and psychological factors in sleep-onset insomnia. J Abnorm Psychol 1982;91:380–9.

66. Adam K, Tomeny M, Oswald L. Physiological and psychological differences between good and poor sleepers. J Psychiatr Res 1986;20:301–16.

67. Varkevisser M, van Dongen HP, Kerkhof GA. Physiological indexes in chronic insomnia during a constant routine: evidence for general hyperarousal? Sleep 2005;28:1588–96.

68. Jurysta F, Languart JP, Sputaels V, et al. The impact of chronic primary insomnia on the heart rate-EEG variability link. Clin Neurophysiol 2009; 120:1054–60.

69. Spiegelhalder K, Fuchs L, Ladwig J, et al. Heart rate and heart rate variability in subjectively reported insomnia. J Sleep Res 2011;20:137–45.

70. Israel B, Buysse DJ, Krafty RT, et al. Short-term stability of sleep and heart rate variability in good sleepers and patients with insomnia: for some measures, one night is enough. Sleep 2012;35: 1285–91.

71. Lack LC, Gradisar M, van Someren EJ, et al. The relationship between insomnia and body temperatures. Sleep Med Rev 2008;12:307–17.

72. Broman JE, Hetta J. Electrodermal activity in patients with persistent insomnia. J Sleep Res 1994; 3:165–70.

73. Vgontzas A, Tsigos C, Bixler EO, et al. Chronic insomnia and activity of the stress system: a preliminary study. J Psychosom Res 1998;45: 21–31.

74. Vgontzas AN, Bixler EO, Lin HM, et al. Chronic insomnia is associated with nyctohemeral activation of the hypothalamic-pituitary-adrenal axis: clinical implications. J Clin Endocrinol Metab 2001;86: 3787–94.

75. Rodenbeck A, Huether G, Rüther E, et al. Interactions between evening and nocturnal cortisol and sleep parameters in patients with severe chronic primary insomnia. Neurosci Lett 2002; 324:159–63.

76. Riemann D, Klein T, Rodenbeck A, et al. Nocturnal cortisol and melatonin secretion in primary insomnia. Psychiatry Res 2002;113:17–27.

77. Backhaus J, Junghanns K, Hohagen F. Sleep disturbances are correlated with decreased morning awakening salivary cortisol. Psychoneuroendocrinology 2004;29:1184–91.

78. Baglioni C, Battagliese G, Feige B, et al. Insomnia as a predictor of depression: a meta-analytic evaluation of longitudinal epidemiological studies. J Affect Disord 2011;135:10–9.

79. Spiegel K, Leproult R, van Cauter E. Impact of sleep debt on metabolic and endocrine function. Lancet 1999;354:1435–9.

80. Smith MT, Perlis ML, Chengazi VU, et al. Neuroimaging of NREM sleep in primary insomnia: a preliminary, Tc-99-HMPAO single photon emission computed tomography study. Sleep 2002;25:325–35.

81. Smith MT, Perlis ML, Chengazi VU, et al. NREM sleep cerebral blood flow before and after behavior therapy for chronic primary insomnia: preliminary single photon emission computed tomography (SPECT) data. Sleep Med 2005;6:93–4.

82. Nofzinger EA, Buysse DJ, Germain A, et al. Functional neuroimaging evidence for hyperarousal in insomnia. Am J Psychiatry 2004;161:2126–9.

83. Cano G, Mochizuki T, Saper CB. Neural circuitry of stress-induced insomnia in rats. J Neurosci 2008; 28:10167–84.

84. Saper CV, Scammell TE, Lu J. Hypothalamic regulation of sleep and circadian rhythms. Nature 2005; 437:1257–63.

85. Nofzinger EA, Nissen C, Germain A, et al. Regional cerebral metabolic correlates of WASO during

NREM sleep in insomnia. J Clin Sleep Med 2006;2: 316–22.

86. Altena E, Van der Werf Y, Sanz-Arigita EJ, et al. Prefrontal hypoactivation and recovery in insomnia. Sleep 2008;31:1271–6.

87. Drummond SP, Walker M, Almklov E, et al. Neural correlates of working memory performance in primary insomnia. Sleep, in press.

88. Huang Z, Liang P, Jia X, et al. Abnormal amygdala connectivity in patients with primary insomnia: evidence from resting state fMRI. Eur J Radiol 2012; 81:1288–95.

89. Plante DT, Jensen JE, Schoerning L, et al. Reduced γ-aminobutyric acid in occipital and anterior cingulate cortices in primary insomnia: a link to major depressive disorder? Neuropsychopharmacology 2012;37:1548–57.

90. Winkelman JW, Buxton OM, Jensen E, et al. Reduced brain GABA in primary insomnia: preliminary data from 4T proton magnetic resonance spectroscopy (1H-MRS). Sleep 2008;31: 1499–506.

91. Morgan PT, Pace-Schott EF, Mason GF, et al. Cortical GABA levels in primary insomnia. Sleep 2012;35:807–14.

92. Taki Y, Hashizume H, Thyreau B, et al. Sleep duration during weekdays affects hippocampal gray matter volume in healthy children. Neuroimage 2012;60:471–5.

93. Neylan TC, Mueller SG, Wang Z, et al. Insomnia severity is associated with a decreased volume of the CA3/dentate gyrus hippocampal subfield. Biol Psychiatry 2010;68:494–6.

94. Riemann D, Voderholzer U, Spiegelhalder K, et al. Chronic insomnia and MRI-measured hippocampal volumes: a pilot study. Sleep 2007;30:955–8.

95. Joo EY, Noh HJ, Kim JS, et al. Brain gray matter deficits in patients with chronic primary insomnia. Sleep, in press.

96. Spiegelhalder K, Regen W, Baglioni C, et al. Insomnia does not appear to be associated with substantial structural brain changes. Sleep 2013; 36:731–7.

97. Noh HJ, Joo EY, Kim ST, et al. The relationship between hippocampal volume and cognition in patients with chronic primary insomnia. J Clin Neurol 2012;8:130–8.

98. Winkelman JW, Benson KL, Buxton OM, et al. Lack of hippocampal volume differences in primary insomnia and good sleeper controls: an MRI volumetric study at 3 Tesla. Sleep Med 2010;11:576–82.

99. Altena E, Vrenken H, van der Werf YD, et al. Reduced orbitofrontal and parietal gray matter in chronic insomnia: a voxel-based morphometric study. Biol Psychiatry 2010;67:182–5.

100. Carp J. On the plurality of (methodological) worlds: estimating the analytic flexibility of fMRI experiments. Front Neurosci 2012;6:149.

101. Ioannidis JP. Excess significance bias in the literature on brain volume abnormalities. Arch Gen Psychiatry 2011;68:773–80.

102. Simmons JP, Nelson LD, Simonsohn U. False-positive psychology: undisclosed flexibility in data collection and analysis allows presenting anything as significant. Psychol Sci 2011;22:1359–66.

103. Ioannidis JP. Why most published research findings are false. PLoS Med 2005;2:e124.

104. Riemann D, Spiegelhalder K, Espie C, et al. Chronic insomnia: clinical and research challenges–an agenda. Pharmacopsychiatry 2011;44: 1–14.

Insomnia With Short Sleep Duration
Nosologic, Diagnostic, and Treatment Implications

Alexandros N. Vgontzas, MD*,
Julio Fernandez-Mendoza, PhD

KEYWORDS

- Insomnia - Short sleep duration - Cardiometabolic - Neurocognitive - Physiologic hyperarousal
- Morbidity - Mortality

KEY POINTS

- The nosology of insomnia is associated with unsatisfactory reliability and validity, whereas current clinical practice guidelines do not recommend the use of objective sleep measures in the diagnosis, evaluation, and treatment of insomnia.
- Recent evidence shows that objective measures of sleep are useful in predicting the biologic severity of insomnia (ie, activation of both limbs of the stress system, cardiometabolic morbidity and mortality, as well as cognitive impairment).
- We propose 2 phenotypes of insomnia, based on objective sleep duration, that differ in terms of physiologic hyperarousal, medical morbidity, psychological profiles, and natural course.
- Objective sleep measures (ie, sleep duration), should be included in the diagnostic criteria for sub-typing insomnia.
- Objective measures of sleep duration obtained with cost-effective and simpler methods than polysomnography may become part of the routine diagnosis and treatment of chronic insomnia in an office setting.
- The 2 phenotypes may respond differentially to treatment, that is, insomnia with short sleep duration may respond better to biologic treatments, whereas insomnia with normal sleep duration may respond primarily to psychological treatments.

NOSOLOGY OF INSOMNIA

The prevalence of insomnia in the general population ranges between 8% and 40%, depending on the definition used. Whereas 20% to 30% of the general population has poor sleep (ie, insomnia symptoms of difficulty initiating or maintaining sleep, early morning awakening, or nonrestorative sleep at any given time), another 8% to 10% of the population suffers from chronic insomnia.[1-3]

Insomnia is a major public health problem, as it is associated with impaired occupational performance, increased absenteeism at work, higher health care costs, and worse quality of life.[4,5] However, the connection of insomnia with cardiometabolic risk and cognitive impairment has not been examined until very recently. This has led some clinicians to view insomnia and its associated mental and physical health complaints as obsessions of otherwise healthy individuals.

Department of Psychiatry, Sleep Research & Treatment Center, Pennsylvania State University College of Medicine, 500 University Drive H073, Hershey, PA 17033, USA
* Corresponding author.
E-mail address: axv3@psu.edu

Sleep Med Clin 8 (2013) 309–322
http://dx.doi.org/10.1016/j.jsmc.2013.04.009
1556-407X/13/$ – see front matter © 2013 Elsevier Inc. All rights reserved.

The diagnostic nosology of insomnia has traditionally faced the dilemma of lumping versus splitting insomnia subtypes. The former view is represented in the Diagnostic and Statistical Manual of Mental Disorders (DSM), which reflects the predominant view of the American Psychiatric Association, whereas the latter is represented in the International Classification of Sleep Disorders (ICSD), which reflects the predominant view of the sleep specialists in North America. In 1987, sleep disorders were included for the first time in the third revised edition of the DSM (DSM-III-R) and overall diagnostic criteria for "insomnia disorders" were included based on the subjective complaints of difficulty initiating or maintaining sleep or of nonrestorative sleep, occurring at least 3 times a week for at least 1 month, and associated daytime functioning complaints. The DSM-III-R[6] allowed the diagnoses of "insomnia related to another mental disorder" or "to a known organic factor," "primary insomnia," and "dysomnia not otherwise specified" (Table 1). The DSM-IV-TR eliminated the definition of "insomnia disorders" and included the diagnoses of "primary insomnia," "dysomnia not otherwise specified," insomnia "related to another mental disorder," "due to a general medical condition," and "substance-induced."[7] The DSM-5 is expected to be published in May 2013, and the diagnoses of "primary insomnia," "sleep disorder related to another mental disorder," and "sleep disorder due to a general medical condition" will most probably be eliminated in favor of "insomnia disorder" with concurrent specification of clinically comorbid mental and/or physical conditions, so that no causal attributions between insomnia and the physical/mental condition are made and the independent clinical attention of insomnia is warranted.[8] The DSM-5 is expected to incorporate the use of self-reported severity measures with the aim of identifying subthreshold sleep disturbances in patients at risk for developing a full-fledged "insomnia disorder" and who may be candidates for preventive interventions.[8] Also, an extension of the duration criterion from 1 month to 3 months is expected. However, no objective measures of the biologic severity of the disorder are expected to be included in the forthcoming DSM-5.

The ICSD (1990), and its revised form, ICSD-R (1997), also defined insomnia based on subjective sleep and daytime functioning complaints but, in contrast, attempted to identify subtypes based on "intrinsic" factors, such as etiology (ie, "psychophysiological"), age of onset (ie, "idiopathic insomnia"), degree of discrepancy between objective sleep findings and subjective perception of sleep (ie, "sleep state misperception") or "extrinsic" environmental factors, such as "inadequate sleep hygiene," "food-allergy," or "altitude insomnia" (see Table 1). However, these subtypes, even when refined in the ICSD-2,[9] have not proven to be clinically useful and their reliability is at best modest.[10–12] For example, although the ICSD-2 diagnosis of "psychophysiological insomnia" is based solely on the subjective reports of the patient, it is presumed to be associated with physiologic hyperarousal and polysomnographic (PSG) disturbances. The diagnostic subtype of "idiopathic insomnia" has produced very little research since it was first proposed[13] and it appears that the proposed differences between "psychophysiological" and "idiopathic insomniacs"[14] are not large enough to determine a true differential treatment approach (eg, medication vs psychotherapy). Finally, the subtype of "paradoxical insomnia" is estimated to represent as few as 5% of all insomnia sufferers according to the ICSD[9]; however, recent epidemiologic studies have shown that insomnia sufferers with clinically significant sleep misperception represent about 50% of all insomnia sufferers.[15] Consequently, large multicenter studies have shown that the current insomnia diagnoses available have low diagnostic reliability and validity.[10–12] Finally, although PSG features are suggested, but not required, for virtually all ICSD subtypes, their usefulness in terms of differential diagnosis or severity assessment have not been demonstrated and are not currently used in clinical practice.

The sleep laboratory is essential for the evaluation of patients with sleep-disordered breathing (SDB), the diagnosis of narcolepsy, and the differential diagnosis of idiopathic versus psychogenic hypersomnia.[16,17] In addition, sleep laboratory measurements provide valuable objective information on the initial effectiveness, continued efficacy or tolerance, and potential withdrawal effects of a hypnotic drug. With the disorder of insomnia, the usefulness of the sleep laboratory has been at best controversial. As mentioned previously, the ICSD-2 includes PSG findings as diagnostic criteria, although not required, for virtually all diagnoses.[9] The validity and clinical utility of sleep laboratory testing for diagnosing insomnia has been evaluated in large studies,[11,18,19] and it has been concluded that (1) PSG is not useful in the evaluation of insomnia, except to confirm or exclude other sleep pathologies when there is reasonable evidence from clinical history (eg, SDB or periodic limb movements),[4,20–22] and (2) sleep integrity measures, such as latency to sleep onset, total sleep time, number of arousals and awakenings, and sleep efficiency, are not useful in the diagnosis or differential diagnosis, including

Table 1
Insomnia diagnoses across DSM and ICSD most recent versions

DSM-III-R (1987)	DSM-IV-TR (2000)	ICSD-R (1997)	ICSD-2 (2005)
Dysomnias	**Primary sleep disorders**	**Dysomnias**	**Insomnias**
Insomnia disorders	*Dysomnias*	*Intrinsic sleep disorders*	Adjustment insomnia
Insomnia related to another mental disorder (nonorganic)	Primary insomnia	Psychophysiologic insomnia	Psychophysiological insomnia
Insomnia related to a known organic factor	Dysomnia not otherwise specified	Sleep state misperception	Paradoxic insomnia
Primary insomnia	**Sleep disorder related to another mental disorder**	Idiopathic insomnia	Idiopathic insomnia
Dysomnia not otherwise specified	Insomnia related to another mental disorder	Intrinsic sleep disorder not otherwise specified	Insomnia due to mental disorder
	Sleep disorder due to a general medical condition	*Extrinsic sleep disorders*	Inadequate sleep hygiene
	Insomnia type	Inadequate sleep hygiene	Behavioral insomnia of childhood
	Substance-induced sleep disorder	Environmental sleep disorder	Insomnia due to drug or substance
	Insomnia type	Altitude insomnia	Insomnia due to medical condition
		Adjustment sleep disorder	Insomnia not due to substance or known physiologic conditions, unspecified
		Limit-setting sleep disorder	Physiologic (organic) insomnia, unspecified
		Sleep-onset association disorder	
		Food allergy insomnia	
		Hypnotic-dependent sleep disorder	
		Stimulant-dependent sleep disorder	
		Alcohol-dependent sleep disorder	
		Toxin-induced sleep disorder	
		Extrinsic sleep disorder not otherwise specified	
		Sleep disorders associated with other disorders	
		Associated with mental disorders	
		Associated with neurologic disorders	
		Associated with other medical disorders	

Abbreviations: DSM-III-R, Diagnostic and Statistical Manual of Mental Disorders, Third edition, revised; DSM-IV-TR, Diagnostic and Statistical Manual of Mental Disorders, Fourth edition, text revision; ICSD-2, International Classification of Sleep Disorders, Second edition; ICSD-R, International Classification of Sleep Disorders, Revised.

subtyping of insomnia.[4,11,18–23] The current consensus is, therefore, that PSG is not recommended for routine, differential diagnosis, or severity assessment of insomnia in clinical practice.[22]

However, we present and discuss evidence, accumulated in the recent years, that objective measures of sleep (1) are useful in predicting the biologic severity of insomnia (ie, cardiometabolic morbidity and mortality as well as cognitive impairment) and (2) should be included in the new nosology of insomnia given their clinical utility for severity assessment and choice of treatment based on relevant clinical outcomes.

PATHOPHYSIOLOGY OF INSOMNIA

In the past 2 decades, several models have been proposed to understand the etiology and pathophysiology of insomnia.[24–30] Most of these models have emphasized the importance of the joint effect of stress and psychological factors in the pathogenesis of insomnia. Kales and Kales[24] early stated that "stressful events when mediated by certain predisposing emotional factors and inadequate coping mechanisms, are indeed closely related to the onset of long-term sleep difficulty." The characteristic psychological profile of insomnia sufferers, consisting of cognitive-emotional hyperarousal (ie, obsessive, anxious, ruminative, and dysthymic personality traits) and emotion-oriented coping strategies,[24,31,32] is thought to be present premorbidly and to play a key role in the etiology of the disorder.[24,33–36] The 3-P model by Spielman and colleagues[25] specified each of the predisposing, precipitating, and perpetuating factors involved in the etiopathogenesis of insomnia and provided with a framework for therapies targeting the cognitive-behavioral factors that perpetuate insomnia after the resolution of the original stressor.

Stress has been associated with the activation of the hypothalamic-pituitary-adrenal (HPA) and the sympatho-adrenal-medullary axes, whereas corticotropin-releasing hormone (CRH) and cortisol (products of the hypothalamus and adrenals, respectively), and catecholamines (products of the sympathetic system) are known to cause arousal and sleeplessness to humans and animals. On the other hand, sleep, and particularly deep sleep, has an inhibitory effect on the stress system, including its main 2 components, the HPA axis and the sympathetic system. Given that insomnia is associated with precipitating stressful life events[37] and cognitive-emotional arousal,[24] it was only natural for researchers to explore the association of this disorder with the stress system. Several studies have shown increased HPA axis, sympathetic, and central activation in insomnia sufferers, including increased cortisol and catecholamine secretion, heart rate and impaired heart rate variability, and 24-hour whole body and brain metabolic rate. Although most early studies reported no difference between subjectively defined "poor sleepers" and controls in the levels of 24-hour cortisol and 17-hydroxysteroid excretion,[38–40] later studies found that 24-hour urinary free cortisol, norepinephrine, and catecholamine metabolite levels were either increased in insomnia sufferers with objective sleep disturbances as compared with controls or were correlated with PSG indices of sleep disturbance in patients with insomnia.[41–47] Only 2 recent studies have not replicated these findings. However, in one of these studies, the objective sleep of insomnia sufferers was very similar to that of controls,[48] whereas in the other study,[49] cortisol levels and other indices of physiologic arousal were increased but not to a statistically significant level because of lack of power and controls not being carefully selected.[50] Finally, of interest is a study that demonstrated that middle-aged healthy individuals are more vulnerable to the sleep-disturbing effects of CRH, which may explain physiologically the increased prevalence of insomnia in older subjects.[51]

Furthermore, although 2 early studies found small differences between subjectively defined good and poor sleepers in heart rate measures,[38,52] 2 more-recent studies that included patients with insomnia who also met objective criteria for sleep disturbances have found significant changes in nocturnal heart rate and heart rate variability.[53,54] Two studies have shown that overall oxygen consumption (V_{O2}), a measure of whole-body metabolic rate, is constantly elevated in patients with insomnia with PSG-documented sleep disturbance as compared with controls, whereas V_{O2} is increased in sufferers of sleep misperception insomnia, but to a lesser degree compared with patients with insomnia with PSG-documented sleep disturbance.[55,56] In a group of patients with insomnia with PSG-verified sleep disturbance, a significantly increased pupil size, indicative of sympathetic system activation, was observed,[57] whereas 2 other studies, in which insomnia diagnosis was based only on subjective measures, showed opposite results (ie, decreased pupil size).[58,59]

Although insomnia sufferers typically complain that they are fatigued and sleepy during the day, and one would expect that during the Multiple Sleep Latency Test (MSLT) they would demonstrate short sleep latencies, they have either similar or increased daytime sleep latencies when compared with controls.[59–62] Importantly, several studies have shown that, within insomnia sufferers, those with shorter objective sleep duration show longer sleep latencies in the MSLT[61,63–65] and are more alert in vigilance tests.[55,56,63] This is in contrast to healthy individuals who, after modest short-term sleep loss, experience significantly reduced sleep latencies on the MSLT and decreased alertness in vigilance tests (ie, physiologic sleepiness).[66,67] Thus, long latencies in the MSLT may represent a reliable marker of physiologic hyperarousal in patients with insomnia.

Finally, evidence about the presence of central nervous system hyperarousal in insomnia comes from studies in human subjects using neuroimaging,[68,69] and spectral,[70–75] arousal,[76,77] and event-related[78,79] electroencephalography analyses, and from studies on the neural circuitry of stress-induced insomnia in rats.[80] Increased cortical arousal during sleep is present to a variable degree in all insomnia sufferers[70–75] and may explain why they perceive their sleep as wake and as nonrestorative.[15,28,81,82]

Collectively, these findings suggest that (1) the activity of the stress system is directly proportional to the degree of objective nighttime sleep disturbance or daytime increased vigilance in insomnia sufferers; (2) physiologic hyperarousal (ie, hyperactivity of both limbs of the stress system) is primarily present in patients with insomnia with objective short sleep duration, whereas cognitive-emotional and cortical arousal is present to a variable degree in all insomnia sufferers; (3) objective short sleep duration appears to be a marker of the physiologic hyperarousal in insomnia and not a measure of cumulative chronic sleep loss; and (4) objective sleep measures (ie, short sleep duration [PSG] or increased daytime sleep latencies [MSLT]) can provide a reliable index of the biologic severity and medical impact of the disorder.[83]

INSOMNIA AND CARDIOMETABOLIC MORBIDITY

Many studies have established that insomnia is highly comorbid with psychiatric disorders and is a risk factor for the development of depression, anxiety, and suicide.[4] However, in contrast to SDB, chronic insomnia has not been linked firmly with significant medical morbidity, such as cardiovascular disease. Several questionnaire-based studies have shown a significant relationship between difficulty falling asleep or poor sleep with cardiometabolic outcomes, such as hypertension[84–86] and diabetes.[87–90] For example, in a prospective study from Japan,[85] persistent (>4 years) complaints of difficulty initiating or maintaining sleep were associated with an increased risk of hypertension (odds ratio [OR] = 1.96). In another prospective study, difficulty falling asleep (hazard ratio [HR] =1.4) and difficulty staying asleep (HR = 1.3) were associated with acute myocardial infarction.[86] Furthermore, other studies have shown that sleep disturbances or complaints are associated with increased incidence of type 2 diabetes.[87–90] However, these studies showed relatively small effect sizes and did not include a PSG evaluation so as to control for SDB or other sleep pathology. The findings of these early studies were dismissed as artifacts or flawed by many clinicians and researchers alike.[91,92] In fact, at least one report showed a reduced mortality rate for those individuals complaining of sleep difficulties after 6 years of follow-up.[93]

Given the well-established association of hypercortisolemia with significant medical morbidity (ie, hypertension, diabetes, metabolic syndrome, osteoporosis, and others) and the findings that hypercortisolemia is primarily associated with insomnia with objective short sleep duration,[41–47] we hypothesized that this type of insomnia is associated with significant cardiometabolic morbidity and mortality. A series of recent epidemiologic studies from the Penn State Adult Cohort,[94,95] which used in-laboratory PSG, have shown that insomnia with objective short sleep duration is associated with a high risk of hypertension,[96] diabetes,[97] and mortality.[98] For example, compared with normal sleepers who slept 6 hours or more per night, the highest odds of hypertension or diabetes was in insomnia sufferers who slept 5 hours or less (OR = 5.1 and OR = 2.95, respectively) and the second highest in insomnia sufferers who slept 5 to 6 hours (OR = 3.5 and OR = 2.07, respectively), whereas insomnia sufferers who slept 6 hours or more were not at significantly increased risk of hypertension or diabetes (OR = 1.3 and OR = 1.1, respectively). Recent longitudinal data from the same cohort has shown that insomnia sufferers who slept less than 6 hours were at a significantly higher risk of incident hypertension (OR = 3.75),[99] suggesting that it is insomnia that causes hypertension and not vice versa. Furthermore, other longitudinal research showed that mortality risk in men was significantly increased in insomnia sufferers who slept less than 6 hours compared with normal sleepers (OR = 4.00), and that there was a marginally significant trend toward higher mortality from insomnia with short sleep duration in men with diabetes or hypertension (OR = 7.17) than in those without these comorbid conditions (OR = 1.45). Thus, the impact of insomnia with short sleep duration was much stronger in those with diabetes and hypertension at baseline versus those who were healthy.[98] In women, mortality was not associated with insomnia with short sleep duration, a finding that might be related to the fact that women were followed-up for a shorter time period and that a smaller number were deceased at the time of follow-up compared with men (5% vs 21%, respectively).

Consistent with the findings of these population-based studies, other recent studies have shown that nighttime systolic blood pressure is higher and day-to-night systolic blood pressure dipping is reduced in insomnia sufferers and that the magnitude of beta electroencephalogram activity correlates with their systolic blood pressure dipping.[100] Also, impaired heart rate variability,[101] lower cardiac pre-ejection period,[102] and poorer indices of glucose metabolism[103] are primarily present in insomnia sufferers with objective short sleep duration. Cumulatively, these data indicate that objective short sleep duration may predict the biologic severity of chronic insomnia.

INSOMNIA AND COGNITIVE IMPAIRMENT

Insomnia is associated with complaints of difficulty concentrating, memory problems, and inattention. However, studies using objective neuropsychological testing have produced inconsistent findings. This has led some researchers to question the existence of true cognitive impairments in insomnia[104] and attribute daytime complaints to excessive attention to the expected consequences of poor sleep.[29]

A recent meta-analysis has shown that individuals with insomnia exhibit performance impairments of small to moderate magnitude in several cognitive functions, including working memory, episodic memory, and some aspects of executive functioning.[105] However, an important factor that has not been examined in meta-analytic research of the neurocognitive literature is the degree of objective sleep disturbance shown by the insomnia sufferers across studies. For example, most of the studies included in meta-analyses have shown that cognitive performance is impaired in insomnia sufferers with objective sleep disturbances[60,106–110] or that it correlates with objective markers of sleep disturbance in insomnia sufferers,[110–116] whereas those studies in which performance was not significantly impaired established insomnia diagnoses using solely subjective criteria.[56,113,117–119] The role of objective sleep measures in the association of insomnia with cognitive impairment has been addressed in a recent study from the Penn State Adult Cohort.[120] This study showed that insomnia sufferers, based solely on a subjective complaint, did not differ significantly from controls on either PSG variables or neurocognitive performance. However, significant interactions between insomnia and objective short sleep duration (ie, <6 hours) on specific neurocognitive tests were found. Specifically, insomnia sufferers with objective short sleep duration showed poorer neuropsychological performance on tests of processing speed, set-switching attention, and number of short-term visual memory errors and omissions compared with control groups with normal or short sleep duration. In contrast, insomnia sufferers with normal sleep duration showed no significant deficits when compared with controls. Based on these findings, it seems that insomnia with objective short sleep duration is associated with deficits in set-switching attention, a key component of the "executive control of attention."[120] Importantly, the presence of a group of good sleepers with short sleep duration allowed to demonstrate that deficits in executive functions were associated with underlying physiologic hyperarousal, a characteristic of chronic insomnia, rather than to short sleep per se.[120] Cumulatively, the data from these studies indicate that objective short sleep duration may predict the biologic severity of chronic insomnia, including its effect on cognitive functions.

Brain functions, such as set-switching attention, working memory, and interference control, have been linked to the activation of the prefrontal and anterior cingulate cortices. Tasks of set-switching attention also require the ability to retain both sets so they are ready to be recalled and, in fact, neuroimaging studies show that set-switching attention and working memory cooperate in the same areas of the prefrontal cortex.[121,122] Together, these findings suggest that insomnia with objective short sleep duration, via hypercortisolemia, may affect brain structures and associated cognitive functions.[123–126] Furthermore, insomnia with objective short sleep duration may be a premorbid risk factor for amnestic and non-amnestic mild cognitive impairment (MCI), an area open to future studies.

NATURAL HISTORY OF INSOMNIA

As mentioned in the introduction, approximately 20% of the general population has poor sleep (ie, insomnia symptoms at any given time) and about another 10% has chronic insomnia. Natural history studies have shown that chronic insomnia is a highly persistent condition, whereas the course of poor sleep is more variable and has a higher remission rate.[33,35,36,127,128] This suggests that insomnia is a disorder, whereas poor sleep is a symptom of underlying mental and physical health problems.[35,36,128] Furthermore, objective short sleep duration has been shown to be a risk factor for poor sleep evolving into the more severe form of chronic insomnia,[36] as well as of chronic insomnia becoming persistent.[128] These latter findings suggest that objective short sleep duration may be a biologic marker of genetic predisposition to chronic insomnia[36] and of the severity and chronicity of the disorder.[128]

CLINICAL IMPLICATIONS

The evidence presented in this article has led us to suggest 2 phenotypes of chronic insomnia that are different in terms of etiology, pathophysiology, biologic severity, natural course, psychological characteristics, and, possibly, treatment response. The first phenotype is primarily associated with physiologic hyperarousal (ie, short sleep duration and activation of both limbs of the stress system), significant medical sequelae (eg, hypertension, diabetes, cognitive impairment, increased mortality), and a persistent course. The second phenotype is associated with cognitive-emotional and cortical arousal, but not with physiologic hyperarousal (ie, normal sleep duration and normal activity of the stress system) or significant medical sequelae, and is more likely to remit over time. Furthermore, the first phenotype is associated with a psychological profile typical of medical outpatients, whereas the second phenotype is associated with sleep misperception, anxious-ruminative traits, and poor coping resources.[83]

Table 2 summarizes the findings of key studies, whereas **Fig. 1** depicts a heuristic model of the underlying pathophysiological mechanisms and clinical characteristics of the 2 insomnia phenotypes.

Our proposed model for the 2 insomnia phenotypes has several implications in terms of nosology, diagnostic procedures, and specificity of treatment for chronic insomnia. As we have stated earlier, previously proposed subtypes of insomnia have been associated with low diagnostic reliability and have not been associated with clinically relevant outcomes. In addition, the current diagnostic procedures used in insomnia are subjective tools, such as clinical interviews, questionnaires, and specific scales. The data reviewed here suggest that objective measures of sleep can be useful in detecting the most severe form of insomnia in terms of its importance on the patient's health. Thus, we propose the inclusion of objective sleep duration as a criterion in future diagnostic manuals for insomnia so as to differentiate these 2 clearly different and clinically relevant subtypes of insomnia.

Further, our data suggest that objective measures of sleep, in addition to a thorough clinical evaluation, should become part of the standard diagnostic procedures for insomnia.[83] Although our studies have focused on the utility of sleep duration, other studies suggest that other variables of sleep efficiency and continuity or of physiologic hyperarousal (ie, MSLT) may also serve as markers of the biologic severity of the disorder.[36,42,106,110,112,129,130] However, a potential disadvantage of biomarkers, such as stage 1, slow-wave sleep, or MSLT, is that they require a full PSG study or daytime laboratory assessment, whereas sleep duration perhaps could be obtained with simpler methods (eg, actigraphy). In

this regard, several studies suggest the potential usefulness of actigraphy to assess sleep patterns for a period of days or weeks in the "habitual home environment," to characterize the severity of the insomnia disorder.[21,131,132] A similar amount of home sleep monitoring with PSG would be difficult and impractical for clinical venues. However, several problems associated with the use of actigraphy, such as lack of an industry standard for the sleep algorithms used in different actigraphic devices and the propensity to overestimate or underestimate sleep time, make its current use limited. Future studies using cost-effective methods should examine whether night-to-night variability in sleep duration may be a stronger predictor of cardiometabolic and neurocognitive morbidity compared with average sleep duration.

Finally, our findings may affect the way we treat both chronic insomnia and poor sleep. The insomnia phenotype with short sleep duration may respond better to treatments that primarily aim at decreasing physiologic hyperarousal and increasing sleep duration, such as medication or other biologic treatments.[46] Previous studies have shown that sedative antidepressants, such as trazodone or doxepin, used at low dosages, downregulate the activity of the HPA axis, decrease cortisol levels, and increase sleep duration.[46,133,134] We should note that biologic treatments should be part of a multidimensional approach that combines behavioral changes (ie, sleep hygiene) and psychological interventions (ie, cognitive-behavioral therapy [CBT]) when indicated from the clinical evaluation. The second phenotype (ie, insomnia with normal sleep duration) is not likely associated with physiologic hyperarousal and hypnotics or sedative antidepressants may be not be warranted. This phenotype may respond better to treatments that primarily aim at decreasing cognitive-emotional arousal, changing sleep-related beliefs and behaviors, and altering sleep misperception, such as CBT.[135,136] In fact, given that insomnia with normal sleep duration is associated with poor coping resources and anxious-ruminative traits that extend beyond sleep-related preoccupation, other psychotherapeutic techniques, such as behavioral experiments or emotion regulation techniques, may be indicated. Of course, use of psychotherapeutic medication may be indicated based on the presence of comorbid psychiatric conditions (ie, anxiety or depressive disorders). The differential treatment response of these 2 phenotypes should be tested in future placebo-controlled clinical trials.

In the prevention of insomnia, treatment strategies for persistent poor sleep should focus on

Table 2
Association of insomnia with short sleep duration with physiologic hyperarousal, cardiometabolic morbidity, neurocognitive impairment, and a persistent course

	Controls	Insomnia With Normal Sleep Duration	Insomnia With Short Sleep Duration
Physiologic hyperarousal			
Cortisol levels (20:00–08:00 h), nmol/L[43]	189.8	172.0	302.0[a]
Cortisol AUC (evening 4 h), μg/mL[44]	15.6	—	24.3[a]
Cortisol AUC (19:00–09:00 h), μg/dL[48]	253.7	214.4	—
Heart rate variability (LHF ratio wake), power[54]	0.8	—	1.2[a]
Heart rate variability (SDNN wake), ms[101]	63.5	64.1	50.5[a]
Whole body metabolic rate (Vo_2), % increased[55,56]	—	6[a]	9[a]
MSLT, minutes[55,56]	9.5	10.2	13.3[a]
Cardiometabolic morbidity			
Hypertension, OR[96]	1.0	1.1	5.1[a]
Incident hypertension, OR[99]	1.0	0.9	3.8[a]
Diabetes, OR[97]	1.0	1.1	2.9[a]
Mortality in men, OR[98]	1.0	0.7	4.0[a]
Mortality in men w/hypertension/diabetes, OR[98]	1.0	0.6	7.2[a]
Neurocognitive Impairment			
SDMT, no. correct[120]	50.6	52.4	46.3[a]
TMT-B, s[120]	75.2	68.0	87.8[a]
TMT B–A, s[120]	43.6	36.0	54.6[a]
SAT, error rate[130]	2.5	3.2	4.5[a]
BVRT, no. omissions[120]	0.4	0.4	0.7[a]
Short-term memory, words[55,56]	7.5	7.2	5.7[a]
Sleep misperception			
Subjective sleep time, h[15]	6.5	5.6[a]	5.0[a]
Objective sleep time, h[15]	6.6	6.6	4.7[a]
Subjective – objective sleep time, h[15]	−0.1	−1.0[a]	0.3
Psychological profile			
MMPI-2 psychasthenia, score[15]	49.1	54.5[a]	51.8
MMPI-2 anxiety, score[15]	48.2	53.8[a]	49.4
MMPI-2 ego strength, score[15]	48.7	44.4[a]	47.8
STAI trait anxiety, score[137]	30.7	37.0[a]	34.9
DBAS effects, score[137]	33.2	44.6[a]	41.5
DBAS needs, score[137]	37.2	46.3[a]	38.3
Natural history			
Persistence vs full remission, OR[128]	1.0	0.2	4.9[a]

Abbreviations: AUC, area under the curve; BVRT, Benton Visual Retention Test; DBAS, Dysfunctional Beliefs and Attitudes about Sleep; LHF, low-high frequency; MMPI-2, Minnesota Multiphasic Personality Invesntory-2; MSLT, Multiple Sleep Latency Test; OR, odds ratio; SAT, Switching Attention Task; SDMT, Symbol Digit Modalities Test; SDNN, standard deviation of RR intervals; STAI, State-Trait Anxiety Inventory; TMT-B, Trail Making Test, part B; TMT B–A, Trail Making Test, part B – part A; Vo_2, overall oxygen consumption.
[a] Value significantly higher or lower as compared with controls.

treating the underlying physical health conditions (eg, cardiovascular disorders, ulcer, or allergy/asthma) as well as the associated psychological distress with, for example, CBT. Given that poor sleepers with shorter objective sleep duration and a family history of sleep problems are at greater risk of developing chronic insomnia,[36] their appropriate detection with objective sleep

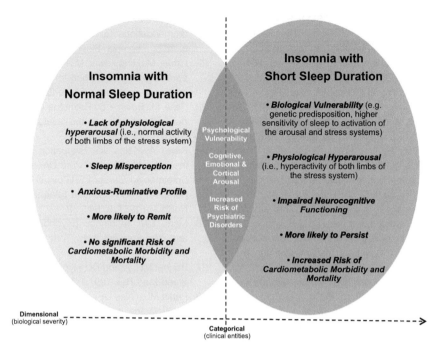

Fig. 1. Heuristic model of the underlying pathophysiological mechanisms and clinical characteristics of the 2 insomnia phenotypes based on objective sleep duration. The common characteristics of the 2 phenotypes are presented in the overlapping area, whereas their unique characteristics are presented in the areas of each phenotype that do not overlap. (*From* Vgontzas AN, Fernandez-Mendoza J, Liao D, et al. Insomnia with objective short sleep duration: the most biologically severe phenotype of the disorder. Sleep Med Rev 2013;17:241–54; with permission.)

measures is warranted and treatment should focus on decreasing physiologic hyperarousal and lengthening sleep duration.

In this article, we present evidence that the degree of objective sleep disturbance in insomnia is directly proportional to the activity of both limbs of the stress system and other indices of physiologic hyperarousal. Evidence suggests that insomnia with objective short sleep duration is associated with a significant risk of cardiometabolic morbidity and mortality and cognitive impairment. In contrast, insomnia with normal sleep duration is associated with cognitive-emotional and cortical arousal and sleep misperception but not with signs of physiologic hyperarousal or cardiometabolic or neurocognitive morbidity. We propose that objective measures of sleep duration may become part of the routine evaluation and diagnosis of chronic insomnia in an office setting. Also, we propose that these insomnia phenotypes may respond differentially to treatment (ie, insomnia with short sleep duration may respond better to biologic treatments, whereas insomnia with normal sleep duration may respond better to psychological treatment alone).

REFERENCES

1. Bixler EO, Vgontzas AN, Lin HM, et al. Insomnia in central Pennsylvania. J Psychosom Res 2002; 53(1):589–92.
2. Ohayon MM. Epidemiology of insomnia: what we know and what we still need to learn. Sleep Med Rev 2002;6:97–111.
3. Morin CM, LeBlanc M, Daley M, et al. Epidemiology of insomnia: prevalence, self-help treatments, consultations, and determinants of help-seeking behaviors. Sleep Med 2006;7:123–30.
4. National Institutes of Health. NIH state of the science statement on manifestations and management of chronic insomnia in adults. J Clin Sleep Med 2005;1:412–21.
5. Léger D, Bayon V. Societal costs of insomnia. Sleep Med Rev 2010;14(6):379–89.
6. Reynolds CF 3rd, Kupfer DJ, Buysse DJ, et al. Subtyping DSM-III-R primary insomnia: a literature review by the DSM-IV Work Group on Sleep Disorders. Am J Psychiatry 1991;148:432–8.
7. American Psychiatric Association. Diagnostic and statistical manual of mental disorders, text revision. 4th edition. Washington, DC: American Psychiatric Association; 2000.

8. Reynolds CF 3rd, Redline S, DSM-V Sleep-Wake Disorders Workgroup, Advisors. The DSM-V sleep-wake disorders nosology: an update and an invitation to the sleep community. Sleep 2010; 33(1):10–1.

9. American Academy of Sleep Medicine. The International Classification of sleep disorders (ICSD-2): diagnostic and coding manual. 2nd edition. Westchester (IL): American Academy of Sleep Medicine; 2005.

10. Soldatos CR, Lugaresi E. Nosology and prevalence of sleep disorders. Semin Neurol 1987;7(3):236–42.

11. Buysse DJ, Reynolds CF III, Hauri PJ, et al. Diagnostic concordance for insomnia patients among sleep specialists using proposed DSM-IV, proposed ICD-10, and ICSD diagnostic systems: report from the APA/NIMH DSM-IV field trial. In: Widiger TA, Frances AJ, Pincus HA, et al, editors. DSM-IV sourcebook, vol. 4. Washington, DC: American Psychiatric Association; 1998. p. 869–89.

12. Edinger JD, Wyatt JK, Stepanski EJ, et al. Testing the reliability and validity of DSM-IV-TR and ICSD-2 insomnia diagnoses. Results of a multitrait-multimethod analysis. Arch Gen Psychiatry 2011; 68(10):992–1002.

13. Hauri P, Olmstead E. Childhood-onset insomnia. Sleep 1980;3(1):59–65.

14. Espie CA, Barrie LM, Forgan GS. Comparative investigation of the psychophysiologic and idiopathic insomnia disorder phenotypes: psychologic characteristics, patients' perspectives, and implications for clinical management. Sleep 2012; 35(3):385–93.

15. Fernandez-Mendoza J, Calhoun SL, Bixler EO, et al. Sleep misperception and chronic insomnia in the general population: role of objective sleep duration and psychological profiles. Psychosom Med 2011;73(1):88–97.

16. Vgontzas AN, Kales A. Sleep and its disorders. Annu Rev Med 1999;50:387–400.

17. Vgontzas AN, Bixler EO, Kales A, et al. Differences in nocturnal and daytime sleep between primary and psychiatric hypersomnia: diagnostic and treatment implications. Psychosom Med 2000;62: 220–6.

18. Vgontzas AN, Bixler EO, Kales A, et al. Validity and clinical utility of sleep laboratory criteria for insomnia. Int J Neurosci 1994;77(1–2):11–21.

19. Vgontzas AN, Kales A, Bixler EO, et al. Usefulness of polysomnographic studies in the differential diagnosis of insomnia. Int J Neurosci 1995;82:47–60.

20. Chesson A Jr, Hartse K, Anderson WM, et al. Practice parameters for the evaluation of chronic insomnia. An American Academy of Sleep Medicine report Standards of Practice Committee of the American Academy of Sleep Medicine. Sleep 2000;23:237–41.

21. Buysse DJ, Ancoli-Israel S, Edinger JD, et al. Recommendations for a standard research assessment of insomnia. Sleep 2006;29:1155–73.

22. Littner M, Hirshkowitz M, Kramer M, et al. Practice parameters for using polysomnography to evaluate insomnia: an update. Sleep 2003;26:754–60.

23. Reite M, Buysse D, Reynolds C, et al. The use of polysomnography in the evaluation of insomnia. Sleep 1995;18:58–70.

24. Kales A, Kales JD. Evaluation and treatment of insomnia. New York: Oxford University Press; 1984.

25. Spielman AJ, Caruso LS, Glovinsky PB. A behavioral perspective on insomnia treatment. Psychiatr Clin North Am 1987;10:541–53.

26. Morin CM. Insomnia: psychological assessment and management. New York: The Guilford Press; 1993.

27. Bonnet MH, Arand DL. Hyperarousal and insomnia. Sleep Med Rev 1997;1:97–108.

28. Perlis ML, Giles DE, Mendelson WB, et al. Psychophysiological insomnia: the behavioural model and a neurocognitive perspective. J Sleep Res 1997;6: 179–88.

29. Harvey AG. A cognitive model of insomnia. Behav Res Ther 2002;40:869–93.

30. Espie CA. Insomnia: conceptual issues in the development, persistence, and treatment of sleep disorder in adults. Annu Rev Psychol 2002;53:215–43.

31. LeBlanc M, Beaulieu-Bonneau S, Mérette C, et al. Psychological and health-related quality of life factors associated with insomnia in a population-based sample. J Psychosom Res 2007;63:157–66.

32. Morin CM, Rodrigue S, Ivers H. Role of stress, arousal, and coping skills in primary insomnia. Psychosom Med 2003;65:259–67.

33. LeBlanc M, Mérette C, Savard J, et al. Incidence and risk factors of insomnia in a population-based sample. Sleep 2009;32:1027–37.

34. Fernández-Mendoza J, Vela-Bueno A, Vgontzas AN, et al. Cognitive-emotional hyperarousal as a premorbid characteristic of individuals vulnerable to insomnia. Psychosom Med 2010;72: 397–403.

35. Singareddy R, Vgontzas AN, Fernandez-Mendoza J, et al. Risk factors for incident chronic insomnia: a general population prospective study. Sleep Med 2012;13(4):346–53.

36. Fernandez-Mendoza J, Vgontzas AN, Bixler EO, et al. Clinical and polysomnographic predictors of the natural history of poor sleep in the general population. Sleep 2012;35(5):689–97.

37. Healey ES, Kales A, Monroe LJ, et al. Onset of insomnia: role of life-stress events. Psychosom Med 1981;43(5):439–51.

38. Monroe LJ. Psychological and physiological differences between good and poor sleepers. J Abnorm Psychol 1967;72(3):255–64.

39. Johns MW, Gay TJ, Masterton JP, et al. Relationship between habits, adrenocortical activity and personality. Psychosom Med 1971;33:499–508.

40. Frankel BL, Buchbinder R, Coursey R, et al. Sleep patterns and psychological test characteristics of chronic primary insomniacs. Sleep Res 1973;2:149.

41. Adam K, Tomeny M, Oswald I. Physiological and psychological differences between good and poor sleepers. J Psychiatr Res 1986;20(4):301–16.

42. Vgontzas AN, Tsigos C, Bixler EO, et al. Chronic insomnia and activity of the stress system: a preliminary study. J Psychosom Res 1998;45: 21–31.

43. Vgontzas AN, Bixler EO, Lin HM, et al. Chronic insomnia is associated with nyctohemeral activation of the hypothalamic-pituitary-adrenal axis: clinical implications. J Clin Endocrinol Metab 2001;86: 3787–94.

44. Rodenbeck A, Huether G, Ruether E, et al. Interactions between evening and nocturnal cortisol secretion and sleep parameters in patients with severe chronic primary insomnia. Neurosci Lett 2002; 324:163–459.

45. Shaver JL, Johnston SK, Lentz MJ, et al. Stress exposure, psychological distress, and physiological stress activation in midlife women with insomnia. Psychosom Med 2002;64:793–802.

46. Rodenbeck A, Cohrs S, Jordan W, et al. The sleep-improving effects of doxepin are paralleled by a normalized plasma cortisol secretion in primary insomnia. A placebo-controlled, double-blind, randomized, cross-over study followed by an open treatment over 3 weeks. Psychopharmacology (Berl) 2003;170(4):423–8.

47. Irwin M, Clark C, Kennedy B, et al. Nocturnal catecholamines and immune function in insomniacs, depressed patients, and controls subjects. Brain Behav Immun 2003;17(5):365–72.

48. Riemann D, Klein T, Rodenbeck A, et al. Nocturnal cortisol and melatonin secretion in primary insomnia. Psychiatry Res 2002;113:17–27.

49. Varkevisser M, Van Dongen HP, Kerkhof GA. Physiologic indexes in chronic insomnia during a constant routine: evidence for general hyperarousal? Sleep 2005;28:1588–96.

50. Bonnet MH. Hyperarousal as the basis for insomnia: effect size and significance. Sleep 2005;28:1500–1.

51. Vgontzas AN, Bixler EO, Wittman AM, et al. Middle-aged men show higher sensitivity of sleep to the arousing effects of corticotropin-releasing hormone than young men: clinical implications. J Clin Endocrinol Metab 2001;86(4):1489–95.

52. Freedman RR, Sattler HL. Physiological and psychological factors in sleep-onset insomnia. J Abnorm Psychol 1982;91(5):380–9.

53. Stepanski E, Glinn M, Zorick F, et al. Heart rate changes in chronic insomnia. Stress Med 1994; 10(4):261–6.

54. Bonnet MH, Arand DL. Heart rate variability in insomniacs and matched normal sleepers. Psychosom Med 1998;60(5):610–5.

55. Bonnet MH, Arand DL. 24-hour metabolic rate in insomniacs and matched normal sleepers. Sleep 1995;18(7):581–8.

56. Bonnet MH, Arand DL. Physiological activation in patients with sleep state misperception. Psychosom Med 1997;59(5):533–40.

57. Lichstein K, Johnson RS. Pupillometric discrimination of insomniacs. Behav Res Ther 1994;32(1): 123–9.

58. Lichstein KL, Johnson RS, Sen Gupta S, et al. Are insomniacs sleepy during the day? A pupillometric assessment. Behav Res Ther 1992;30(3):283–92.

59. Lichstein KL, Wilson NM, Noe SL, et al. Daytime sleepiness in insomnia: behavioral, biological and subjective indices. Sleep 1994;17(8):693–702.

60. Seidel WF, Ball S, Cohen S, et al. Daytime alertness in relation to mood, performance, and nocturnal sleep in chronic insomniacs and noncomplaining sleepers. Sleep 1984;7(3):230–8.

61. Stepanski E, Zorick F, Roehrs T, et al. Daytime alertness in patients with chronic insomnia compared with asymptomatic control subjects. Sleep 1988; 11(1):54–60.

62. Bonnet MH, Arand DL. Activity, arousal, and the MSLT in patients with insomnia. Sleep 2000;23(2): 205–12.

63. Sugerman JL, Stern JA, Walsh JK. Daytime alertness in subjective and objective insomnia: some preliminary findings. Biol Psychiatry 1985;20(7): 741–50.

64. Dorsey CM, Bootzin RR. Subjective and psychophysiologic insomnia: an examination of sleep tendency and personality. Biol Psychiatry 1997;41(2): 209–16.

65. Roehrs TA, Randall S, Harris E, et al. MSLT in primary insomnia: stability and relation to nocturnal sleep. Sleep 2011;34(12):1647–52.

66. Bonnet MH, Arand DL. Clinical effects of sleep fragmentation versus sleep deprivation. Sleep Med Rev 2003;7(4):297–310.

67. Vgontzas AN, Zoumakis E, Bixler EO, et al. Adverse effects of modest sleep restriction on sleepiness, performance, and inflammatory cytokines. J Clin Endocrinol Metab 2004;89(5):2119–26.

68. Nofzinger EA, Nissen C, Germain A, et al. Regional cerebral metabolic correlates of WASO during NREM sleep in insomnia. J Clin Sleep Med 2006; 2(3):316–22.

69. Winkelman JW, Buxton OM, Jensen JE, et al. Reduced brain GABA in primary insomnia: preliminary data from 4T proton magnetic resonance

spectroscopy (1H-MRS). Sleep 2008;311(11): 1499–506.

70. Hall M, Buysse DJ, Nowell PD, et al. Symptoms of stress and depression as correlates of sleep in primary insomnia. Psychosom Med 2000;62(2): 227–30.

71. Hall M, Thayer JF, Germain A, et al. Psychological stress is associated with heightened physiological arousal during NREM sleep in primary insomnia. Behav Sleep Med 2007;5(3):178–93.

72. Perlis ML, Smith MT, Andrews PJ, et al. Beta/ Gamma EEG activity in patients with primary and secondary insomnia and good sleeper controls. Sleep 2001;24(1):110–7.

73. Krystal AD, Edinger JD, Wohlgemuth WK, et al. NREM sleep EEG frequency spectral correlates of sleep complaints in primary insomnia subtypes. Sleep 2002;25:630–40.

74. Corsi-Cabrera M, Figueredo-Rodríguez P, del Río-Portilla Y, et al. Enhanced frontoparietal synchronized activation during the wake-sleep transition in patients with primary insomnia. Sleep 2012; 35(4):501–11.

75. Spiegelhalder K, Regen W, Feige B, et al. Increased EEG sigma and beta power during NREM sleep in primary insomnia. Biol Psychol 2012;91(3):329–33.

76. Feige B, Al-Shajlawi A, Nissen C, et al. Does REM sleep contribute to subjective wake time in primary insomnia? A comparison of polysomnographic and subjective sleep in 100 patients. J Sleep Res 2008; 17:180–90.

77. Parrino L, Milioli G, De Paolis F, et al. Paradoxical insomnia: the role of CAP and arousals in sleep misperception. Sleep Med 2009;10:1139–45.

78. Turcotte I, St-Jean G, Bastien CH. Are individuals with paradoxical insomnia more hyperaroused than individuals with psychophysiological insomnia? Event-related potentials measures at the peri-onset of sleep. Int J Psychophysiol 2011; 81(3):177–90.

79. Bastien CH, Turcotte I, St-Jean G, et al. Information processing varies between insomnia types: measures of N1 and P2 during the night. Behav Sleep Med 2013;11(1):56–72.

80. Cano G, Mochizuki T, Saper CB. Neural circuitry of stress-induced insomnia in rats. J Neurosci 2008; 28(40):10167–84.

81. Harvey AG, Tang NK. (Mis)perception of sleep in insomnia: a puzzle and a resolution. Psychol Bull 2012;138(1):77–101.

82. Stone KC, Taylor DJ, McCrae CS, et al. Nonrestorative sleep. Sleep Med Rev 2008;12(4):275–88.

83. Vgontzas AN, Fernandez-Mendoza J, Liao D, et al. Insomnia with objective short sleep duration: the most biologically severe phenotype of the disorder. Sleep Med Rev 2013. [Epub ahead of print].

84. Bonnet MH, Arand DL. Cardiovascular implications of poor sleep. Sleep Med Clin 2007;2:529–38.

85. Suka M, Yoshida K, Sugimori H. Persistent insomnia is a predictor of hypertension in Japanese male workers. J Occup Health 2003;45:344–50.

86. Laugsand LE, Vatten LJ, Platou C, et al. Insomnia and the risk of acute myocardial infarction: a population study. Circulation 2011;124:2073–81.

87. Kawakami N, Takatsuka N, Shimizu H. Sleep disturbance and onset of type 2 diabetes. Diabetes Care 2004;27:282–3.

88. Nilsson PM, Rööst M, Engström G, et al. Incidence of diabetes in middle-aged men is related to sleep disturbances. Diabetes Care 2004;27: 2464–9.

89. Meisinger C, Heier M, Loewel H, MONICA/KORA Augsburg Cohort Study. Sleep disturbance as a predictor of type 2 diabetes mellitus in men and women from the general population. Diabetologia 2005;48:235–41.

90. Mallon L, Broman JE, Hetta J. High incidence of diabetes in men with sleep complaints or short sleep duration: a 12-year follow-up study of a middle-aged population. Diabetes Care 2005;28: 2762–7.

91. Phillips B, Mannino DM. Do insomnia complaints cause hypertension or cardiovascular disease? J Clin Sleep Med 2007;3:489–94.

92. Bonnet MH. Evidence for the pathophysiology of insomnia. Sleep 2009;32:441–2.

93. Kripke DF, Garfinkel L, Wingard DL, et al. Mortality associated with sleep duration and insomnia. Arch Gen Psychiatry 2002;59:131–6.

94. Bixler EO, Vgontzas AN, Ten Have T, et al. Effects of age on sleep apnea in men: I. Prevalence and severity. Am J Respir Crit Care Med 1998;157: 144–8.

95. Bixler EO, Vgontzas AN, Lin HM, et al. Prevalence of sleep-disordered breathing in women: effects of gender. Am J Respir Crit Care Med 2001;163: 608–13.

96. Vgontzas AN, Liao D, Bixler EO, et al. Insomnia with objective short sleep duration is associated with a high risk for hypertension. Sleep 2009; 32(4):491–7.

97. Vgontzas AN, Liao D, Pejovic S, et al. Insomnia with objective short sleep duration is associated with type 2 diabetes: a population-based study. Diabetes Care 2009;32(11):1980–5.

98. Vgontzas AN, Liao D, Pejovic S, et al. Insomnia with short sleep duration and mortality: the Penn State cohort. Sleep 2010;33(9):1159–64.

99. Fernandez-Mendoza J, Vgontzas AN, Liao D, et al. Insomnia with objective short sleep duration and incident hypertension: the Penn State Cohort. Hypertension 2012;60:929–35. http://dx.doi.org/10.1161/HYPERTENSIONAHA.112.193268.

100. Lanfranchi PA, Pennestri MH, Fradette L, et al. Nighttime blood pressure in normotensive subjects with chronic insomnia: implications for cardiovascular risk. Sleep 2009;32:760–6.

101. Spiegelhalder K, Fuchs L, Ladwig J, et al. Heart rate and heart rate variability in subjectively reported insomnia. J Sleep Res 2011;20(1 Pt 2):137–45.

102. De Zambotti M, Covassin N, De Min Tona G, et al. Sleep onset and cardiovascular activity in primary insomnia. J Sleep Res 2011;20(2):318–25.

103. Knutson KL, Van Cauter E, Zee P, et al. Cross-sectional associations between measures of sleep and markers of glucose metabolism among subjects with and without diabetes: the Coronary Artery Risk Development in Young Adults (CARDIA) Sleep Study. Diabetes Care 2011;34(5):1171–6.

104. Riedel BW, Lichstein KL. Insomnia and daytime functioning. Sleep Med Rev 2000;4(3):277–98.

105. Fortier-Brochu E, Beaulieu-Bonneau S, Ivers H, et al. Insomnia and daytime cognitive performance: a meta-analysis. Sleep Med Rev 2012;16(1):83–94.

106. Edinger JD, Glenn DM, Bastian LA, et al. Slow-wave sleep and waking cognitive performance II: findings among middle-aged adults with and without insomnia complaints. Physiol Behav 2000;70(1–2):127–34.

107. Szelenberger W, Niemcewicz S. Severity of insomnia correlates with cognitive impairment. Acta Neurobiol Exp (Wars) 2000;60(3):373.

108. Varkevisser M, Kerkhof GA. Chronic insomnia and performance in a 24-h constant routine study. J Sleep Res 2005;14(1):49–59.

109. Haimov I, Hanuka E, Horowitz Y. Chronic insomnia and cognitive functioning among older adults. Behav Sleep Med 2008;6(1):32–54.

110. Edinger JD, Means MK, Carney CE, et al. Psychomotor performance deficits and their relation to prior nights' sleep among individuals with primary insomnia. Sleep 2008;31(5):599–607.

111. Rosa RR, Bonnet MH. Reported chronic insomnia is independent of poor sleep as measured by electroencephalography. Psychosom Med 2000;62(4):474–82.

112. Bastien CH, Fortier-Brochu E, Rioux I, et al. Cognitive performance and sleep quality in the elderly suffering from chronic insomnia. Relationship between objective and subjective measures. J Psychosom Res 2003;54(1):39–49 [Erratum in: J Psychosom Res 2003;55(5):475].

113. Orff HJ, Drummond SP, Nowakowski S, et al. Discrepancy between subjective symptomatology and objective neuropsychological performance in insomnia. Sleep 2007;30(9):1205–11.

114. Fang SC, Huang CJ, Yang TT, et al. Heart rate variability and daytime functioning in insomniacs and normal sleepers: preliminary results. J Psychosom Res 2008;65(1):23–30.

115. Backhaus J, Junghanns K, Born J, et al. Impaired declarative memory consolidation during sleep in patients with primary insomnia: influence of sleep architecture and nocturnal cortisol release. Biol Psychiatry 2006;60(12):1324–30.

116. Nissen C, Kloepfer C, Feige B, et al. Sleep-related memory consolidation in primary insomnia. J Sleep Res 2011;20(1 Pt 2):129–36.

117. Broman JE, Lundh LG, Aleman K, et al. Subjective and objective performance in patients with persistent insomnia. Scand J Behav Ther 1992;21(3):115–26.

118. Lundh LG, Froding A, Gyllenhammar L, et al. Cognitive bias and memory performance in patients with persistent insomnia. Scand J Behav Ther 1997;26(1):27–35.

119. Varkevisser M, Van Dongen HP, Van Amsterdam JG, et al. Chronic insomnia and daytime functioning: an ambulatory assessment. Behav Sleep Med 2007;5(4):279–96.

120. Fernandez-Mendoza J, Calhoun S, Bixler EO, et al. Insomnia with objective short sleep duration is associated with deficits in neuropsychological performance: a general population study. Sleep 2010;33(4):459–65.

121. Ríos M, Periáñez JA, Muñoz-Céspedes JM. Attentional control and slowness of information processing after severe traumatic brain injury. Brain Inj 2004;18(3):257–72.

122. Sánchez-Cubillo I, Periáñez JA, Adrover-Roig D, et al. Construct validity of the Trail Making Test: role of task-switching, working memory, inhibition/interference control, and visuomotor abilities. J Int Neuropsychol Soc 2009;15(3):438–50.

123. Riemann D, Voderholzer U, Spiegelhalder K, et al. Chronic insomnia and MRI-measured hippocampal volumes: a pilot study. Sleep 2007;30(8):955–8.

124. Altena E, Van Der Werf YD, Sanz-Arigita EJ, et al. Prefrontal hypoactivation and recovery in insomnia. Sleep 2008;31(9):1271–6.

125. Altena E, Vrenken H, Van Der Werf YD, et al. Reduced orbitofrontal and parietal gray matter in chronic insomnia: a voxel-based morphometric study. Biol Psychiatry 2010;67(2):182–5.

126. Winkelman JW, Benson KL, Buxton OM, et al. Lack of hippocampal volume differences in primary insomnia and good sleeper controls: an MRI volumetric study at 3 Tesla. Sleep Med 2010;11:576–82.

127. Morin CM, Bélanger L, LeBlanc M, et al. The natural history of insomnia: a population-based 3-year longitudinal study. Arch Intern Med 2009;169(5):447–53.

128. Vgontzas AN, Fernandez-Mendoza J, Bixler EO, et al. Persistent insomnia: the role of objective short

sleep duration and mental health. Sleep 2012; 35(1):61–8.

129. Fung MM, Peters K, Redline S, et al. Decreased slow wave sleep increases risk of developing hypertension in elderly men. Hypertension 2011; 58(4):596–603.

130. Edinger JD, Means MK, Krystal AS. Does physiological hyperarousal enhance error rates among insomnia sufferers? Sleep, in press.

131. Sánchez-Ortuño MM, Edinger JD, Means MK, et al. Home is where sleep is: an ecological approach to test the validity of actigraphy for the assessment of insomnia. J Clin Sleep Med 2010;6(1):21–9.

132. Ancoli-Israel S, Cole R, Alessi C, et al. The role of actigraphy in the study of sleep and circadian rhythms. Sleep 2003;26:342–92.

133. Deuschle M, Schmider J, Weber B, et al. Pulse-dosing and conventional application of doxepin: effects on psychopathology and hypothalamus-pituitary-adrenal (HPA) system. J Clin Psychopharmacol 1997;17(3):156–60.

134. Monteleone P. Effects of trazodone on plasma cortisol in normal subjects. A study with drug plasma levels. Neuropsychopharmacology 1991; 5(1):61–4.

135. Morin CM, Colecchi C, Stone J, et al. Behavioral and pharmacological therapies for late-life insomnia: a randomized controlled trial. JAMA 1999;281(11):991–9.

136. Edinger JD, Wohlgemuth WK, Radtke RA, et al. Cognitive behavioral therapy for treatment of chronic primary insomnia: a randomized controlled trial. JAMA 2001;285(14):1856–64.

137. Edinger JD, Fins AI, Glenn DM, et al. Insomnia and the eye of the beholder: are there clinical markers of objective sleep disturbances among adults with and without insomnia complaints? J Consult Clin Psychol 2000;68(4):586–93.

The Role of Genes in the Insomnia Phenotype

Philip R. Gehrman, PhD, CBSM[a],[*], Cory Pfeiffenberger, PhD[b],
Enda M. Byrne, PhD[c]

KEYWORDS

• Insomnia • Genetics • GWAS • Animal models

KEY POINTS

- With the development of genetic model systems for sleep, it seems logical to use them to screen human insomnia genetic studies for bona fide hits and to further characterize the mechanisms behind insomnia.
- Studies on the genetics of insomnia must be an important component of future research on the disorder.
- Understanding of the role of genes in the insomnia phenotype is limited.
- There are several molecular genetic tools available that were not in existence even a few years ago.
- The time is ripe for research on the genetics of insomnia that may finally shed light on the mechanisms of this common sleep disorder.

Current conceptualizations of insomnia are largely based on the 3 Ps (Predisposing, Precipitating, and Perpetuating factors) model[1] in its original or adapted form. According to this model, the onset of acute insomnia is due to the interaction between 1 or more precipitating factors and premorbid predisposing factors. Predisposing factors can increase vulnerability to developing insomnia or, when low, may confer a degree of resiliency. There is no universally agreed-on set of predisposing factors, but virtually all presentations of the model suggest that genetic factors may play a role. Yet, there has been little research in the genetic basis of insomnia. This is beginning to change, and investigations are starting to take advantage of the powerful tools that are part of the genomics revolution currently under way. The goal of this article is to summarize current understanding of the role of genetics in the pathophysiology of insomnia.

WHAT IS THE INSOMNIA PHENOTYPE?

To study the genetics of insomnia, the phenotype of interest must be defined. Insomnia research has long been plagued by the use of a wide range of phenotypic definitions of insomnia. Efforts have been made to create a more standardized assessment approach to create greater uniformity[2,3] but substantial heterogeneity continues. At the most fundamental level, insomnia can be assessed with the single question: Do you have trouble sleeping? Although this question has face validity, it is associated with several difficulties, including interindividual variation in beliefs about what constitutes trouble. Clinical[4,5] and research[3] diagnostic systems require that the insomnia be associated with some degree of associated distress or impairment. In clinical settings, this requirement is almost always met

Funded by: National Institutes of Health.
[a] Department of Psychiatry, Perelman School of Medicine, University of Pennsylvania, 3535 Market Street, Suite 670, Philadelphia, PA 19104, USA; [b] Translational Research Laboratories, Center for Sleep and Circadian Neurobiology, Perelman School of Medicine, University of Pennsylvania, 125 South 31st Street, Suite 2100, Philadelphia, PA 19104-3403, USA; [c] Queensland Brain Institute, University of Queensland, Upland Road, St Lucia, Queensland 4072, Australia
* Corresponding author.
E-mail address: gehrman@exchange.upenn.edu

because an individual is not likely to seek treatment if there are no perceived negative consequences. In community samples, there is a portion of the population who report difficulty initiating or maintaining sleep but who do not report associated consequences.[6] It is not known if those without impairment should be considered insomnia cases for genetic studies, but it seems clear that neither are they true controls. Current diagnostic systems divide insomnia into several specific subtypes, including psychophysiologic, idiopathic, and paradoxic forms that are thought to reflect subtypes in the population; however, the upcoming revisions of the *Diagnostic and Statistical Manual of Mental Disorders* and *International Classification of Sleep Disorders* have eliminated most of these distinctions due to lack of supporting evidence.[7]

Objective measures of sleep can also be used to define the insomnia phenotype and have the advantage of reduced influence by self-report biases. The gold standard for the objective measurement of sleep is polysomnography (PSG), which involves the measurement of multiple physiologic signals (electroencephalographic [EEG], electromyographic, and electroocculgraphic) over the course of the night. PSG can provide highly detailed information on sleep architecture and the time course of sleep patterns. Sleep architecture variables seem to represent individual traits that are highly heritable, suggesting that PSG may be an optimal strategy for genetics studies of insomnia.[8] Two practical limitations of PSG are that it is time consuming and expensive, hindering its applicability for the types of large-scale studies needed for many genetic approaches. More importantly, PSG studies have often failed to find objective evidence of disturbed sleep in individuals with subjective reports of insomnia.[9] This discrepancy may be due to inherent limitations in using standard visual methods for determining sleep and wake on PSG. An alternative approach is to use computer-based spectral analysis methods of the EEG signal to provide a finer-grained analysis of the microarchitecture of sleep. Compared with good sleepers, individuals with insomnia frequently demonstrate increased EEG activity in the beta frequency range during sleep.[10] Beta EEG is thought indicative of increased cortical processing, leading to the hypothesis that insomnia can be associated with a mixed state of wakefulness and sleep that an individual perceives as wakefulness. This explains the discrepancy between subjective and objective assessments of sleep found in many insomnia studies. Beta EEG power would be an ideal phenotype for genetic studies of insomnia, but spectral analysis methods can be cumbersome to implement on any large scale.

ARE INSOMNIA PHENOTYPES HERITABLE?

The first step in studying the genetics of any trait is to establish that variability in its manifestation is attributable in part to genetic factors. Several approaches can be used to estimate the narrow-sense heritability of a trait (h^2) (ie, the proportion of variation in the trait that can be explained by additive genetic factors). The goal is to tease apart the relative contributions of genetic and nongenetic (environmental) factors. The 2 strategies most frequently used to establish heritability are twin studies and family studies.

In family history studies, family members of individuals affected with the condition of interest are compared with family members of unaffected individuals. If genetic factors contribute to the condition, the family members of affected individuals are more likely to also report the condition than those of unaffected individuals, given that they have shared genes. The greater the degree of genetic similarity between individuals, the more they should be alike on phenotypic measures. In an early family study of insomnia, Abe and Shimakawa[11] compared the sleep patterns of parents with their 3-year-old children. Parents who reported sleeping poorly as children tended to have children with similar patterns. Although somewhat methodologically crude, this study demonstrates that the idea that insomnia may run in families is not new.

Hauri and Olmstead[12] conducted one of the only studies of childhood-onset insomnia, which is characterized by early age of onset and a relative absence of clear precipitating factors and is thought more likely due to genetic causes. Individuals whose insomnia originated in childhood reported a positive family history of sleep complaints at a higher rate (55%) than those with adult-onset insomnia (39%). In a study of patients with insomnia presenting to a sleep disorders clinic, 35% of those with insomnia reported 1 or more family members also experiencing some form of sleep disturbance, and there was a trend toward higher rates in the families of those with an earlier age of onset.[13] In a second clinic sample from this group, there was a positive family history of insomnia in 72.7% of individuals with primary insomnia, 43.4% of those with psychiatric insomnia, and 24.1% of controls.[14]

In a larger cohort study,[15] there was almost no difference in a positive family history of insomnia in those categorized as good sleepers, as having symptoms of insomnia, and as meeting criteria for a full insomnia syndrome (32.7%, 36.7%, and 38.1%, respectively). Significant differences were found only when the good sleepers were separated into those with and without a personal history of insomnia; those without a personal history had a significantly lower rate of family history (29.0%) than those without a past history (48.9%). This pattern of results highlights a difficulty of studying insomnia, a disorder whose clinical state can vary over time such that individuals who are good sleepers at the time of assessment may have a prior history of insomnia, making it unclear if they are truly controls.

The small body of family history studies of insomnia phenotypes suggests that there is familial aggregation. A limit of these types of studies is that family members share both genes and environment. Familial aggregation could be due to

shared effects in either domain. Twin studies seek to disentangle these effects by comparing monozygotic (MZ) and dizygotic (DZ) twins raised together. The rationale for twin studies is that each twin pair is raised together and thus the family-specific environmental effects are assumed to not contribute to phenotypic differences between twins. MZ twins share 100% and DZ twins share approximately 50% of their genes, so if there are higher rates of similarity in MZ twins compared with DZ twins, it should be due to these differences in common genes. Several twin studies have investigated the genetic and environmental etiology of insomnia phenotypes (summarized in **Table 1**). The first of these was conducted in 14 MZ and 14 DZ good sleeper twin pairs who completed 1 night of PSG.[16] The participants did not have insomnia, but the study is noteworthy in

Table 1
Twin studies of insomnia phenotypes

Authors	Sample	Phenotypes	Heritability
Webb & Campbell,[16] 1983	14 MZ, 14 DZ Young adults	Sleep latency Wake time	N/A
Partinen et al,[17] 1983	2238 MZ, 4545 DZ Adults	Sleep length Sleep quality	$h^2 = 0.44$ $h^2 = 0.44$
Heath et al,[18] 1990	1792 MZ, 2101 DZ Adults	Sleep quality Initial insomnia Sleep latency Anxious insomnia Depressed insomnia	$h^2 = 0.32$ $h^2 = 0.32$ $h^2 = 0.44\ ♂, 0.32\ ♀$ $h^2 = 0.36$ $h^2 = 0.33$
Heath et al,[19] 1998	1792 MZ, 2101 DZ Adults	Composite score	12.1% of Variance in ♀, 8.3% in ♂
McCarren et al,[20] 1994	1605 MZ, 1200 DZ Male veterans	Trouble falling asleep Trouble staying asleep Waking up several times Waking up tired Composite score	$h^2 = 0.28$ $h^2 = 0.42$ $h^2 = 0.26$ $h^2 = 0.21$ $h^2 = 0.28$
de Castro,[50] 2002	86 MZ, 129 DZ Adult good sleepers	Sleep duration Number of wake-ups	$h^2 = 0.30$ $h^2 = 0.21$
Watson et al,[21] 2006	1042 MZ, 828 DZ Young adults	Insomnia	$h^2 = 0.64$
Boomsma et al,[22] 2008	548 Twins, 265 siblings Adults	Insomnia factor	$h^2 = 0.20$
Gregory et al,[23] 2004	2162 MZ, 4229 DZ Age 3–7 y	Sleep problems scale	$h^2 = 0.18\ ♂, 0.20\ ♀$
Gregory et al,[24] 2006	100 MZ, 200 DZ Age 8	Sleep onset delay Night wakings	$h^2 = 0.17$ for Child report, 0.79 for parental report $h^2 = 0.27$ for Child report, 0.32 for parental report
Gregory,[25] 2008	100 MZ, 200 DZ Age 8	Dyssomnia scale	$h^2 = 0.71$
Gregory et al,[24] 2006	192 MZ, 384 DZ Age 8	Sleep problems score	$h^2 = 0.61$

that there were significant dominant genetic effects for both sleep-onset latency and several measures of time spent awake during the night. Partinen and colleagues[17] collected self-reported sleep data from a much larger sample of 2238 MZ and 4545 DZ adult twin pairs and found significant heritability for sleep length ($h^2 = 0.44$) and sleep quality ($h^2 = 0.44$). It may be that individuals with insomnia are simply those at one end of the distribution of these traits in the population, in which case studying the genetics of sleep-wake traits in general may provide insight into the pathophysiology of insomnia.

The twin study with the broadest assessment of sleep and insomnia phenotypes was conducted with the Australian Twin Registry.[18] Their survey of 1792 MZ and 2101 DZ twin pairs included several questions related to sleep quality, disturbance, and overall patterns. Of most relevance for insomnia, additive genetic influences were found for sleep quality ($h^2 = 0.32$), initial insomnia ($h^2 = 0.32$), sleep latency ($h^2 = 0.44$ for men and 0.32 for women), anxious insomnia ($h^2 = 0.36$), and depressed insomnia ($h^2 = 0.33$). In a subsequent report based on this twin registry,[19] genetic influences accounted for 12.1% of the variance in a composite sleep disturbance factor for women and 8.3% for men. In a study of twin pairs from the Vietnam Era Twin Registry,[20] heritability estimates were trouble falling asleep ($h^2 = 0.28$), trouble staying asleep ($h^2 = 0.42$), waking up several times per night ($h^2 = 0.26$), waking up feeling tired and worn out ($h^2 = 0.21$), and a composite sleep score ($h^2 = 0.28$). A questionnaire item, "How often do you have trouble falling asleep of staying asleep?" from the University of Washington Twin Registry yielded a heritability of 0.64.[21] Lastly, a survey of twins and siblings found that the insomnia-related questions clustered on a single factor, which had a heritability of 0.20.[22]

Several studies have been conducted by Gregory and colleagues[23] examining sleep problems in youth. Total scores on a 4-item sleep problem scale showed modest evidence of additive genetic influence ($h^2 = 0.18$ for boys and 0.20 for girls). A second study of 8-year old twin pairs involved both the childrens' self-ratings of their sleep and their parents' ratings of how well they perceived that their children slept.[24] Parental ratings are commonly used to account for children not having developed good skills for observing their own sleep patterns, but a drawback of this approach is that the parents are not observing all aspects of their children's sleep. Estimates of additive genetic influences on the sleep-onset delay subscale were different for parental ($h^2 = 0.79$) compared with child ($h^2 = 0.17$) ratings. Estimates for the

night wakings subscale were more comparable, with estimates of 0.32 and 0.27 for parental and child reports, respectively. A dyssomnia scale was computed based on 10 items from the parental rating scale that showed evidence of substantial heritability ($h^2 = 0.71$).[25]

In summary, family and twin studies demonstrate that insomnia phenotypes tend to aggregate in families, with a greater degree of genetic similarity correlating with greater phenotypic similarity. With few exceptions, heritability estimates in adults were consistently in the range of 0.25 to 0.45, regardless of the exact question or phenotype used. In children, parental estimates of sleep problems demonstrate substantially greater heritability, with estimates across studies ranging from 0.60 to 0.80. Mild sleep problems may be more likely to go unnoticed by parents, so their ratings capture mostly the more severe cases that likely have stronger genetic underpinnings than when the full spectrum of severity is considered. Thus, insomnia, broadly defined, is moderately heritable when rated by individuals, with approximately one-third of the variance in symptoms attributable to genetic factors.

GENES RELATED TO INSOMNIA

Now that it is established that insomnia phenotypes are partially due to genetic factors, the next question is, Which genes are involved? One approach to identifying specific genes related to insomnia is to select candidate genes based on a priori knowledge about the mechanisms underlying regulation of sleep and wake. A reasonable starting point is genes involved in the generation of circadian rhythms because there is strong interplay between circadian and sleep mechanisms. These so-called clock genes have been well characterized, as have the transcriptional-translational feedback loops through which these genes produce circadian rhythms.[26] Several studies have examined the relationships among sleep-wake characteristics and clock genes, which may be of relevance for insomnia.

In one study, Laposky and colleagues[27] created mice carrying a null allele for a core circadian clock gene: BMAL1/Mop3. These mice demonstrated alterations in sleep-wake characteristics, including greater sleep fragmentation, reduced duration of sleep bouts, and altered total sleep time. In a human study, Viola and colleagues[28] focused on the PER3 gene and compared individuals homozygous for either the short ($PER3^{4/4}$) or long ($PER3^{5/5}$) alleles. The group with the long allele, compared with those with the short allele, had shorter sleep latency and spent a greater proportion of the night in slow-wave sleep. Several studies have examined the relationships between clock genes and sleep-wake characteristics in patients with mood disorders. For example, Serretti and colleagues[29] found an association between the 3111T/C CLOCK gene polymorphisms and insomnia symptoms in patients with major depression. In a larger cohort study in Finland, Utge and colleagues[30] examined the associations between 113 single nucleotide polymorphisms (SNPs) across 18 clock genes and sleep disturbance in individuals with depression and controls. They found that the TIMELESS gene was associated with early morning awakenings in the depressed group, but that this effect was different for men and women.

In addition to the clock genes, several studies have examined genes related to the various neurotransmitter systems involved in sleep-wake regulation.

Serotonin

The serotonin transporter-linked polymorphic region (5HTTLPR) gene has been extensively studied in psychiatric genetics. The short allele is associated with reduced efficiency of transcription and has been shown to confer risk for several psychiatric disorders. One pharmacogenetic study of patients with major depression found that the short allele was associated with an increased likelihood of developing new or worsening insomnia in response to fluoxetine treatment.[31] Brummett and colleagues[32] examined the relationship between sleep quality and the serotonin transporter gene in caregivers of individuals with dementia. They found a significant gene × environment interaction with caregiving, such that caregivers with the short allele were more likely to report poor sleep quality than those with the long allele, but there was no relationship for non-caregivers. The availability of serotonin in the brain is influenced by monoamine oxidase A, and 2 studies have found relationships between monoamine oxidase A polymorphisms and insomnia phenotypes.[33,34]

GABA

Sedative hypnotic medications almost universally act through the inhibitory γ-aminobutyric acid (GABA) system. Buhr and colleagues[35] reported a case study of a patient with a missense mutation of the β_3 subunit of the GABA$_A$ receptor. The patient had insomnia, as did several members of his family, suggesting that this mutation may have affected sleep. Drosophila with the mutant GABA$_A$ receptor Rdl^{A302S}, which is associated with increased channel current, exhibited decreased sleep latency.[36]

Adenosine

Adenosine is thought to play a role in the regulation of sleep homeostasis, so genes affecting adenosine activity could influence sleep-wake dynamics and hence insomnia. Individuals with the G/A allele of the adenosine deaminase gene had fewer awakenings at night, spent more time in slow wave sleep, and had higher delta power than those with the G/G allele.[37] Gass and colleagues[38] focused on 117 SNPs from 13 genes related to adenosine transporters, receptors, and metabolism enzymes in cases with depression and controls. Polymorphisms in the SLC29A3 gene, which is related to adenosine metabolism, were associated with early morning awakenings only in women.

Hypocretin/Orexin

There has been an increased interest in the role that hypocretins/orexins play in sleep regulation. Prober and colleagues[39] created zebrafish that overexpressed hypocretin that led to a phenotype characterized by hyperarousal and reduced ability to initiate and maintain sleep.

Taken together, these candidate gene studies provide preliminary evidence that genes affecting both circadian mechanisms and neurotransmitters known to be involved in sleep-wake regulation may have some bearing on insomnia phenotypes; however, more work needs to be done in this area.

A limitation of the candidate genes approach is knowing which genes to examine, but the mechanisms underlying insomnia and sleep-wake regulation are not fully known. An alternate strategy is to perform a hypothesis-free search through the use of gene discovery strategies, such as linkage and genome-wide association studies (GWAS). The first gene discovery study of sleep-related phenotypes examined a subset of the Framingham Heart Study Offspring Cohort.[40] The phenotypes of interest were usual bedtime and sleep duration. Linkage analysis failed to find any associations with log odds greater than 3 (a standard criterion for significance), but 5 peaks with log odds greater than 2 were found, including a linkage between usual bedtime and CSNK2A2, a gene known to be a component of the circadian clock. In a population-based test, usual bedtime was associated with the SNP rs324981, located in the gene NPSR1, which encodes the neuropeptide S receptor.

Allebrandt and colleagues[41] pooled data from several cohorts to conduct a GWAS of self-reported sleep duration. With a discovery sample of 4251 individuals and replication sample of 5949, they identified an associated intronic variant in the *ABCC9* gene, which is related to K_{ATP} channels. What is interesting about this study is that rather than stopping after the GWAS, the investigators took this finding into a model system by interfering with this gene in *Drosophila* neurons using RNA interference, which resulted in flies that did not sleep for the first 3 hours of the night, validating the importance of this gene for sleep regulation.

The only other GWAS of insomnia phenotypes conducted to date included 10,038 individuals in Korea.[42] Cases with insomnia and controls were defined based on responses to a series of questions about their sleep patterns. A GWAS found associations between case-control status on the ROR1 gene, which modulates synapse formation, although this association did not reach genome-wide significance.

Animal models provide opportunities for methodological approaches not possible in humans, such as experimental breeding. Wu and colleagues[43] conducted a forward genetic screen in *Drosophila* of approximately 3000 lines to identify short-sleeping mutants. Short-sleeping flies tended to sleep in shorter bouts compared with longer-sleeping flies, suggesting that they may have had difficulty with sleep maintenance, a possible insomnia phenotype. The short-sleeping flies also exhibited reduced arousal thresholds and were more easily awoken. It is not known whether these flies were short sleepers because of impaired sleep ability (ie, insomnia) or reduced sleep need, but the reduced arousal threshold of these mutants suggests some degree of overlap with insomnia. The sleep changes were associated with a novel allele of the dopamine transporter gene.

Seugnet and colleagues[44] selectively bred flies with shorter sleep durations and were able to produce flies they referred to as insomnia-like whose total sleep time was only 60 minutes per day. The flies had difficulties with initiating and maintaining sleep, increased waking activity levels, and impairments in learning on an avoidance task and in motor coordination. The investigators propose that this animal model captures both the nighttime and daytime characteristics of insomnia. Gene profiling identified 1350 genes that were differentially expressed in the insomnia-like flies compared with wild-type flies, many of which fell into categories related to metabolism, neuronal activity, behavior, and sensory perception.

This collection of studies is noteworthy in the degree to which they represent some of the various research strategies that can be used for discovery of genes that may relate to insomnia. Few studies have been conducted, several of which involved phenotypes of only marginal significance for insomnia. A great deal of work needs to be done.

FUTURE DIRECTIONS

The research described in this article indicates that insomnia phenotypes are heritable, with approximately 30% to 40% of the variability in insomnia related to genetic factors. In terms of the search for specific genes that relate to the pathophysiology of insomnia, the sleep field is 10 to 20 years behind the work that has been accomplished for mood disorders and schizophrenia. Furthermore, compared with the attention received by mood disorders and schizophrenia, there are few investigators pursuing the genetics of insomnia, so progress is likely to be slow for the foreseeable future. Nevertheless, a research agenda for some of the next steps that are needed is laid out:

1. There is a need for more consistent phenotyping of insomnia in genetic studies of humans. As described previously in this review, the existing studies have primarily used a wide range of homemade sleep questions rather than validated measures. Most of these questions did not include assessments of daytime impairment due to poor sleep, which is necessary for determining whether some may meet diagnostic criteria for an insomnia disorder.[4,5] Thus, much of the literature to date is more related to insomnia symptoms rather than to insomnia itself. It may be that the genetic architecture of insomnia disorder is such that it is not merely one end of the distribution of scores on these symptom-related traits and requires validated case and control definitions to determine underlying genes. Efforts to create a more standardized assessment of insomnia[2] should facilitate greater homogeneity across studies in the future.

2. Additional GWAS are needed to identify genetic variants that contribute to insomnia phenotypes. The advantage of this approach is that it requires no prior hypothesis about which genes are likely to influence the trait and is instead considered hypothesis generating. GWAS studies may lead to the discovery of novel pathways and mechanisms involved not only in insomnia phenotypes but also in sleep-wake regulation in general. GWAS is predicated on the common-variant hypothesis, which states that disease is related to genetic variants (alleles) that are common in the population,

each of which explains a small proportion of the variance. Although this approach has been fruitful in identifying risk genes for a wide range of conditions,[45] the past decade of GWAS research has highlighted the critical need for replication because many significant findings from one study are not confirmed in subsequent investigations.

3. An alternative to the common-variant view is the rare-variant hypothesis, which states that genetic variants that are rare in the population (<1% minor allele frequency) are more likely to have large effects and explain the majority of variation in risk to disease in the population. The extreme of the rare-variant hypothesis is mendelian mutations, in which a single variant is sufficient to produce disease, as in Huntington disease. Several tools have emerged in the past few years to facilitate the search for rare variants. Efforts, such as the 1000 Genomes project (www.1000genomes.org), have created databases of normative genetic variation against which the results of individual studies can be compared. Next-generation sequencing technologies, such as exome and even whole-genome sequencing, are more practical due to the rapid decline in costs for these methods. To the authors' knowledge, there have been no studies using these approaches in the search for insomnia-related genes.

4. Although studies have begun to identify genes that are associated with insomnia, the molecular underpinnings of this disease remain unclear for 3 primary reasons. First, insomnia is a broad disease composed of both primary (direct) and secondary (ie, stress, diet, and so forth) causes, ranging from environmental factors to single-gene polymorphisms to combinatorial resultd of 10s if not 100s of genetic polymorphisms. Second, human studies are messy, often relying on subjective rather than objective data, making it difficult to correlate phenotype with genotype. Third, human studies are limited to single-gene polymorphisms that cause insomnia but no other behavioral or developmental disorders. Finally, the best studies in humans often localize a disease to a chromosomal region that includes 100s of genes—How best to shave this number down to 1 or at most a handful of genes?

A simple answer to these problems is one that has been successfully offered to unravel many of medicine's seemingly intractable questions, such as, How do we develop from a single cell into a complex organism? How do our bodies maintain a 24-hour rhythm even in the absence of external cues? and How do our cells regulate gene expression? The solution time and again has been to use functional genetics in powerful model systems.

For a model system to be useful, it must meet several criteria that make it superior to direct genetic studies in humans. Practically, it must be cheap and have a short lifespan, a short generation time, and moderate to high fecundity. It must also be useful as a genetic system, with a fully sequenced genome and tools available to target disruption of specific genes. Finally, it must be capable of reproducing the human behavior or disease state, in this case an inability to initiate or maintain quality sleep. To this end, several model systems have been developed to study the genetics of sleep that can easily be used to better understanding of the mechanisms underlying insomnia.

Mice are the most obvious choice for an insomnia model system. They are mammals with a nervous system that resembles humans— approximately 90% genome conservation and rapid eye movement and non–rapid eye movement sleep states as determined by EEG. They also have a powerful genetic tool kit that allows researchers to target disruption or overexpression of specific genes and to do so in defined subsets of the brain during discrete temporal windows, such as in adultd or only after sleep deprivation. These tools have been used in the study of narcolepsy by creating mice with altered orexin signaling[46] as well as by identifying a novel narcolepsy-like gene, the glutamate receptor-binding protein, *homer1*.[47] Insomnia studies have lagged, but recent work by De Boer and colleagues[48] has demonstrated that disinhibition of the calcium channel, *CACNA1A*, results in reduced sleep, likely by disrupting adenosine signaling.

Although mice offer a powerful genetic system, they do have drawbacks, in particular, a long generation time that can translate into a gap of years between an experimental idea and meaningful data. To streamline the process, 2 models with high fecundity and short generation times have been developed to study the genetics of sleep: the fruit fly *Drosophila melanogaster* and the nematode *Caenorhabditis elegans*. Like mice, both systems offer powerful genetic tool kits that permit researchers to disrupt or overexpress genes in subsets of the nervous system in defined temporal windows. These tools have been used most successfully in *Drosophila* in which Hendricks and colleagues[49] first demonstrated that altering cyclic adenosine monophosphate signaling could lead to insomnia-like reductions in sleep. Since that time, 10s of genes have been identified and characterized with similar phenotypes, with more genes likely to be identified in the future.

With the development of these powerful and fast genetic model systems for sleep in general, it seems only logical to use them to screen human insomnia genetic studies for bona fide hits and to further characterize the mechanism behind insomnia. Inclusion of these models must be an important component of future research on the genetics of insomnia. As this summary of the extant research demonstrates, understanding of the role of genes in the insomnia phenotype is limited. On a more positive side, there are several molecular genetic tools available that were not in existence even a few years ago. The time is ripe for research on the genetics of insomnia that may finally shed light on the mechanisms of this common sleep disorder.

REFERENCES

1. Spielman A, Caruso L, Glovinsky P. A behavioral perspective on insomnia treatment. Psychiatr Clin North Am 1987;10:541–53.
2. Buysse DJ, Ancoli-Israel S, Edinger JD, et al. Recommendations for a standard research assessment of insomnia. Sleep 2006;29(9):1155–73.
3. Edinger JD, Bonnet MH, Bootzin RR, et al. Derivation of research diagnostic criteria for insomnia: report of an American Academy of Sleep Medicine Work Group. Sleep 2004;27(8):1567–96.
4. American Psychiatric Association. Diagnostic and statistical manual of mental disorders. 4th edition, text revision. Washington, DC: American Psychiatric Association; 2000.
5. American Academy of Sleep Medicine. International classification of sleep disorders. 2nd edition. Westchester, IL: American Academy of Sleep Medicine; 2005.
6. Fichten CS, Creti L, Amsel R, et al. Poor sleepers who do not complain of insomnia: myths and realities about psychological and lifestyle characteristics of older good and poor sleepers. J Behav Med 1995;18(2):189–223.
7. Reynolds CF 3rd, Redline S, DSM-V Sleep-Wake Disorders Workgroup and Advisors. The DSM-v sleep-wake disorders nosology: an update and an invitation to the sleep community. J Clin Sleep Med 2010;6(1):9–10.
8. Ambrosius U, Lietzenmaier S, Wehrle R, et al. Heritability of sleep electroencephalogram. Biol Psychiatry 2008;64(4):344–8.
9. Perlis M, Smith M, Andrews P, et al. Beta/gamma EEG activity in patients with primary and secondary insomnia and good sleeper controls. Sleep 2001;24:110–7.
10. Perlis M, Merica H, Smith M, et al. Beta EEG activity and insomnia. Sleep Med Rev 2001;5:365–76.
11. Abe K, Shimakawa M. Genetic-constitutional factor and childhood insomnia. Psychiatr Neurol (Basel) 1966;152(6):363–9.
12. Hauri P, Olmstead E. Childhood-onset insomnia. Sleep 1980;3(1):59–65.
13. Bastien CH, Morin CM. Familial incidence of insomnia. J Sleep Res 2000;9(1):49–54.
14. Dauvilliers Y, Morin C, Cervena K, et al. Family studies in insomnia. J Psychosom Res 2005; 58(3):271–8.
15. Beaulieu-Bonneau S, LeBlanc M, Merette C, et al. Family history of insomnia in a population-based sample. Sleep 2007;30(12):1739–45.
16. Webb WB, Campbell SS. Relationships in sleep characteristics of identical and fraternal twins. Arch Gen Psychiatry 1983;40(10):1093–5.
17. Partinen M, Kaprio J, Koskenvuo M, et al. Genetic and environmental determination of human sleep. Sleep 1983;6(3):179–85.
18. Heath A, Kendler K, Eaves L, et al. Evidence for genetic influences on sleep disturbance and sleep pattern in twins. Sleep 1990;13:318–35.
19. Heath A, Eaves L, Kirk K, et al. Effects of lifestyle, personality, symptoms of anxiety and depression, and genetic predisposition on subjective sleep disturbance and sleep pattern. Twin Res 1998;1:176–88.
20. McCarren M, Goldberg J, Ramakrishnan V, et al. Insomnia in Vietnam era veteran twins: influence of genes and combat experience. Sleep 1994; 17(5):456–61.
21. Watson NF, Goldberg J, Arguelles L, et al. Genetic and environmental influences on insomnia, daytime sleepiness, and obesity in twins. Sleep 2006;29(5): 645–9.
22. Boomsma DI, van Someren EJ, Beem AL, et al. Sleep during a regular week night: a twin-sibling study. Twin Res Hum Genet 2008;11(5):538–45.
23. Gregory AM, Eley TC, O'Connor TG, et al. Etiologies of associations between childhood sleep and behavioral problems in a large twin sample. J Am Acad Child Adolesc Psychiatry 2004;43(6): 744–51.
24. Gregory AM, Rijsdijk FV, Eley TC. A twin-study of sleep difficulties in school-aged children. Child Dev 2006;77(6):1668–79.
25. Gregory AM. A genetic decomposition of the association between parasomnias and dyssomnias in 8-year-old twins. Arch Pediatr Adolesc Med 2008; 162(4):299–304.
26. Lowrey PL, Takahashi JS. Mammalian circadian biology: elucidating genome-wide levels of temporal organization. Annu Rev Genomics Hum Genet 2004;5:407–41.
27. Laposky A, Easton A, Dugovic C, et al. Deletion of the mammalian circadian clock gene BMAL1/Mop3 alters baseline sleep architecture and the response to sleep deprivation. Sleep 2005;28(4):395–409.

28. Viola AU, Archer SN, James LM, et al. PER3 polymorphism predicts sleep structure and waking performance. Curr Biol 2007;17(7):613–8.

29. Serretti A, Benedetti F, Mandelli L, et al. Genetic dissection of psychopathological symptoms: insomnia in mood disorders and CLOCK gene polymorphism. Am J Med Genet B Neuropsychiatr Genet 2003;121B(1):35–8.

30. Utge SJ, Soronen P, Loukola A, et al. Systematic analysis of circadian genes in a population-based sample reveals association of TIMELESS with depression and sleep disturbance. PLoS One 2010;5(2):e9259.

31. Perlis RH, Mischoulon D, Smoller JW, et al. Serotonin transporter polymorphisms and adverse effects with fluoxetine treatment. Biol Psychiatry 2003; 54(9):879–83.

32. Brummett BH, Krystal AD, Ashley-Koch A, et al. Sleep quality varies as a function of 5-HTTLPR genotype and stress. Psychosom Med 2007;69(7): 621–4.

33. Brummett BH, Krystal AD, Siegler IC, et al. Associations of a regulatory polymorphism of monoamine oxidase-A gene promoter (MAOA-uVNTR) with symptoms of depression and sleep quality. Psychosom Med 2007;69(5):396–401.

34. Craig D, Hart DJ, Passmore AP. Genetically increased risk of sleep disruption in Alzheimer's disease. Sleep 2006;29(8):1003–7.

35. Buhr A, Bianchi MT, Baur R, et al. Functional characterization of the new human GABA(A) receptor mutation beta3(R192H). Hum Genet 2002;111(2): 154–60.

36. Agosto J, Choi JC, Parisky KM, et al. Modulation of GABAA receptor desensitization uncouples sleep onset and maintenance in Drosophila. Nat Neurosci 2008;11(3):354–9.

37. Retey JV, Adam M, Honegger E, et al. A functional genetic variation of adenosine deaminase affects the duration and intensity of deep sleep in humans. Proc Natl Acad Sci U S A 2005;102(43): 15676–81.

38. Gass N, Ollila HM, Utge S, et al. Contribution of adenosine related genes to the risk of depression with disturbed sleep. J Affect Disord 2010; 126(1–2):134–9.

39. Prober DA, Rihel J, Onah AA, et al. Hypocretin/ orexin overexpression induces an insomnia-like phenotype in zebrafish. J Neurosci 2006;26(51): 13400–10.

40. Gottlieb DJ, O'Connor GT, Wilk JB. Genome-wide association of sleep and circadian phenotypes. BMC Med Genet 2007;8(Suppl 1):S9.

41. Allebrandt KV, Amin N, Muller-Myhsok B, et al. A K(ATP) channel gene effect on sleep duration: from genome-wide association studies to function in Drosophila. Mol Psychiatry 2013;18(1):122–32.

42. Ban HJ, Kim SC, Seo J, et al. Genetic and metabolic characterization of insomnia. PLoS One 2011;6(4):e18455.

43. Wu MN, Koh K, Yue Z, et al. A genetic screen for sleep and circadian mutants reveals mechanisms underlying regulation of sleep in Drosophila. Sleep 2008;31(4):465–72.

44. Seugnet L, Suzuki Y, Thimgan M, et al. Identifying sleep regulatory genes using a Drosophila model of insomnia. J Neurosci 2009;29(22):7148–57.

45. McCarthy MI, Hirschhorn JN. Genome-wide association studies: potential next steps on a genetic journey. Hum Mol Genet 2008;17(R2):R156–65.

46. Chemelli RM, Willie JT, Sinton CM, et al. Narcolepsy in orexin knockout mice: molecular genetics of sleep regulation. Cell 1999;98(4):437–51.

47. Naidoo N, Ferber M, Galante RJ, et al. Role of Homer proteins in the maintenance of sleep-wake states. PLoS One 2012;7(4):e35174.

48. De Boer T, van Diepen HC, Ferrari MD, et al. Reduced sleep and low adenosinergic sensitivity in Cacna1a R192Q mutant mice. Sleep 2013; 36(1):127–36.

49. Hendricks JC, Williams JA, Panckeri K, et al. A noncircadian role for cAMP signaling and CREB activity in Drosophila rest homeostasis. Nat Neurosci 2001;4(11):1108–15.

50. de Castro JM. The influence of heredity on self-reported sleep patterns in free-living humans. Physiol Behav 2002;76(4–5):479–86. PubMed PMID: 12126983.

Section 2: Challenges and Methods in Insomnia Management

Optimizing the Pharmacologic Treatment of Insomnia
Current Status and Future Horizons

Jared Minkel, PhD[a,b], Andrew D. Krystal, MD, MS[a,*]

KEYWORDS

- Insomnia • Pharmacotherapy • Prescription agents • Over-the-counter remedies

KEY POINTS

- Several different types of medications are available for treating patients with insomnia.
- Medications available for treating insomnia differ in their properties.
- Insomnia patients differ as to the risk/benefit ratio associated with the use of the available insomnia medications.
- Optimizing the medication treatment of insomnia for a given patient requires that the clinician select an agent with characteristics that make it most likely to effectively and safely address the type of sleep difficulty experienced by that individual.

INTRODUCTION

Several different types of medications are currently available for the treatment of insomnia. These agents include: (1) a group approved by the US Food and Drug Administration (FDA) for this purpose; (2) agents approved by the FDA for the treatment of another condition but are used off-label for the treatment of insomnia; and (3) agents available "over the counter" (OTC) for insomnia treatment.

The use of these medications is often performed as a "one-size-fits-all" endeavor whereby clinicians identify a medication that they prefer and administer it to all individuals who complain of disturbed sleep. However, this approach does a disservice to insomnia sufferers. The nature of the sleep problem experienced by those with insomnia varies. The medications available for treating insomnia also vary in their characteristics and,

as a result, in their suitability for patients with the different presentations of insomnia encountered in practice.

One of the ways in which patients with insomnia differ is the time of night when their sleep problems occur (problems with onset, maintenance, and/or early morning sleep difficulty). Another such factor distinguishing patients is the temporal pattern of their sleep problems across nights (nightly, intermittent and frequent, intermittent and occasional). A final factor that must be addressed to optimize pharmacotherapy for insomnia is the presence of comorbidities such as mood disorders, anxiety disorders, pain, and substance use/dependence.

Optimizing the medication management of insomnia for a given patient requires that the clinician select an agent with characteristics that make it most likely to effectively and safely address the sleep difficulty experienced by that individual. Carrying out this process requires awareness of: (1) the

Disclosure Information: Dr Krystal Grants/research support: NIH, Teva/Cephalon, Pfizer, Sunovion/Sepracor, Transcept, Phillips-Respironics, Astellas, Abbott, Neosynch, Brainsway.
Consultant: Abbott, Astellas, AstraZeneca, BMS, Teva/Cephalon, Eisai, Eli Lilly, GlaxoSmithKline, Jazz, Johnson and Johnson, Merck, Neurocrine, Novartis, Ortho-McNeil-Janssen, Respironics, Roche, Sanofi-Aventis, Somnus, Sunovion/Sepracor, Somaxon, Takeda, Transcept, Kingsdown Inc.

[a] Department of Psychiatry and Behavioral Sciences, Duke University School of Medicine, Trent Drive, Durham, NC, USA; [b] Department of Psychiatry, University of North Carolina School of Medicine, NC, USA
* Corresponding author.
E-mail address: andrew.krystal@duke.edu

Sleep Med Clin 8 (2013) 333–350
http://dx.doi.org/10.1016/j.jsmc.2013.06.002
1556-407X/13/$ – see front matter © 2013 Elsevier Inc. All rights reserved.

basic characteristics of all of the insomnia medications; (2) the fundamental ways that insomnia may differ among individuals that can affect the optimal choice of treatment; and (3) the available data that provide guidance regarding how to match characteristics of insomnia medication to the nature of an individual's sleep complaint.

This article provides the information required to optimize the management of insomnia through medication. It begins by reviewing the basic characteristics of the medications used to treat insomnia, followed by a review of fundamental patient characteristics that affect the choice of medication therapy. The review addresses how to best choose a medication based on the characteristics of the available medications, the key differences among patients with insomnia, and the available research literature. Lastly, the authors consider the types of studies needed to further optimize pharmacologic approaches to the management of insomnia.

AVAILABLE TYPES OF PHARMACOLOGIC TREATMENT FOR INSOMNIA
Prescription Agents Approved by the FDA for Treatment of Insomnia

Benzodiazepines
Pharmacology The benzodiazepines are a class of chemically related medications known for their sedative-hypnotic properties, and include triazolam, temazepam, flurazepam, alprazolam, clonazepam, and lorazepam (among many others). These medications are sedating because of their effects on γ-aminobutyric acid (GABA), the primary inhibitory neurotransmitter throughout the brain. Benzodiazepines bind to the GABA-A receptor and promote its inhibitory effects by causing conformational changes in the proteins that form channels through which chloride ions flow across neuronal membranes.[1] The change facilitates the inward flow of negative ions, which results in hyperpolarization, thus biasing the neuron away from depolarization, and ultimately reducing neuronal firing. The activity in GABAergic projections to wake-promoting regions of the brain are thus increased, decreasing arousal and facilitating sleep. GABA-A receptors, however, are also found outside of brain areas involved in sleep/wake function. Benzodiazepines therefore have additional effects beyond sleep enhancement, including anxiolytic effects, reward, memory impairment, motor impairment, anticonvulsant effects, and myorelaxation. Adverse effects may therefore include sedation, cognitive impairment (anterograde short-term memory loss), motor impairment and the potential for abuse. Anxiolytic

and myorelaxant effects, however, may be beneficial in the treatment of insomnia because anxiety and/or pain are frequent comorbidities.[2]

The most commonly prescribed benzodiazepines in the treatment of insomnia are triazolam, flurazepam, temazepam, estazolam, quazepam, clonazepam, lorazepam, and alprazolam.[3] Of these, only triazolam, flurazepam, and temazepam are approved by the FDA in the United States for the treatment of insomnia. Although benzodiazepines differ in their effects on GABA-A receptors in different brain regions to a degree, the primary factors that distinguish the benzodiazepines are route of metabolism and elimination half-life. Longer half-life and higher dosage tend to produce longer-lasting clinical effects. Shorter half-life and lower dosage tends to produce fewer next-day effects. Of the benzodiazepines commonly prescribed for insomnia, triazolam has the shortest half-life and is least likely to produce next-day effects. Some benzodiazepines have half-lives that exceed 24 hours, including flurazepam, quazepam and clonazepam. These medications are relatively likely to lead to next-day effects, such as daytime sedation.

Evidence base Several controlled trials have established the efficacy of benzodiazepines for the treatment of insomnia. Triazolam, temazepam, flurazepam, quazepam, and estazolam have been found to have beneficial effects on sleep onset and maintenance for patients aged 18 to 65 years with insomnia.[3] In older adults ($\geq$65 years), triazolam and flurazepam have been found to benefit sleep onset and maintenance. Temazepam has been found to be helpful for sleep maintenance only. Although there have been fewer trials in patients with insomnia and co-occurring medical or psychiatric conditions, the available evidence suggests that they can provide sleep-improving benefits in these populations as well.

Three placebo-controlled studies were performed evaluating the addition of clonazepam to fluoxetine in subjects with major depression.[4–6] In all 3 studies clonazepam improved sleep, whereas 2 of the studies showed greater improvement in depression symptoms with combined therapy than with fluoxetine alone. However, the results also suggest that improvement in depression symptoms with clonazepam may not be sustained with longer duration of therapy.

There has also been a placebo-controlled study in which patients with rheumatoid arthritis and disturbed sleep were treated with a benzodiazepine. In this study patients reported a benefit of triazolam relative to placebo for both sleep and morning stiffness.[7]

Nonbenzodiazepines

Pharmacology The nonbenzodiazepines include some of the most commonly prescribed sleep-promoting medications, including zolpidem, zaleplon, and eszopiclone.[3] These agents are chemically unrelated to benzodiazepines (hence the term "nonbenzodiazepines"), but have similar effects by acting through related pharmacologic mechanisms. Although they bind to the same site on the GABA-A receptor complex as the benzodiazepines, they bind more specifically to subtypes of GABA-A receptors.[8] In contrast to benzodiazepines, which tend to have broad effects at the receptors containing the α_1-, α_2-, α_3-, and α_5-subunit–containing GABA receptors, the nonbenzodiazepines tend to selectively bind to a subset of these subunit-containing GABA-A receptors.[8,9] On this basis, zolpidem and zaleplon, which bind relatively preferentially to α_1-containing GABA receptors, would be expected to have effects limited to anticonvulsant, amnestic, and motor-impairing effects as well as sleep enhancement.[10] Eszopiclone, on the other hand, would be expected to have anxiolytic and myorelaxant effects in addition to sleep enhancement, owing to its relatively greater effects at α_2- and α_3-subunit–containing GABA-A receptors.

The nonbenzodiazepine agents also differ in terms of elimination half-lives. All of these agents have shorter half-lives than most benzodiazepines (with the exception of triazolam) and may, therefore, have fewer next-day effects. However, the limited data on head-to-head comparisons of these 2 classes of medication cannot confirm this prediction. Zaleplon and zolpidem each have a relatively short half-life, and therefore can be expected to be most effective in facilitating sleep onset.[3] Indeed, both of these agents are approved by the FDA only for treating sleep-onset problems. Longer-acting agents such as eszopiclone and a controlled-release version of zolpidem are useful for maintaining sleep as well as facilitating sleep onset, and are approved by the FDA for treating both onset and maintenance difficulties.[3]

Evidence base A substantial body of literature supports the efficacy of the nonbenzodiazepines in the treatment of insomnia. Zolpidem and zaleplon have been shown to be effective in the treatment of sleep-onset problems in younger and older adults with primary insomnia.[3] Controlled-release (CR) zolpidem has demonstrated efficacy for improving sleep onset and maintenance in adults aged 18 to 65 years.[3] Eszopiclone has been shown to be effective for treating sleep onset and maintenance difficulties in older adults ($\geq$65) as well.[3]

In contrast to benzodiazepines, the nonbenzodiazepines have been evaluated for longer-term efficacy and safety. Eszopiclone has been evaluated over 6 months in a 2 placebo-controlled trials[11,12] and for up to 12 months in an open-label extension.[13] Zaleplon has been shown to be safe in 6- to 12-month open-label studies of older adults.[14] Zolpidem CR has not been evaluated in a placebo-controlled study of nightly treatment of more than 3 weeks in duration; however, it has been found to have sustained efficacy over 6 months in a placebo-controlled study wherein patients received doses 3 to 7 nights per week.[15]

The nonbenzodiazepines have also been evaluated in patients with comorbid psychiatric disorders. A controlled trial of patients with insomnia and major depression compared fluoxetine plus eszopiclone with fluoxetine plus placebo. Patients with the active insomnia medication demonstrated better sleep, and greater and faster reductions in depression symptoms.[16] A similar study of patients with insomnia and generalized anxiety disorder (GAD) found that eszopiclone plus escitalopram improved both sleep and anxiety outcomes over eszopiclone plus escitalopram.[17] Of interest, essentially identical trials were performed with zolpidem CR and, unlike eszopiclone, sleep was improved but no effects on depression or GAD outcomes were found.[18,19] Both eszopiclone and zolpidem were found to improve sleep in menopausal insomnia.[20,21] Two placebo-controlled studies have also been performed with eszopiclone, establishing that it has therapeutic effects on sleep and pain in those with chronic pain syndromes. One was performed in patients with rheumatoid arthritis; eszopiclone was also evaluated in a placebo-controlled trial as an add-on therapy to open-label naproxen in 54 patients with chronic low back pain, and was found to significantly improve sleep and pain outcomes.[22] A placebo-controlled trial of eszopiclone was also performed in patients with rheumatoid arthritis, and indicated that this agent significantly improved sleep, ratings of daytime functions, and some pain outcomes in comparison with placebo.[23] Lastly, a placebo-controlled cross-over study performed in 24 patients with insomnia occurring comorbid to post-traumatic stress disorder (PTSD) indicated that patients receiving eszopiclone 3 mg had significantly greater improvements in both sleep disturbance and PTSD symptoms than did those receiving placebo.[24]

Overall, the strong evidence base for the nonbenzodiazepines makes them an attractive option in the treatment of insomnia. The side-effect profile of nonbenzodiazepines has been found to be similar to the benzodiazepines and includes sedation, dizziness, and psychomotor impairment. Nonbenzodiazepines appear to have lower abuse potential at recommended doses, but may still have a significant risk at higher doses.[25] Zaleplon and zolpidem both have relatively lower risks of unwanted daytime sedation while still providing effective treatment of sleep-onset difficulties. The longer-acting agents eszopiclone and zolpidem CR are effective for the treatment of sleep-maintenance problems as well as sleep initiation. These agents are the only ones other than benzodiazepines that are currently approved by the FDA for the treatment of both sleep-onset and sleep-maintenance problems.

Melatonin receptor agonists

Pharmacology Melatonin is an endogenous hormone produced by the pineal gland that is intimately involved in circadian rhythms. Two melatonin agonists are currently available in the United States: melatonin (available as an OTC supplement), and ramelteon (FDA approved for the treatment of insomnia). Unlike benzodiazepines and nonbenzodiazepines, the sleep-enhancing effects of melatonin agonists have not been found to vary with dose.

Ramelteon is melatonin receptor agonist (MT1 and MT2) that was introduced in 2005. It has a strong affinity for the MT1 receptor, which is believed to regulate drowsiness by dampening wake-promoting signals from the suprachiasmatic nucleus.[26] The half-life of melatonin is very short, between 1 and 3 hours, making it useful for sleep-onset insomnia, but not for sleep-maintenance insomnia.[26] There is no evidence that ramelteon carries any risk of tolerance or abuse and, therefore, it is one of only two FDA-approved medications for insomnia that has not been designated by the US Drug Enforcement Administration as having a significant potential for abuse (the other being doxepin).[25]

Evidence base Exogenous melatonin is available as a supplement that is not regulated by the FDA and is therefore available in a wide range of doses. Controlled studies have not found it to have substantive therapeutic effects in patients with insomnia.[26] However, it does show some promise in some populations, including children with neurodevelopmental disorders.[27–41] Unfortunately, a limitation in interpreting the results of studies performed with melatonin is that the dose in the studies has ranged from 0.1 to 75 mg and timing has varied from 30 minutes to 3 hours before bedtime, making the application of their findings to clinical practice somewhat challenging.[42,43] Studies that have attempted to establish a dose-response curve have been unsuccessful, finding no relationship between serum blood levels of melatonin agonists and therapeutic effects.[43] The efficacy of ramelteon for treating insomnia has been demonstrated in several randomized, placebo-controlled trials. Most studies have evaluated a dose of 8 mg administered 30 minutes before lights out.[3] Studies have been done in older adults (age $\geq$65 years) as well as in those between the ages of 18 and 65. The effects have been limited to improvements in sleep-onset latency, with larger effects shown by polysomnography than by subjective measures of sleep. The most commonly reported side effects were headache, somnolence, and sore throat, but these were not significantly elevated relative to placebo.

Ramelteon and melatonin have favorable profiles of adverse effects and no significant potential for abuse (although they have not been studied in populations at high risk for substance abuse). The most common adverse effects of melatonin are headache, sedation, and slowed reaction times.[34,44–46] There is some evidence that it may temporarily affect fertility in both men and women[47–50] and is, therefore, not the treatment of choice for individuals trying to conceive. Ramelteon has also been associated with somnolence, dizziness, nausea, and fatigue, but no effects on fertility have been reported. It has also been found to be safe for use in patients with mild to moderate sleep apnea[51] and moderate to severe obstructive pulmonary disease.[52] Placebo-controlled trials have also demonstrated that ramelteon is safe and effective over a long period (up to 6 months) with nightly use.[53]

H1 antagonists (antihistamines)

Pharmacology The term antihistamine is typically used for agents that were developed for the treatment of allergies, but many other agents are significant antagonists of H1 histamine receptors, and could therefore also be referred to as antihistamines. For the sake of clarity, in this article the term "antihistamine" is used only to refer to agents that were intended to treat allergies but also have been used to treat insomnia. H1 antagonists are believed to exert therapeutic effects on sleep by blocking the wake-promoting effects of histamine.[54] Among the antihistamines, diphenhydramine and doxylamine are the most commonly used. Both are available OTC, alone and in combination with nonprescription analgesics (eg, Tylenol PM). Both medications have similar properties, and the usual dose for each is 25 to 50 mg. Both have significant muscarinic cholinergic antagonist effects that are believed to contribute to their effects on sleep and be the primary source of side effects.

Evidence base There have been no placebo-controlled trials in patients with insomnia to evaluate the safety or efficacy of doxylamine, but a few exist for diphenhydramine.[55–59] Unlike benzodiazepines and nonbenzodiazepines, diphenhydramine appears to have stronger effects on sleep maintenance than on sleep onset in the few available studies. Doxylamine has only been evaluated for the treatment of insomnia in one large double-blind trial of postoperative patients. Results indicated a significant benefit on subjective measures of sleep.[60] One study of diphenhydramine suggests that benefits from daytime dosing are lost over consecutive days of administration, and similar studies are needed to determine if tolerance occurs to nighttime dosing as well.[61]

The only selective H1 antagonist that has been studied for the treatment of insomnia is doxepin, a tricyclic antidepressant that has FDA approval for the treatment of depression in dosages from 75 to 150 mg and for the treatment of insomnia in doses from 3 to 6 mg.[54] Of note, doxepin is a more potent and selective H1 antagonist than any agent referred to as an antihistamine currently available in the United States. As with diphenhydramine, low-dose doxepin has stronger effects on sleep maintenance than it has on sleep onset. The therapeutic effect on sleep maintenance has been demonstrated for both younger and older adults, and it is approved by the FDA for treating sleep-maintenance but not sleep-onset problems.[3,54] Of particular note, doxepin is the only agent available that has been demonstrated to have therapeutic effects in the last third of the night, including the final hour of an 8-hour sleep period, without significant adverse effects in the morning.[54,62,63]

The most common adverse effects associated with antihistamines are anticholinergic effects such as dry mouth, blurred vision, constipation, urinary retention, and delirium, and should therefore be avoided in patients at risk for complications attributable to anticholinergic effects, such as those with dementia, urinary retention, and narrow-angle glaucoma. Other adverse effects include sedation, dizziness, and weight gain. Less frequent side effects of diphenhydramine include agitation and insomnia. Case reports have suggested that doxylamine may be associated with coma and rhabdomyolysis.[64] It is important to bear in mind that doxepin is without any anticholinergic side effects in the approved 3- to 6-mg dose range because of its H1 selectivity, and appears to be without risk for weight gain or other adverse effects commonly associated with the antihistamines, nearly all of which are due to receptor

effects other than H1 antagonism.[54] The abuse potential of antihistamines is relatively negligible, making them appropriate for abuse-prone patients with insomnia. The benefits for allergies make antihistamines particularly well suited to insomnia occurring with allergies or nasal congestion.

Prescription Agents Used Off-Label for the Treatment of Insomnia

Antidepressants

Antidepressants are often used in the treatment of insomnia, but relatively few data exist on their efficacy and safety when used for this purpose.[3,65] Trazodone, in particular, is prescribed for the treatment of insomnia much more frequently that one would expect given the evidence base.[3] Of note, trazodone has been one of the most frequently prescribed agents for the treatment of insomnia for many years and yet has only been evaluated in a single large-scale placebo-controlled trial in patients with insomnia, in which it failed to have significant sustained therapeutic effects in comparison with placebo.[66]

Because of the paucity of placebo-controlled trials with these agents, their use cannot be recommended except in those individuals who fail or for some reason are precluded from the usual treatments. Antidepressants are typically prescribed at lower doses for the treatment of insomnia than for the treatment of major depression. These agents enhance sleep through antagonism of wake-promoting systems including serotonin, norepinephrine, acetylcholine, and histamine, although the relative degree of these effects differs among the antidepressants. Here the pharmacology and limited evidence base for the tricyclic antidepressants doxepin (doses >6 mg), amitriptyline, and trimipramine, as well as trazodone and mirtazapine, are reviewed.

Tricyclic antidepressants These agents promote sleep by antagonism of norepinephrine, histamine, and acetylcholine, all of which are involved in maintaining wakefulness and arousal. Most data on the sleep effects of these agents come from trials of patients with major depression.[67] Only 2 tricyclic antidepressants have been investigated in the treatment of primary insomnia. Trimipramine dosed at 50 to 200 mg has been found to improve sleep quality and sleep efficiency, but not sleep-onset latency.[68,69] Doxepin has been evaluated in 3 studies in a range of 25 to 50 mg. Findings from these studies support its efficacy for improving sleep quality, sleep onset, and sleep maintenance.[68,70–72] Tricyclic antidepressants have several side effects including sedation, weight gain, orthostatic hypotension, and anticholinergic side effects (dry mouth, blurred vision, constipation, urinary retention, exacerbation of narrow-angle glaucoma, and risk of delirium).[73,74] More severe side effects include impairment of cardiac electrical conduction, resulting in heart block and/or seizures, but these effects are not common. All of these side effects are dose dependent and are derived from antihistaminergic, anticholinergic, antiserotinergic, and antiadrenergic effects. The abuse potential for tricyclic antidepressants is negligible, so these agents may be useful in the treatment of insomnia among patients at high risk for substance abuse. In addition, they may be useful in treating insomnia in the context of comorbid conditions such as anxiety disorders or chronic pain.[75] Owing to a lack of data, it is unclear as to how effective these agents are in treating both depression and insomnia in a single patient. The safety and efficacy of combining these agents with nonsedating antidepressants is also unknown, so better established combined treatments are generally preferred. Caution should be exercised when administering these agents to patients with significant heart disease and/or sensitivity to anticholinergic effects of these medications. Finally, these agents must be prescribed with great caution for those at risk of suicide, as they can be lethal in overdose.

Trazodone Trazodone is approved by the FDA for the treatment of major depression in doses from 200 to 600 mg, but is also frequently used off-label to treat insomnia at lower doses (25–150 mg). Despite a relative lack of controlled trials demonstrating efficacy for insomnia, trazodone has been among the most frequently administered treatments for insomnia over the last 20 years.[65] Its sleep-enhancing effects are believed to derive from its antagonism of serotonin (5-HT2 receptors), norepinephrine (α_1 receptors), and histamine (H1) receptors. Trazodone is metabolized into a wake-promoting molecule (methyl-chlorophenylpiperazine or mCPP) to a highly variable degree, owing to a genetic polymorphism that is not rare in the population.[76,77] This feature may undermine the therapeutic effects of trazodone for some patients and lead them to have distressing levels of anxiety. It is helpful to inform patients about this possibility before prescribing the medication. Genetic polymorphisms that affect the metabolism of trazodone into an active, sedating, metabolite and the elimination of that metabolite also exist. As a result, some individuals experience prohibitive daytime sedation with this agent.

Given its frequency of use, it is perhaps surprising that there has been only one placebo-controlled study of trazodone for insomnia,[66] a 2-week study wherein trazodone was dosed at 50 mg. The group receiving active medication reported better sleep than placebo-treated subjects for the first week, but there were no differences between groups in the second week of treatment. Two smaller placebo-controlled studies, one in abstinent alcoholics and another in patients with major depression,[78,79] reported sleep-promoting effects of trazodone, but did not evaluate the treatment of insomnia per se.

The most common adverse effects associated with trazodone are sedation, dizziness, headache, dry mouth, blurred vision, and orthostatic hypotension.[3,66] Trazodone has rarely been associated with priapism, a prolonged erection associated with pain, that can lead to irreversible impotence.[80] Trazodone does not appear to have significant abuse potential and may be appropriate for use in abuse-prone patients with insomnia. The small placebo-controlled trial in abstinent alcoholics did not show any problems with abuse of the medication.[78] Because trazodone has antidepressant properties, it is possible that there would be a benefit for mood in individuals with comorbid anxiety and depression, but given the difference in dosage used for each disorder, this cannot be assumed and has not been systematically evaluated. Preliminary evidence suggests that trazodone can be safely used to treat insomnia in conjunction with fluoxetine and bupropion, but its use with other antidepressants has not been evaluated.[79]

Mirtazapine Mirtazapine is believed to have sleep-promoting effects related to its antagonism of serotoninergic (5-HT2 and 5-HT3), adrenergic (α_1), and histaminergic (H1) receptors.[81] In addition, it is thought to antagonize adrenergic α_2 receptors, which are presynaptic and inhibit the release of norepinephrine.[82] As a result of this property, the sleep-enhancing effects of mirtazapine are thought to decrease as the dose increases. Although the range for antidepressant dosing is 7.5 to 45 mg, doses below 30 mg are generally used to promote sleep.

There have been no placebo-controlled trials of mirtazapine for the treatment of insomnia. The evidence that mirtazapine may benefit sleep comes from a double-blind evaluation of mirtazapine versus fluoxetine in patients with major depression, an open-label study of healthy volunteers without sleep complaints, preoperative patients at risk for insomnia after surgery, and a pilot study of depressed patients.[83–85]

Based on trials treating major depression, the most common side effects associated with mirtazapine are sedation, increased appetite, weight gain, dry mouth, and constipation.[82] As with other antidepressants, mirtazapine is appropriate for use with patients prone to substance abuse, owing to its low potential for abuse. Because of the overlap in dosages used to treat insomnia and depression, mirtazapine can be considered for single-agent therapy for those with insomnia and comorbid depression. Future studies will be needed to evaluate this agent's effectiveness relative to combining a nonsedating antidepressant with an established insomnia therapy.

Antipsychotics

Pharmacology Similar to the antidepressants used to enhance sleep, some antipsychotics are used off-label to treat insomnia. The antipsychotics most commonly used for this purpose are quetiapine (dosed at 25–250 mg) and olanzapine (dosed at 2.5–20 mg).[65,86] The doses used for insomnia are somewhat lower than would be used to treat disorders of thought or mood. These agents enhance sleep through antagonism of dopamine, histamine (H1 receptors), serotonin (5-HT2 receptors), acetylcholine (muscarinic receptors), and norepinephrine (α_1 receptors).[3] Olanzapine has a t_{max} of 4 to 6 hours, making it better suited for the treatment of sleep-maintenance problems than for sleep-onset problems. Quetiapine, on the other hand, has a t_{max} of 1 to 2 hours and a half-life of 7 hours,[3] making it well suited for both sleep-onset problems and sleep-maintenance problems.

Evidence base No placebo-controlled trials have been completed with these agents for the treatment of insomnia specifically, therefore the risk/benefit profile is difficult to assess. Evidence for a sleep-enhancing effect of quetiapine (25–75 mg) was reported from open-label studies of patients with primary insomnia and healthy volunteers,[87] whereas olanzapine has been noted to enhance sleep in an open-label study of healthy volunteers only.[86] Evidence for effects on sleep is greater for patients with comorbid thought disorders or mood disorders.[86,88,89]

The most common side effects associated with antipsychotic agents in the treatment of insomnia are sedation, dizziness, anticholinergic side effects (dry mouth, blurred vision, constipation, urinary retention), and increased appetite,[86] with some agents having better side-effect profiles than others. Other potential side effects associated with dopamine antagonism can result, including parkinsonism, acute dystonic reactions, akathisia, and tardive dyskinesia.[87] These extrapyramidal side effects are less common with atypical antipsychotics than with typical antipsychotics.

Olanzapine has been found to increase the risk of insulin resistance, impaired cognition, and mortality in dementia patients. All of these agents should be used with caution in older adults because of the increased risk of cardiac-related mortality.[90]

Antipsychotic agents are not generally used in patients with insomnia who do not have a co-occurring psychotic or mood disorder, but may be particularly useful in this population. In addition to the effects already mentioned, many of these agents have mood-stabilizing properties useful in the treatment of mania. Quetiapine is also approved by the FDA for the treatment of depression. Antipsychotic agents can also be considered for use in abuse-prone patients with insomnia because of their low abuse potential.

Anticonvulsants

Pharmacology Anticonvulsants such as gabapentin, pregabalin, and tiagabine are sometimes used in the treatment of insomnia. Gabapentin and pregabalin bind to the $\alpha2$-δ subunit of N-type voltage-gated calcium channels, which decreases the activity of wake-promoting glutamate and norepinephrine systems. Tiagabine enhances sleep by inhibiting the reuptake of GABA.[91,92] Gabapentin has a relatively long t_{max} of 3 to 3.5 hours, making it relatively unlikely to facilitate sleep onset.

Evidence base Gabapentin and pregabalin have been demonstrated to have sleep-enhancing effects in a variety of populations including healthy volunteers, patients with restless legs syndrome, patients with chronic pain, and patients with partial seizures.[93–96] A smaller study demonstrated a benefit of gabapentin on time to relapse in patients with alcohol dependence, but found no benefit over placebo on sleep parameters.[97] In placebo-controlled trials of patients with primary insomnia, tiagabine has been found to increase slow-wave sleep, but has not been shown to improve sleep onset or sleep maintenance consistently.[98–101]

The most common side effects associated with gabapentin are ataxia and diplopia, whereas pregabalin is associated with dry mouth, cognitive impairment, peripheral edema, and increased appetite. Tiagabine is most commonly associated with nausea. Of these medications, only pregabalin is associated with abuse potential and should be used with caution in patients who are prone to substance abuse.[102] Preliminary evidence suggests gabapentin to be effective for the treatment of insomnia in patients with alcohol-use disorders. For insomnia that is comorbid with pain, gabapentin and pregabalin may be particularly useful. Pregabalin should be considered in the treatment of insomnia in patients with fibromyalgia because available evidence suggests it is effective for both conditions. Preliminary evidence also suggests that gabapentin may be indicated for patients with restless legs syndrome and periodic movements of sleep.

Antihypertensives

Pharmacology Prazosin is an antihypertensive medication with relatively recently discovered benefits for sleep, primarily in those who experience frequent nightmares and sleep disturbance associated with PTSD.[103] It is an α_1-adrenoreceptor antagonist, but it is not yet possible to propose a pharmacologic mechanism that explains the basis of the therapeutic effect on nightmares in PTSD.[104] Studies to date have generally prescribed 2 to 6 mg for most patients, with an upper limit of 15 to 20 mg. The recommended starting dose is 1 mg to prevent hypotension, then the dose is slowly titrated upward until a therapeutic effect is achieved.[105] In addition, it is important to warn patients that orthostatic hypotension is most likely to occur the morning after dose increases.

Evidence base Placebo-controlled trials have reported benefits of prazosin in the treatment of sleep disturbance and trauma-related nightmares in military veterans and civilians with PTSD.[105–108] Evidence to date has consistently shown prazosin to reduce nightmares and improve sleep overall, and results have been similar for samples of military veterans and civilians. Improvements in self-reported symptoms associated with prazosin include nightmare frequency, insomnia severity, and PTSD symptom severity; symptom improvement as measured by home polysomnography has also been found for total sleep time, rapid eye movement (REM) sleep time, and REM duration.[105–108] One study found comparable rates of improvement in prazosin and a behavioral sleep intervention, both of which outperformed placebo.[108]

Prazosin has been found to be well tolerated in all trials to date. Although studies thus far have not been powered to detect adverse effects in prazosin relative to placebo, the following symptoms have been reported in the trials mentioned herein: transient dizziness, nasal congestion, initial insomnia, dry mouth, sweating, depression, and lower extremity edema.[103–108] It is likely that some of these symptoms are not related to medication as they were also reported by patients in the placebo condition, but further study is needed to more adequately characterize adverse events associated with this agent. Prazosin is the only sleep-enhancing agent that has been shown to reduce sleep impairment caused by nightmares, and is therefore particularly useful in sleep disturbances associated with PTSD.

FACTORS TO BE CONSIDERED FOR OPTIMIZING MEDICATION MANAGEMENT OF INSOMNIA
Time of Night of Sleep Problem

As reviewed in the previous section, the medications used to treat insomnia differ as regards the time of night during which they have been established to have therapeutic effects. Some have been found only to improve problems with sleep onset, some have reliable therapeutic effects on sleep maintenance without onset effects, and some have reliable effects on both sleep onset and sleep maintenance. Among those with sleep-maintenance effects, some agents maintain these effects to the end of the night while others do not. The time of night during which sleep problems occur differs among insomnia sufferers. Treatment optimization therefore depends on selecting a medication that has therapeutic effects at the time of night during which an individual's sleep problem occurs. The following discussion reviews how to match the choice of medication to the patient's specific type of sleep problem.

Patients with only sleep-onset difficulties
For those who have difficulties falling asleep without difficulties staying asleep, the optimal strategy is to choose a medication that has been demonstrated to have therapeutic effects on sleep onset with the fewest associated adverse effects; this would include those agents that have been demonstrated to have therapeutic effects on sleep onset without having effects on sleep maintenance. These medications include:

> Ramelteon
> Zaleplon
> Zolpidem

Any of these might be appropriate for treating a patient with sleep-onset difficulties. However, optimizing the choice among these agents requires considering the patient's history with medications (have they failed to improve with 1 or more of these agents in the past? Did they have problems with side effects with 1 or more of these agents in the past?) and the other patient-specific factors that affect medication choice, including the temporal pattern of sleep problems and the presence of comorbidities (see later discussion). Although not a factor related to optimizing the matching of medication to the patient's sleep problem, cost may affect what medication can practically be obtained or which is tried first. If any of the aforementioned factors precludes the use of all 3 of the medications best suited for treating those with sleep-onset problems, the following agents, which have been demonstrated to have therapeutic effects on both sleep onset and sleep maintenance, could be considered for second-line use with the understanding that they are likely to have a greater risk of adverse effects.

> Eszopiclone
> Temazepam
> Zolpidem CR

Patients with only sleep-maintenance difficulties

For those who have difficulties staying asleep without difficulties falling asleep, the optimal strategy is to choose a medication that has been demonstrated to have therapeutic effects on sleep maintenance with the fewest associated adverse effects; this would include the agents that have been demonstrated to have therapeutic effects on sleep maintenance without having effects on sleep onset. These medications include:

> Doxepin 3 to 6 mg
> Sublingual zolpidem (Intermezzo) dosed during a middle-of-the-night awakening
> Zaleplon dosed during a middle-of-the-night awakening

For those individuals who have difficulties in the last 2 hours of the night, the only option is doxepin 3 to 6 mg.[62,63,70,72,109]

If factors such as prior experience with the medications, temporal pattern of the sleep problem, comorbidities, or cost factors precludes the use of all 3 of the medications listed, the following agents, which have therapeutic effects on both sleep onset and sleep maintenance, could be considered for second-line use with the understanding that they are likely to have a greater risk of adverse effects.

> Eszopiclone
> Zolpidem CR
> Temazepam

A final consideration is that doxepin is the only agent demonstrated to have therapeutic effects in the last 2 hours of the night without substantively increasing the risks of daytime impairment.[109] As a result, for those with this type of sleep difficulty, there is no satisfactory second-line therapy.

Patients with both sleep-onset and sleep-maintenance difficulties

A subset of the agents used in the treatment of insomnia has been demonstrated to have therapeutic effects in patients with both sleep-onset and sleep-maintenance problems. These medications are:

> Eszopiclone
> Temazepam
> Zolpidem CR

In those with difficulties in the last 2 hours of the night, the only option is to use doxepin to address this problem and combine it with an agent with therapeutic effects only for sleep-onset problems, such as:

> Ramelteon
> Zaleplon
> Zolpidem

The need to administer 2 medications in this circumstance, owing to the absence of a single medication that improves sleep at the end of the night and also improves sleep onset, suggests an unmet need in the treatment of insomnia.

Temporal Pattern of Sleep Problem

Another factor that is necessary to consider in the optimization of the medication management of insomnia is the patient's temporal pattern of sleep difficulties over nights. Some individuals have their problems nightly, whereas others have their problems intermittently. Among those with intermittent insomnia, the problem can occur anywhere from rarely to nearly every night. The temporal pattern has important implications for determining the optimal strategy for medication management.

Patients with nightly problems falling asleep

For patients with nightly difficulties falling asleep, nightly administration of an agent targeting sleep onset is generally indicated (see earlier discussion). However, a challenge that arises is that nightly use of an effective sleep medication may make it difficult to determine if the insomnia ceases at some point such that the medication is no longer needed. This situation can make both patients and prescribers uncomfortable because it raises the possibility that once treatment with a sleep medication begins, it continues indefinitely.

Further contributing to this problem is the concern that rebound insomnia occurring with discontinuation after a period of nightly use may falsely reinforce a sense of an ongoing need for nightly medication. Of note, a substantial number of relatively recent studies have indicated that significant rebound insomnia did not occur with nightly treatment for 6 months with eszopiclone; up to 1 year with zaleplon (open-label study); 1 year with zolpidem; 6 months with ramelteon;

and 3 months with doxepin.[11,12,14,53,110] However, rebound insomnia does at times occur, as was observed on the first night after discontinuing treatment after 3 weeks of nightly therapy with zolpidem CR.[111] Although rebound insomnia can occur, the authors' experience suggests it is more commonly the case that reluctance to discontinue nightly use of medications for insomnia reflects either the return of sleep problems after elimination of an effective therapy or anxiety about not sleeping well without medication. Without systematic data collection, such experiences can create the perception among clinicians that rebound insomnia is nearly universal, which can lead practitioners to avoid treating patients with nightly insomnia with medications or to require that their patients use the medications non-nightly.

In the authors' experience, the most effective means for addressing this challenge is to have an a priori strategy for stopping medications in those with nightly sleep problems. The most effective strategy has been to agree, before starting medications, that after a fixed period of time (typically 3 months), a trial medication taper will be instituted. This taper is nearly always effective in allowing patients to discontinue medications if they are warned to expect a transitory worsening of sleep following medication discontinuation and if the taper is performed slowly enough. Once the patient has discontinued use of the medication, an assessment can be made about whether the patient was better off using the medication or not using it. If the former is the case, the medication is restarted with a plan to institute another trial taper in 3 months. If the latter turns out to be true, the medication is discontinued. This type of exit strategy tends to make both patients and prescribers less anxious about the nightly use of medications for insomnia in those with nightly sleep problems, and ensures that medication use will persist for roughly the period required.

All 3 of the medications that have been reported to have therapeutic effects on sleep onset without effects on sleep maintenance, namely ramelteon, zaleplon, and zolpidem, have all been demonstrated to be safe and effective for at least 6 months of nightly treatment, and could all be used in individuals with nightly difficulties falling asleep. When the use of these medications is precluded, eszopiclone, which has also been demonstrated to have a good efficacy/safety profile over 6 months of nightly use, may also be considered.

Patients with nightly problems staying asleep

There are 2 options for treating patients with problems staying asleep. One is to administer a medication at bedtime in an attempt to prevent the awakening from occurring. The other is to have the patient take a medication if he or she wakes up in the middle of the night to speed the return to sleep. When the problem with middle-of-the-night awakenings occurs on a nightly basis, however, the best strategy is to take medication nightly at bedtime to prevent the awakening from occurring, rather than having to suffer from awakening nightly and then waiting for the medication to take effect. If nightly sleep-maintenance problems occur in the absence of problems falling asleep, doxepin, which has been demonstrated to be efficacious and safe over 3 months of nightly use, could be used. If problems in both falling asleep and staying asleep are present, the best choice from the point of view of long-term safety and efficacy is eszopiclone. As with nightly sleep-onset problems, when prescribing these medications nightly it is necessary to have a plan for stopping the medication, such as instituting periodic trial medication tapers.

Patients with intermittent problems falling asleep

When trouble falling asleep occurs intermittently, the optimal treatment strategy depends on whether the affected individual is able to tell before going to bed whether he or she is likely to have a "bad night." In those able to predict difficulties falling asleep, medication therapy can be administered on nights when problems are anticipated. Where prediction is not possible, one option is to have patients try to sleep and then take a medication if they fail to do so. However, for patients prone to developing a worsening of insomnia if they have nights wherein they try to sleep and fail, this strategy is best avoided, and implementation of cognitive behavioral insomnia therapy should be considered.

Patients with intermittent problems staying asleep

For those with difficulty staying asleep occurring nightly or nearly nightly, nightly treatment at bedtime in an attempt to prevent the awakening is generally the best strategy. However, for those with relatively infrequent difficulties waking up in the middle of the night, optimal treatment would involve providing an intervention to take in the middle of the night only on those nights when the awakening occurs. If it were possible to predict the nights when the middle-of-the-night awakenings were most likely to occur, a strategy of using a medication before bedtime to prevent those awakenings would be optimal. However, these awakenings are generally not predictable at bedtime. As a result, the strategy of taking a medication in the middle of the night has the substantial advantage over nightly bedtime dosing in that it only requires medication use on nights when the sleep problem occurs, thereby reducing the number of nights when medication is used. This strategy decreases the cost and associated risks of the medication used.

Data demonstrating that this strategy can be used effectively and safely have been reported for sublingual zolpidem (Intermezzo) and zaleplon, when these are taken up to 4 hours before getting out of bed in the morning.[112,113] These agents could therefore be considered for those patients who experience intermittent unpredictable middle-of-the-night awakenings. There are no studies demonstrating the safe and effective use of a medication for a middle-of-the-night awakening that occurs less than 4 hours before getting out of bed. This sort of practice, therefore, cannot be recommended.

Comorbidities

One additional consideration in optimizing the medication management of insomnia is the presence of comorbidities such as mood disorders, anxiety disorders, pain, and substance use/dependence. This factor is highly important because patients with comorbid medical and psychiatric conditions constitute the majority of patients with insomnia.[2] The available agents vary in their therapeutic effects and risks in patients with comorbidities. As a result, failure to consider the presence of such comorbidities can lead to suboptimal or adverse treatment outcomes. The following discussion provides guidance for optimizing the treatment of those comorbid conditions for which the most data are available and which are most commonly associated with insomnia. These comorbidities include major depression, GAD, PTSD, chronic pain, and alcoholism.

Insomnia comorbid with major depression
The long-standing view of insomnia occurring in those with major depression has been that insomnia is a secondary symptom of the depression that does not merit specific treatment. It was assumed that effective antidepressant therapy would eliminate insomnia just as it improves other symptoms. However, the available data clearly indicate that this view is incorrect, and speak to the need to provide insomnia-targeted treatment along with administration of antidepressant therapy.[114] Options for treating insomnia in those with comorbid major depression include administering a nonsedating antidepressant along with a medication targeting insomnia, or administering a

single agent that has antidepressant and sleep-enhancing properties.

As already described, 5 studies have been performed in which patients with insomnia comorbid with major depression were treated with an antidepressant medication along with an agent used in the treatment of insomnia or placebo. These studies provide some support for the utility of adding clonazepam to selective serotonin reuptake inhibitor therapy in patients with depression and insomnia. Sleep was improved in 3 of the studies conducted, and in 2 it was associated with greater improvement in symptoms of depression.[4–6]

In all 3 studies performed with clonazepam, this agent improved sleep and in 2 it was associated with greater improvement in depression symptoms, although it appears that with longer duration of treatment the improvement in depression symptoms with clonazepam may not be sustained. A study of patients with insomnia and rheumatoid arthritis reported a benefit of triazolam relative to placebo for both sleep and morning.[7]

As described earlier, a study in which patients with insomnia and comorbid depression were randomized to receive eszopiclone or placebo along with fluoxetine indicated that eszopiclone improved not only sleep but also was associated with more rapid and greater improvement in depression symptoms (sleep items were removed from the depression rating scale).[16] Of note, essentially the identical trial was performed with zolpidem (Ambien CR), and this agent was found to improve sleep but not depression symptoms in comparison with placebo.[18]

In terms of single-agent therapy, a few placebo-controlled studies have assessed the therapeutic sleep effects of antidepressants (a small study of tricyclic antidepressants and one study of mirtazapine) in therapeutic antidepressant dosages in patients with comorbid insomnia and depression.[67,83] These studies provide some support for the use of single-agent therapy for such patients, but it must be kept in mind that this is based on a relative paucity of data, and the relative utility of single-agent therapy versus combining a hypnotic agent and a nonsedating antidepressant remains unknown.

Overall, the available data most strongly suggest the use of eszopiclone along with a nonsedating antidepressant for initial therapy for those with insomnia comorbid with major depression. However, it should be noted that data exist only for combining eszopiclone with fluoxetine, and it remains unknown whether similar effects would be seen with other antidepressants. Clonazepam could be considered for use in these patients, but the relatively higher risk of daytime sedation and possibility of loss of antidepressant benefit over time suggests that it should be reserved for second-tier use. Zolpidem CR could also be considered, although eszopiclone would be preferred because of its relatively greater benefit for depression symptoms. Lastly, using single-agent therapy with mirtazapine is also a supported option. Although a small amount of data supports the use of single-agent therapy with tricyclic antidepressants, the risk/benefit for these agents is far inferior to the other options. Data are needed to evaluate the utility of single-agent therapy with mirtazapine versus the combination of eszopiclone and a nonsedating antidepressant.

Another consideration relevant to those with depression and comorbid insomnia is the choice of treatment when an individual is treated with an antidepressant and improves, but has sustained insomnia that has not been treated. Studies have been performed using trazodone and zolpidem in this circumstance.[79,115] Trazodone was found to improve sleep in a placebo-controlled trial of 15 patients treated with several different antidepressants. Zolpidem was observed to improve sleep to a greater extent than placebo in a larger study (N = 110) of patients who had achieved remission of depression with paroxetine, fluoxetine, or sertraline. Based on these studies, zolpidem and perhaps trazodone could be considered for patients with insomnia who have remitted to nonsedating antidepressant therapy.

Insomnia comorbid with generalized anxiety disorder

As with major depression, it has long been assumed that it was not necessary to administer insomnia-specific treatment to those with GAD. However, relatively recent guidelines recommend administering insomnia-targeted therapy along with anxiolytic therapy in individuals with GAD.[114] As already described, only 2 placebo-controlled trials have been performed to assess the therapeutic effects of adding insomnia therapy (eszopiclone 3 mg) rather than placebo to anxiolytic therapy (escitalopram).[17] As with the similar study in those with major depression, eszopiclone led to greater improvement not only in sleep but also anxiety, whereas an essentially identical study performed with zolpidem CR found improvements in sleep but not anxiety with this agent.[19] Clearly more data on the treatment of insomnia comorbid with GAD are needed. However, based on available data, eszopiclone would be the treatment of choice when adding a sleep-targeted therapy to treatment with a selective serotonin reuptake inhibitor. Zolpidem CR could also be considered for improving sleep, but should be considered as a second choice based on the lesser improvement in anxiety symptoms.

Insomnia comorbid with posttraumatic stress disorder

Few studies have been performed on the pharmacologic treatment of sleep problems occurring in the setting of PTSD. As reviewed earlier, the only agents that have been evaluated in placebo-controlled trials are eszopiclone and prazosin. Eszopiclone improved both sleep disturbance and PTSD symptoms in a cross-over study conducted with 24 patients.[24] Four placebo-controlled studies have been performed with prazosin in PTSD patients with sleep disturbance, all of which show significant improvement in sleep disturbance and nightmares.[105–108] Given the larger evidence base supporting the therapeutic effects of prazosin, the fact that it is the only agent that has been found to reduce nightmares in addition to disturbed sleep, and that it is well tolerated, this agent should be considered for first-line use in patients with PTSD-related sleep disturbance. Eszopiclone should also be considered for use in these patients, based on results of the relevant small cross-over study.

Insomnia comorbid with chronic pain

The available evidence suggests that individuals with insomnia comorbid with chronic pain are best treated by administering both pain-targeted and insomnia-targeted therapies.[114] As outlined earlier, 3 placebo-controlled trials with insomnia pharmacotherapy evaluating this paradigm have been performed. Triazolam was found to improve sleep and morning stiffness in those with rheumatoid arthritis,[7] and eszopiclone led to improvement in sleep and some pain ratings in this same population.[23] There is also evidence that eszopiclone has therapeutic effects when added to naproxen treatment in patients with chronic low back pain.[22] These studies provide a modest evidence base for influencing treatment decisions in patients with insomnia and chronic pain conditions. However, they indicate that eszopiclone has potential as a sleep-targeted therapy in this setting, and that triazolam could also be considered. Studies with other insomnia medications are needed to establish whether the therapeutic effects seen in patients with pain are specific to eszopiclone and triazolam, or would be seen with other medications.

Insomnia comorbid with alcoholism

The pharmacologic treatment of sleep problems occurring in patients with alcoholism have been the subject of little research. As already reviewed, in only one small placebo-controlled trial has trazodone been found to have therapeutic effects on sleep in patients with alcoholism (recently abstinent).[78] In general, benzodiazepines and non-benzodiazepines are avoided in this population because of abuse risk. Trazodone, which appears to have minimal abuse potential, should be considered in this population, but more studies are needed with agents without significant abuse potential to help guide the management of insomnia in patients with alcoholism.

FUTURE DIRECTIONS

As should be evident from the foregoing review, there is a need for more studies aimed at identifying how to optimally manage patients with insomnia, particularly among patients with comorbid conditions. Additional studies are also needed to define how to best manage patients with nightly sleep-onset problems. Although agents with established therapeutic effects on sleep onset and sleep maintenance are available for use in clinical practice, a need remains for the development of new agents that have therapeutic effects at the end of the night without increasing the risks of daytime sedation, and that have this effect alongside a therapeutic effect on sleep onset. Two agents under development are worthy of note in this regard. One is the S-isomer of the antidepressant mirtazapine discussed earlier. This agent has a pharmacologic profile comparable with that of the racemate, with predominant, highly potent, and selective H1 antagonist effects. Based on its pharmacology, this agent administered in relatively low doses, as have been evaluated, would be expected to have properties similar to those of the selective H1 antagonist doxepin. Preliminary data from 4 placebo-controlled studies with S-mirtazapine suggest that this is essentially the case, although effects on sleep onset may be more evident. These studies suggest that S-mirtazapine has consistent therapeutic effects on sleep maintenance, and tends to have therapeutic effects on sleep onset, although these effects are not as large or consistent and are dose dependent. In addition, there appears to be a dose-dependent risk of daytime sedation.[116–119]

Another agent with potential to make a significant contribution to the armamentarium of insomnia medications is the dual hypocretin/orexin receptor antagonist suvorexant, which has potential to improve both sleep onset and sleep maintenance, including at the end of the night, without prohibitive daytime adverse effects. Hypocretin/orexin is a relatively recently discovered set of peptidergic neurons arising in the lateral hypothalamus that play an important role in maintaining wakefulness.[120] Blocking these hypocretin/orexin receptors therefore has the potential to offer sleep-enhancing effects. Preliminary data from several trials suggest that this agent has therapeutic effects on sleep onset and maintenance (including in the last third of the night), and has sustained therapeutic effects with long-term nightly use without significant withdrawal or rebound insomnia on discontinuation, and overall appears to have a favorable adverse-effect profile.[121–124]

These agents have the potential to add to the options available for providing individualized insomnia pharmacotherapy that best meets the needs of patients with insomnia. The clinical availability of such agents, and the completion of more studies to help define how to best tailor the choice of treatment for each patient, promise to continue the steady evolution of the field toward greater capacity to select insomnia medications that optimize outcomes and thereby improve the treatment of the many who suffer from insomnia.

REFERENCES

1. Sieghart W, Sperk G. Subunit composition, distribution and function of GABA(A) receptor subtypes. Curr Top Med Chem 2002;2:795–816.
2. Ford D, Kamerow D. Epidemiologic study of sleep disturbances in psychiatric disorders. JAMA 1989; 262:1479–84.
3. Krystal AD. A compendium of placebo-controlled trials of the risks/benefits of pharmacological treatments for insomnia: the empirical basis for US clinical practice. Sleep Med Rev 2009;13(4):265.
4. Londborg P, Smith WT, Glaudin V, et al. Short-term cotherapy with clonazepam and fluoxetine: anxiety, sleep disturbance and core symptoms of depression. J Affect Disord 2000;61:73–9.
5. Smith W, Londborg PD, Glaudin V, et al. Short-term augmentation of fluoxetine with clonazepam in the treatment of depression: a double-blind study. Am J Psychiatry 1998;155(10):1339–45.
6. Smith W, Londborg P, Glaudin V, et al. Is extended clonazepam cotherapy of fluoxetine effective for outpatients with major depression? J Affect Disord 2002;70(3):251–9.
7. Walsh J, Muehlbach MJ, Lauter SA, et al. Effects of triazolam on sleep, daytime sleepiness, and morning stiffness in patients with rheumatoid arthritis. J Rheumatol 1996;23(2):245–52.
8. Sanna E, Busonero F, Talani G, et al. Comparison of the effects of zaleplon, zolpidem, and triazolam at various GABA(A) receptor subtypes. Eur J Pharmacol 2002;451(2):103–10.
9. Jia F, Goldstein PA, Harrison NL. The modulation of synaptic GABA(A) receptors in the thalamus by

eszopiclone and zolpidem. J Pharmacol Exp Ther 2009;328(3):1000–6.

10. Crestani F, Assandri R, Tauber M, et al. Contribution of the alpha1-GABA(A) receptor subtype to the pharmacological actions of benzodiazepine site inverse agonists. Neuropharmacology 2002; 43:679–84.

11. Walsh J, Krystal AD, Amato DA. Nightly treatment of primary insomnia with eszopiclone for six months: effect on sleep, quality of life and work limitations. Sleep 2007;30(8):959–68.

12. Krystal AD, Walsh JK, Laska E, et al. Sustained efficacy of eszopiclone over six months of nightly treatment: results of a randomized, double-blind, placebo controlled study in adults with chronic insomnia. Sleep 2003;26:793–9.

13. Roth T, Walsh JK, Krystal A, et al. An evaluation of the efficacy and safety of eszopiclone over 12 months in patients with chronic primary insomnia. Sleep Med 2005;6(6):487.

14. Ancoli-Israel S, Richardson GS, Mangano RM, et al. Long-term use of sedative hypnotics in older patients with insomnia. Sleep Med 2005; 6(2):107–13.

15. Krystal AD, Erman M, Zammit GK, et al. Long-term efficacy and safety of zolpidem extended-release 12.5 mg, administered 3 to 7 nights per week for 24 weeks, in patients with chronic primary insomnia: a 6-month, randomized, double-blind, placebo-controlled, parallel-group, multicenter study. Sleep 2008;31(1):79–90.

16. Fava M, McCall WV, Krystal A, et al. Eszopiclone co-administered with fluoxetine in patents with insomnia co-existing with major depressive disorder. Biol Psychiatry 2006;59:1052–60.

17. Pollack M, Kinrys G, Krystal A, et al. Eszopiclone co-administered with escitalopram in patients with insomnia and comorbid generalized anxiety disorder. Arch Gen Psychiatry 2008;65(5):551–62.

18. Fava M, Asnis GM, Shrivastava RK, et al. Improved insomnia symptoms and sleep-related next-day functioning in patients with comorbid major depressive disorder and insomnia following concomitant zolpidem extended-release 12.5 mg and escitalopram treatment: a randomized controlled trial. J Clin Psychiatry 2011;72(7):914–28.

19. Fava M, Asnis GM, Shrivastava R, et al. Zolpidem extended-release improves sleep and next-day symptoms in comorbid insomnia and generalized anxiety disorder. J Clin Psychopharmacol 2009; 29(3):222–30.

20. Soares C, Rubens R, Caron J, et al. Eszopiclone treatment during menopausal transition: sleep effects, impact on menopausal symptoms, and mood. Sleep 2006;29:A239.

21. Dorsey C, Lee KA, Scharf MB. Effect of zolpidem on sleep in women with perimenopausal and postmenopausal insomnia: a 4-week, randomized, multicenter, double-blind, placebo-controlled study. Clin Ther 2004;26(10):1578–86.

22. Goforth H, Preud'homme X, Krystal A. A randomized, double-blind, placebo-controlled trial of eszopiclone for the treatment of insomnia in patients with chronic low back pain. Sleep, in press.

23. Roth T, Price JM, Amato DA, et al. The effect of eszopiclone in patients with insomnia and coexisting rheumatoid arthritis: a pilot study. Prim Care Companion J Clin Psychiatry 2009;11(6):292.

24. Pollack MH, Hoge EA, Worthington JJ, et al. Eszopiclone for the treatment of posttraumatic stress disorder and associated insomnia: a randomized, double-blind, placebo-controlled trial. J Clin Psychiatry 2011;72(7):892–7.

25. Griffiths R, Johnson M. Relative abuse liability of hypnotic drugs: a conceptual framework and algorithm for differentiating among compounds. J Clin Psychiatry 2005;66(Suppl 9):31–41.

26. Richey S, Krystal A. Pharmacological advances in the treatment of insomnia. Curr Pharm Des 2011; 17(15):1471–5.

27. Hughes R, Sack RL, Lewy AJ. The role of melatonin and circadian phase in age-related sleep-maintenance insomnia: assessment in a clinical trial of melatonin replacement. Sleep 1998;21:52–68.

28. Singer C, Tractenberg RE, Kaye J, et al. A multicenter, placebo-controlled trial of melatonin for sleep disturbance in Alzheimer's disease. Sleep 2003;26(7):893–901.

29. Smits M, Nagtegaal EE, van der Heijden J, et al. Melatonin for chronic sleep onset insomnia in children: a randomized placebo-controlled trial. J Child Neurol 2001;16(2):86–92.

30. Zhdanova I, Wurtman RJ, Morabito C, et al. Effects of low oral doses of melatonin, given 2-4 hours before habitual bedtime, on sleep in normal young humans. Sleep 1996;19(5):423–31.

31. Zhdanova I, Wurtman RJ, Wagstaff J. Effects of a low dose of melatonin on sleep in children with Angelman syndrome. J Pediatr Endocrinol 1999; 12(1):57–67.

32. Zhdanova I, Wurtman R, Regan M, et al. Melatonin treatment for age-related insomnia. J Clin Endocrinol Metab 2001;86:4727–30.

33. Waldhauser F, Saletu B, Trinchard-Lugan I. Sleep laboratory investigations on hypnotic properties of melatonin. Psychopharmacology 1990;100(2): 222–6.

34. Dalton E, Rotondi D, Levitan RD, et al. Use of slow-release melatonin in treatment-resistant depression. J Psychiatry Neurosci 2000;25(1):48–52.

35. Andrade C, Srihari B, Reddy K, et al. Melatonin in medically ill patients with insomnia: a double-blind, placebo-controlled study. J Clin Psychiatry 2001;62(1):41–5.

36. Serfaty M, Kennell-Webb S, Warner J, et al. Double blind randomised placebo controlled trial of low dose melatonin for sleep disorders in dementia. Int J Geriatr Psychiatry 2002;17(12):1120–7.

37. Suresh Kumar P, Andrade C, Bhakta SG, et al. Melatonin in schizophrenic outpatients with insomnia: a double-blind, placebo-controlled study. J Clin Psychiatry 2007;68(2):237–41.

38. Van der Heijden K, Smits MG, Van Someren EJ, et al. Effect of melatonin on sleep, behavior, and cognition in ADHD and chronic sleep-onset insomnia. J Am Acad Child Adolesc Psychiatry 2007;46(2):233–41.

39. Wasdell M, Jan JE, Bomben MM, et al. A randomized, placebo-controlled trial of controlled release melatonin treatment of delayed sleep phase syndrome and impaired sleep maintenance in children with neurodevelopmental disabilities. J Pineal Res 2008;44(1):57–64.

40. Braam W, Didden R, Smits M, et al. Melatonin treatment in individuals with intellectual disability and chronic insomnia: a randomized placebo-controlled study. J Intellect Disabil Res 2008;52(3):256–64.

41. Haimov I, Lavie P, Laudon M, et al. Melatonin replacement therapy of elderly insomniacs. Sleep 1995;18(7):598–603.

42. Mendelson WB. Efficacy of melatonin as a hypnotic agent. J Biol Rhythms 1997;12(6):651–6.

43. Sack R, Hughes RJ, Edgar DM, et al. Sleep-promoting effects of melatonin: at what dose, in whom, under what conditions, and by what mechanisms? Sleep 1997;20(10):908–15.

44. Graw P, Werth E, Krauchi K, et al. Early morning melatonin administration impairs psychomotor vigilance. Behav Brain Res 2001;121:167–72.

45. Dollins A, Zhdanova IV, Wurtman RJ, et al. Effect of inducing nocturnal serum melatonin concentrations in daytime on sleep, mood, body temperature and performance. Proc Natl Acad Sci U S A 1994;91:1824–8.

46. Krystal A. The possibility of preventing functional impairment due to sleep loss by pharmacologically enhancing sleep. Sleep 2005;28:16–7.

47. Lerchl A. Melatonin administration alters semen quality in normal men. J Androl 2004;25(2):185–6.

48. Ianas O, Manda D, Câmpean D, et al. Effects of melatonin and its relation to the hypothalamic-hypophyseal-gonadal axis. Adv Exp Med Biol 1999;460:321–8.

49. Partonen T. Melatonin-dependent infertility. Med Hypotheses 1999;52(3):269–70.

50. Pang S, Li L, Ayre E, et al. Neuroendocrinology of melatonin in reproduction: recent developments. J Chem Neuroanat 1998;14(3–4):157–66.

51. Kryger M, Wang-Weigand S, Roth T. Safety of ramelteon in individuals with mild to moderate obstructive sleep apnea. Sleep Breath 2007;11(3):159–64.

52. Kryger M, Roth T, Wang-Weigand S, et al. The effects of ramelteon on respiration during sleep in subjects with moderate to severe chronic obstructive pulmonary disease. Sleep Breath 2009;13(1):79–84.

53. Mayer G, Wang-Weigand S, Roth-Schechter B, et al. Efficacy and safety of 6-month nightly ramelteon administration in adults with chronic primary insomnia. Sleep 2009;32(3):351.

54. Krystal AD, Richelson E, Roth T. Review of the histamine system and the clinical effects of H1 antagonists: basis for a new model for understanding the effects of insomnia medications. Sleep Med Rev 2013;17(4):263–72.

55. Kudo Y, Kurihara MC. Clinical evaluation of diphenhydramine hydrochloride for the treatment of insomnia in psychiatric patients: a double-blind study. J Clin Pharmacol 1990;30(11):1041–8.

56. Rickels K, Morris RJ, Newman H, et al. Diphenhydramine in insomniac family practice patients: a double-blind study. J Clin Pharmacol 1983;23(5–6):234–42.

57. Morin C, Koetter U, Bastien C, et al. Valerian-hops combination and diphenhydramine for treating insomnia: a randomized placebo-controlled clinical trial. Sleep 2005;28(11):1465–71.

58. Meuleman J, Nelson RC, Clark RL. Evaluation of temazepam and diphenhydramine as hypnotics in a nursing-home population. Drug Intell Clin Pharm 1987;21(9):716–20.

59. Glass JR, Sproule BA, Herrmann N, et al. Effects of 2-week treatment with temazepam and diphenhydramine in elderly insomniacs: a randomized, placebo-controlled trial. J Clin Psychopharmacol 2008;28(2):182–8.

60. Smith G, Smith PH. Effects of doxylamine and acetaminophen on postoperative sleep. Clin Pharmacol Ther 1985;5:549–57.

61. Richardson G, Roehrs TA, Rosenthal L, et al. Tolerance to daytime sedative effects of H1 antihistamines. J Clin Psychopharmacol 2002;22(5):511–5.

62. Roth T, Rogowski R, Hull S, et al. Efficacy and safety of doxepin 1 mg, 3 mg, and 6 mg in adults with primary insomnia. Sleep 2007;30(11):1555–61.

63. Scharf M, Rogowski R, Hull S, et al. Efficacy and safety of doxepin 1 mg, 3 mg, and 6 mg in elderly patients with primary insomnia: a randomized, double-blind, placebo-controlled crossover study. J Clin Psychiatry 2008;69(10):1557.

64. Koppel C, Tenczer J, Ibe K. Poisoning with over-the-counter doxylamine preparations: an evaluation of 109 cases. Hum Toxicol 1987;6(5):355–9.

65. Walsh JK. Drugs used to treat insomnia in 2002: regulatory-based rather than evidence-based medicine. Sleep 2004;27(8):14441–2.

66. Walsh JK, Erman M, Erwin CW, et al. Subjective hypnotic efficacy of trazodone and zolpidem in DSM-III-R primary insomnia. Hum Psychopharmacol 1998;13:191–8.

67. Dunleavy D, Brezinova V, Oswald I, et al. Changes during weeks in effects of tricyclic drugs on the human sleep brain. Br J Psychiatry 1972; 120:663–72.

68. Riemann D, Voderholzer U, Cohrs S, et al. Trimipramine in primary insomnia: results of a polysomnographic double-blind controlled study. Pharmacopsychiatry 2002;35(5):165–74.

69. Hohagen F, Montero RF, Weiss E. Treatment of primary insomnia with trimipramine: an alternative to benzodiazepine hypnotics? Eur Arch Psychiatry Clin Neurosci 1994;244(2):65–72.

70. Rodenbeck A, Cohrs S, Jordan W, et al. The sleep-improving effects of doxepin are paralleled by a normalized plasma cortisol secretion in primary insomnia. Psychopharmacology (Berl) 2003;170: 423–8.

71. Hajak G, Rodenbeck A, Adler L, et al. Nocturnal melatonin secretion and sleep after doxepin administration in chronic primary insomnia. Pharmacopsychiatry 1996;29(5):187–92.

72. Hajak G, Rodenbeck A, Voderholzer U, et al. Doxepin in the treatment of primary insomnia: a placebo-controlled, double-blind, polysomnographic study. J Clin Psychiatry 2001;62(6):453–63.

73. Richelson E, Nelson A. Antagonism by antidepressants of neurotransmitter receptors of normal human brain in vitro. J Pharmacol Exp Ther 1984; 230(1):94–102.

74. Ziegler V, Biggs JT, Ardekani AB, et al. Contribution to the pharmacokinetics of amitriptyline. J Clin Pharmacol 1978;18(10):462–7.

75. Murphy D, Siever LJ, Insel TR. Therapeutic responses to tricyclic antidepressants and related drugs in non-affective disorder patient populations. Prog Neuropsychopharmacol Biol Psychiatry 1985; 9(1):3–13.

76. Caccia S, Ballabio M, Fanelli R, et al. Determination of plasma and brain concentrations of trazodone and its metabolite, 1-m-chlorophenylpiperazine, by gas-liquid chromatography. J Chromatogr 1981;5(210):311–8.

77. Greenblatt DJ, Friedman H, Burstein ES, et al. Trazodone kinetics: effects of age, gender and obesity. Clin Pharmacol Ther 1987;42:193–200.

78. Le Bon O, Murphy JR, Staner L, et al. Double-blind, placebo-controlled study of the efficacy of trazodone in alcohol post-withdrawal syndrome: polysomnographic and clinical evaluations. J Clin Psychopharmacol 2003;23(4):377–83.

79. Nierenberg A, Adler L, Peselow E, et al. Trazodone for antidepressant-associated insomnia. Am J Psychiatry 1994;151:1069–72.

80. Warner M, Peabody CA, Whiteford HA, et al. Trazodone and priapism. J Clin Psychiatry 1987;48(6): 244–5.

81. de Boer T. The pharmacologic profile of mirtazapine. J Clin Psychiatry 1996;57(Suppl 4):19–25.

82. Fawcett J, Barkin RL. Review of the results from clinical studies on the efficacy, safety and tolerability of mirtazapine for the treatment of patients with major depression. J Affect Disord 1998; 51(3):267–85.

83. Winokur A, Sateia MJ, Hayes JB, et al. Acute effects of mirtazapine on sleep continuity and sleep architecture in depressed patients: a pilot study. Biol Psychiatry 2000;48(1):75–8.

84. Winokur A, DeMartinis NA 3rd, McNally DP, et al. Comparative effects of mirtazapine and fluoxetine on sleep physiology measures in patients with major depression and insomnia. J Clin Psychiatry 2003;64(10):1224–9.

85. Sørensen M, Jørgensen J, Viby-Mogensen J, et al. A double-blind group comparative study using the new anti-depressant Org 3770, placebo and diazepam in patients with expected insomnia and anxiety before elective gynaecological surgery. Acta Psychiatr Scand 1985;71(4):331–46.

86. Krystal A, Goforth HW, Roth T. Effects of antipsychotic medications on sleep in schizophrenia. Int Clin Psychopharmacol 2008;23(3):150–60.

87. Wiegand MH, Landry F, Brückner T, et al. Quetiapine in primary insomnia: a pilot study. Psychopharmacology (Berl) 2008;196(2):337–8.

88. Moreno R, Hanna MM, Tavares SM, et al. A double-blind comparison of the effect of the antipsychotics haloperidol and olanzapine on sleep in mania. Braz J Med Biol Res 2007;40(3):357–66.

89. Todder D, Caliskan S, Baune BT. Night locomotor activity and quality of sleep in quetiapine-treated patients with depression. J Clin Psychopharmacol 2006;26(6):638–42.

90. Kirshner H. Controversies in behavioral neurology: the use of atypical antipsychotic drugs to treat neurobehavioral symptoms in dementia. Curr Neurol Neurosci Rep 2008;8(6):471–4.

91. Rose M, Kam CA. Gabapentin: pharmacology and its use in pain management. Anaesthesia 2002;57: 451–62.

92. Gajraj N. Pregabalin: its pharmacology and use in pain management. Anesth Analg 2007;105(6): 1805–15.

93. Gilron I. Gabapentin and pregabalin for chronic neuropathic and early postsurgical pain: current evidence and future directions. Curr Opin Anaesthesiol 2007;20(5):456–72.

94. Hindmarch I, Dawson J, Stanley N. A double-blind study in healthy volunteers to assess the effects on sleep of pregabalin compared with alprazolam and placebo. Sleep 2005;28(2):187–93.

95. de Haas S, Otte A, de Weerd W, et al. Exploratory polysomnographic evaluation of pregabalin on sleep disturbance in patients with epilepsy. J Clin Sleep Med 2007;3(5):473–8.

96. Garcia-Borreguero D, Larrosa O, de la Llave Y, et al. Treatment of restless legs syndrome with gabapentin: a double-blind, cross-over study. Neurology 2002;59(10):1573–9.

97. Brower K, Myra Kim H, Strobbe S, et al. A randomized double-blind pilot trial of gabapentin versus placebo to treat alcohol dependence and comorbid insomnia. Alcohol Clin Exp Res 2008; 32(8):1429–38.

98. Walsh J, Zammit G, Schweitzer PK, et al. Tiagabine enhances slow wave sleep and sleep maintenance in primary insomnia. Sleep Med 2006; 7(2):155–61.

99. Roth T, Wright KP Jr, Walsh J. Effect of tiagabine on sleep in elderly subjects with primary insomnia: a randomized, double-blind, placebo-controlled study. Sleep 2006;29(3):335–41.

100. Walsh J, Perlis M, Rosenthal M, et al. Tiagabine increases slow-wave sleep in a dose-dependent fashion without affecting traditional efficacy measures in adults with primary insomnia. J Clin Sleep Med 2006;2(1):35–41.

101. Walsh J, Randazzo AC, Frankowski S, et al. Dose-response effects of tiagabine on the sleep of older adults. Sleep 2005;28(6):673–6.

102. Guay D. Pregabalin in neuropathic pain: a more "pharmaceutically elegant" gabapentin? Am J Geriatr Pharmacother 2005;3(4):274–87.

103. Taylor F, Raskind MA. The [alpha] 1-adrenergic antagonist prazosin improves sleep and nightmares in civilian trauma posttraumatic stress disorder. J Clin Psychopharmacol 2002;22(1):82–5.

104. Krystal AD, Davidson J. The use of prazosin for the treatment of trauma nightmares and sleep disturbance in combat veterans with post-traumatic stress disorder. Biol Psychiatry 2007;61(8):925.

105. Taylor FB, Martin P, Thompson C, et al. Prazosin effects on objective sleep measures and clinical symptoms in civilian trauma PTSD: a placebo-controlled study. Biol Psychiatry 2008;63(6):629.

106. Raskind MA, Peskind ER, Kanter ED, et al. Reduction of nightmares and other PTSD symptoms in combat veterans by prazosin: a placebo-controlled study. Am J Psychiatry 2003;160(2):371–3.

107. Raskind MA, Peskind ER, Hoff DJ, et al. A parallel group placebo controlled study of prazosin for trauma nightmares and sleep disturbance in combat veterans with post-traumatic stress disorder. Biol Psychiatry 2007;61(8):928–34.

108. Germain A, Richardson R, Moul DE, et al. Placebo-controlled comparison of prazosin and cognitive-behavioral treatments for sleep disturbances in US military veterans. J Psychosom Res 2012; 72(2):89–96.

109. Krystal AD, Lankford A, Durrence HH, et al. Efficacy and safety of doxepin 3 and 6 mg in a 35-day sleep laboratory trial in adults with chronic primary insomnia. Sleep 2011;34(10):1433.

110. Roehrs TA, Randall S, Harris E, et al. Twelve months of nightly zolpidem does not lead to rebound insomnia or withdrawal symptoms: a prospective placebo-controlled study. J Psychopharmacol 2012; 26(8):1088–95.

111. Roth T, Soubrane C, Titeux L, et al. Efficacy and safety of zolpidem-MR: a double-blind, placebo-controlled study in adults with primary insomnia. Sleep Med 2006;7(5):397–406.

112. Roth T, Krystal A, Steinberg FJ, et al. Novel sublingual low-dose zolpidem tablet reduces latency to sleep onset following spontaneous middle-of-the-night awakening in insomnia in a randomized, double-blind, placebo-controlled, outpatient study. Sleep 2013;36(2):189–96.

113. Zammit G, Corser B, Doghramji K, et al. Sleep and residual sedation after administration of zaleplon, zolpidem, and placebo during experimental middle-of-the-night awakening. J Clin Sleep Med 2006;2(4):417–23.

114. NIH State of the Science Conference statement on Manifestations and Management of Chronic Insomnia in Adults statement. Sleep 2005;28(9): 1049–57.

115. Asnis GM, Chakraburtty A, DuBoff EA, et al. Zolpidem for persistent insomnia in SSRI-treated depressed patients. J Clin Psychiatry 1999;60:668–76.

116. Krystal A, Roth T, Pong A, et al. Efficacy and safety of esmirtazapine in elderly patients with primary insomnia in a 2-week sleep laboratory trial. Sleep 2012;35:A222.

117. Ivgy-May N, Roth T, Amari N, et al. Efficacy and safety of esmirtazapine in non-elderly adult patients with primary insomnia. A 2-week outpatient trial. Sleep 2012;35:A222–3.

118. Ivgy-May N, Amari N, Pathirajaj K, et al. Efficacy and safety of esmirtazapine in a six-week sleep laboratory study in patients with primary insomnia. Sleep 2012;35:A223.

119. Ruwe F, Ivgy-May N, Ijzerman-Boon P, et al. A phase II randomized, 4-way crossover, double-blind, placebo-controlled, multi-center, dose-finding trial with esmirtazapine in patients with primary insomnia. Sleep 2012;35:A224–5.

120. Mignot E. The perfect hypnotic? Science 2013; 340(6128):36–8.

121. Sun H, Kennedy W, Wilbraham D, et al. Phase II randomized, 4-way crossover, double-blind, placebo-controlled, multi-center, dose-finding trial with esmirtazapine in patients with primary insomnia. Sleep 2013;36:259–67.

122. Herring WJ, Snyder E, Budd K, et al. Orexin receptor antagonism for treatment of insomnia: a randomized clinical trial of suvorexant. Neurology
2012;79(23):2265–74.

123. Connor K, Budd K, Snavely D, et al. Efficacy and
safety of suvorexant, an orexin receptor

antagonist, in patients with primary insomnia: a
3-month phase 3 trial (trial# 1). J Sleep Res
2012;21:97.

124. Herring W, Snyder E, Paradis E, et al. Long term
safety and efficacy of suvorexant in patients with
primary insomnia. Sleep 2012;35:A217.

The Role of Bright Light Therapy in Managing Insomnia

Nicole Lovato, PhD*, Leon Lack, PhD

KEYWORDS

- Circadian rhythms • Bright light • Insomnia • Melatonin • Delayed sleep phase
- Advanced sleep phase

KEY POINTS

- Two types of insomnia, sleep-onset insomnia and early-morning-awakening insomnia, have been associated with delayed and advanced circadian rhythms, respectively.
- These circadian rhythm abnomalies can be treated with the use of morning bright light in the case of sleep-onset insomnia, and evening bright light in the case of early-morning-awakening insomnia.
- Although robust evidence shows that appropriately timed light therapy can retime the body clock, evidence of the therapeutic value of bright light therapy for these types of insomnia needs further development.
- Large randomized controlled trials of bright light and behavior therapies, alone and in combination, are needed to improve the treatment of these debilitating disorders.

INTRODUCTION

Some types of insomnia have been associated with abnormalities in the timing of circadian rhythms.[1,2] These difficulties are often chronic and are accompanied by decreased total sleep, impaired daytime functioning,[3,4] and depressed mood and anxiety.[5,6] Insomnia, with the main symptom being difficulty initiating sleep at conventional bedtime, is associated with a circadian rhythm timed later than normal. In contrast, early-morning-awakening insomnia is associated with an advanced or earlier-than-normal timed circadian rhythm. Thus, a cause of 2 types of insomnia symptoms, sleep-onset and early-morning-awakening insomnia, may be an abnormally timed circadian rhythm.

REGULATION OF SLEEP

Sleep and wake periods across the 24-hour day are regulated by the complex interaction between 2 biologic mechanisms: the homeostatic and circadian procesess.[7]

The homeostatic process refers to the increase in the propensity or pressure for sleep with continued wakefulness. This process is similar to the increase in hunger as one goes without food. Put simply, the need for sleep increases throughout wakefulness, so that the longer an individual is awake, the sleepier they will become.[7,8] Once asleep, the need for sleep decreases, rapidly in the initial stages before continuing to decline at a slower rate throughout the remainder of the sleep period. Sleeping reduces the drive for sleep the same way that eating reduces the drive to eat.[9]

The second process involved in the regulation of sleep is the circadian process that is largely independent of prior wake time and is therefore distinct from the homeostatic process. The circadian process regulates sleep propensity through self-sustaining cycles of physiologic activity, referred to as *circadian rhythms*. These rhythms are

School of Psychology, Faculty of Social and Behavioural Sciences, Flinders University, Sturt Road, Bedford Park, Adelaide, South Australia 5042, Australia
* Corresponding author.
E-mail address: nicole.lovato@flinders.edu.au

Sleep Med Clin 8 (2013) 351–359
http://dx.doi.org/10.1016/j.jsmc.2013.06.003
1556-407X/13/$ – see front matter © 2013 Elsevier Inc. All rights reserved.

generated and regulated by the body clock located in the suprachiasmatic nuclei (SCN). The SCN is a group of neural cells located in the anterior hypothalamus of the brain a few centimeters behind the eyes that receives direct input from the retinas of the eyes. The SCN controls the timing of slave clocks throughout the body and the synthesis of melatonin in the pineal gland.[10] The concentration of melatonin circulating in the blood feeds back to the SCN, helping to maintain the stability of circadian rhythm timing.[11,12] The SCN produces rhythms that take approximately 24.2 hours on average to complete a full cycle in humans.[13] The time needed for the circadian rhythms to complete a full cycle is referred to as *period length* or *tau*. Circadian rhythms are endogenous because they originate from within the organism. However, they are affected significantly by behavior and exogenous environmental cues that serve as zeitgebers, or "time givers."

Circadian rhythms play an important role in determining the timing of sleep and wakefulness across the 24-hour day. It has been well established that the circadian rhythms of core body temperature and melatonin are synchronized and offer reliable indicators of the timing of the circadian system, including the circadian propensity for sleep. **Fig. 1** shows the relationship between the sleep period and the circadian rhythms of core body temperature and melatonin for a normally entrained individual (ie, a person with normally timed circadian rhythms). The sleep period begins at approximately 11:00 PM when core body temperature is falling and about an hour or two after melatonin secretion begins.

A reliable biological marker for the timing of the melatonin rhythm is the dim light melatonin onset (DLMO) that can be determined from melatonin concentrations assayed from saliva samples taken regularly from about 7:00 PM to 1:00 AM under dim light conditions.[14] The determination of the DLMO has been increasingly recommended for suspected circadian rhythm timing abnormalities to confirm and optimize circadian re-timing therapy.[15] Maximum circadian sleep propensity then occurs between approximately 1:00 and 6:00 AM, coinciding with high melatonin concentration and the minimum core body temperature.[16–18] Wake-up usually occurs as core body temperature rises and melatonin secretion ends.

In addition to playing a crucial role in regulating sleep, circadian rhythms are also heavily involved in maintaining alertness during certain periods of the 24-hour day. Two periods of the day exist during which sleep is very difficult to initiate and maintain.[19,20] These periods are indicated as the wake-maintenance zone and wake-up zone in **Fig. 1**. The wake-maintenance zone spans 2 to 3 hours, normally from about 6:00 to 9:00 PM for someone who usually sleeps from about 11:00 PM to 7:00 AM. During the wake-maintenance zone it is very difficult to fall asleep. After sleep, the wake-up zone normally occurs from approximately 9:00 AM to noon for a conventionally timed sleeper, when staying asleep becomes difficult. The wake-maintenance and wake-up zones are particularly relevant to sleep-onset and early-morning-awakening insomnia, respectively.

INSOMNIAS RELATED TO CIRCADIAN MIS-TIMING

Chronic difficulties sleeping can occur when the timing of an individual's endogenous circadian

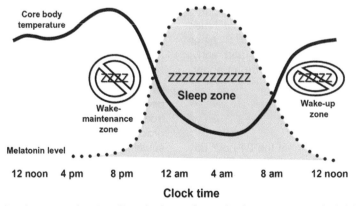

Fig. 1. The relationship between the circadian rhythms of core body temperature (*solid line*) and melatonin (*dotted line*) for a good sleeper who normally sleeps between 11:00 PM and 7:00 AM. The circadian "bed" or sleep zone (*gray shading*) occurs when temperature is low and melatonin is high. However, it is bracketed by 2 zones of alertness: a wake-maintenance zone (6:00–9:00 PM) and a wake-up zone (8:00 AM–noon). (*From* Lack L, Wright H. The use of bright light in the treatment of insomnia. In: Perlis M, Aloia M, Kuhn K, editors. Behavioral treatments for sleep disorders. London: Elsevier; 2011. p. e2; with permission.)

sleep-wake rhythm does not coincide with their preferred sleep-wake schedule.[1,2] If an individual has a delayed or late-timed circadian rhythm but is attempting to sleep at the earlier "normal" time, they will be doing so during their evening wake-maintenance zone, and therefore experience difficulty falling asleep. This difficulty initiating sleep coupled with the need to adhere to a normal waking time (eg, for work or social obligations) results in reduced sleep time. Likewise, if an individual has an advanced or earlier-timed circadian rhythm, their wake-up zone may occur as early as 3:00 AM, resulting in reduced sleep time with difficulty maintaining sleep beyond this point. In both instances, reduced sleep, particularly when occurring over several nights, will result in daytime impairments and associated distress.[3,4]

Sleep-Onset Insomnia and Circadian Rhythm Delay

A delayed circadian rhythm can lead to chronic difficulty falling asleep at night and difficulty waking in the morning at a conventional time to meet work and social commitments. Chronic difficulty initiating sleep at the start of the night is a core characteristic of sleep-onset insomnia. If trouble falling asleep persists over a prolonged period, the bedroom can quickly become associated with negative emotions, such as frustration, anger, and anxiety. These emotions in turn increase arousal and delay sleep onset further. Numerous associations of sleeping difficulty with the bedroom environment, time of night, and even the intention to sleep can produce learned or psychophysiologic insomnia.[1,2] Once developed, this chronic learned insomnia can exacerbate the circadian rhythm delay.

Substantial evidence shows that sleep-onset insomnia is associated with delays of the circadian rhythm of approximately 2 to 3 hours. Morris and colleagues[21] reported that individuals with sleep-onset insomnia, who took an average of 45 minutes to fall asleep, had a 2.5-hour delay of their core body temperature rhythm compared with healthy, good sleepers. Wright and colleagues[22] found a 2-hour delay in the melatonin rhythm of a group of sleep-onset insomniacs compared with a control group of good sleepers. In a recent study, Van Veen and colleagues[23] assessed the DLMOs of a group of sleep-onset insomniacs and good-sleeper controls. The individuals with sleep-onset insomnia fell asleep an average of 53 minutes later than the good sleepers, and had a DLMO of approximately 2 hours and 45 minutes later than the good sleepers. In a similar study, the DLMO

of a group of sleep-onset insomniacs was reported to be more than 3 hours later than in a control group of good sleepers.[24]

Later sleep-onset times increase individuals' tendency to sleep later into the morning in attempt to obtain sufficient sleep. However, when required to rise for work or social obligations (eg, at 7:00 AM), an individual with a delayed circadian rhythm will experience extreme difficulty, because they are attempting to rise at the time of maximum circadian sleepiness. The negative experience of this physiologically based difficulty, coupled with insufficient sleep, can amplify the negative consequences of difficulty falling asleep and feed back into the cycle of chronic insomnia. Although later rising time can provide more sleep and an easier awakening, it also avoids or delays exposure to morning bright light and allows the longer-than-24-hour tau circadian rhythms to drift later or delay further.[25,26] This effect subsequently increases the sleep-onset difficulty at a conventional bedtime. Therefore, regardless of the initial cause, the sleep-onset difficulty combined with sleeping later in the morning perpetuates the circadian delay and the conditioned arousal in response to the nightly sleep challenge.

Clinical example of an individual with sleep-onset insomnia

The 7-day sleep/wake diary shown in **Fig. 2** illustrates the typical sleep pattern of a man with a moderately delayed circadian rhythm who experienced sleep-onset insomnia.

On weeknights, he tended to go to bed at approximately midnight but was not falling asleep for 60 to 90 minutes on most nights. However, once asleep, he had no problem staying asleep throughout the night. He set his alarm for 7:15 AM to be out of bed by 8:00 AM to meet his study commitments. However, on most occasions he slept through the alarm. On mornings when he rose shortly after his alarm (eg, Wednesday morning), he had only obtained approximately 5 hours of sleep. On the weekend, he stayed up later on Friday and Saturday nights and slept in very late on Saturday and Sunday mornings. Sleeping late resulted in great difficulty falling asleep on Sunday night and waking on Monday morning.

This man also reported feeling anxious and frustrated when attempting to initiate sleep after going to bed. He reported difficulty "switching off" his racing mind and felt he had lost control over his ability to fall asleep. He had experienced these feelings repeatedly over several months. As mentioned earlier, the repeated and prolonged experience of these feelings can result in a conditioned arousal or learned insomnia.

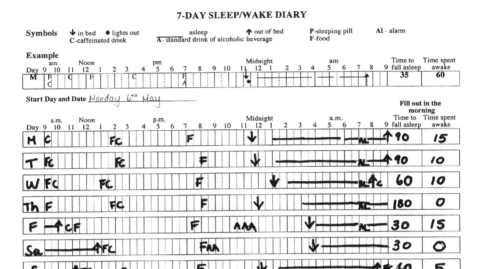

Fig. 2. Seven-day sleep/wake diary of an individual with sleep-onset insomnia who shows evidence of a delayed circadian rhythm.

Early-Morning-Awakening Insomnia and Circadian Rhythm Phase Advance

An advanced or early-timed circadian rhythm can result in difficulties maintaining sleep during the latter half of the sleep period and waking earlier than intended.[20,27] Early-morning-awakening insomnia is characterized by a pattern of routinely waking much earlier than desired. This form of sleep difficulty is attributed to an advanced timing of the wake-up zone. Even if an individual has not yet obtained sufficient sleep before entering the wake-up zone, a premature final awakening can occur because of circadian arousal mechanisms overriding the remaining homeostatic sleep drive. The distress and daytime impairments caused by obtaining an insufficient amount of sleep can lead to feelings of frustration or helplessness when awakening too early in the morning. This type of arousal response can become habitual and perpetuate the difficulties maintaining sleep or waking too early in the morning.

Compelling evidence shows that a phase advance can lead to sleep maintenance and/or early-morning-awakening insomnia.[20,27–29] Lack and colleagues[30] compared the phase timing of good sleepers and individuals with early-morning-awakening insomnia. Despite similar lights-out and sleep-onset times, wake-up time differed significantly between the groups. The mean wake-up time for the insomnia group (4:49 AM) was earlier than for the good sleeper group (7:24 AM). The insomnia group was waking after only 5 hours of sleep, whereas the good sleepers were waking after 7.75 hours of sleep.

The insomnia group was phase-advanced by 2 to 4 hours, with their mean core body temperature minimum occurring at 12:20 AM. Similar research has confirmed these findings, with several studies reporting advanced temperature minima and DLMO in individuals with early-morning-awakening insomnia.[31,32]

Clinical example of an individual with early-morning-awakening insomnia

Fig. 3 illustrates the typical sleep pattern of a woman with early-morning-awakening insomnia with indications of an advanced circadian rhythm.

This individual experienced overwhelming sleepiness in the evening and, as a result, unintentionally fell asleep in front of the television on most nights. She reported no difficulty falling sleep after getting into bed, which occurred between 9:30 and 10:00 PM. However after only 5 to 6 hours of sleep, she woke and experienced difficulty falling back to sleep. On most mornings she lay awake in bed for an hour or more before getting out of bed. She reported frustration, anxiety, and feelings of helplessness about waking earlier than intended and being unable to get sufficient sleep, as evidenced mainly by daytime fatigue.

RETIMING THE CIRCADIAN RHYTHM

The timing of the circadian rhythm can be altered by zeitgebers that include bright light, exogenous melatonin, and melatonin agonists. The most potent and powerful zeitgeber is bright light entering the eye. In the clinical setting, the light source is typically sunlight or an artificial light,

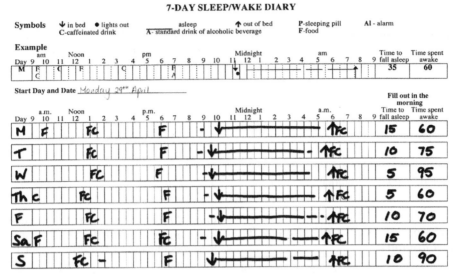

Fig. 3. Seven-day sleep/wake diary of a typical client with early-morning-awakening insomnia, suggesting an advanced circadian rhythm.

such as commercially available light boxes or more recently developed portable light devices. Bright light therapy has certain characteristics, such as the timing, intensity, and duration of light exposure, and the wavelength (or color) of the light, that must be considered to ensure its efficacy in resetting the circadian rhythm.

The timing of bright light visual exposure greatly influences the direction and magnitude of the circadian phase shift, described as the *phase response curve*.[33] **Fig. 4** illustrates typical phase response curves to light. If exposure to bright light occurs before the core body temperature minimum, the circadian rhythm is delayed or retimed to later. On the contrary, if exposure to bright light is timed to occur after the temperature minimum, the circadian rhythm is advanced or shifted to an earlier time. A multitude of studies have shown that the closer the light exposure is to the temperature minimum, the greater the phase change.[34–36] Therefore, bright morning light (after temperature minimum) is recommended for people with delayed or late-timed circadian rhythms, whereas evening bright light (before temperature minimum)

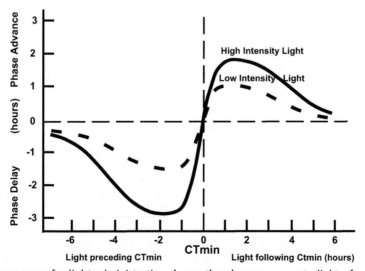

Fig. 4. Phase response curve for light administration shown the phase-response to light of varying intensity.

is appropriate for those with advanced or early-timed circadian rhythms.

The magnitude of the retiming effect of bright light on the circadian rhythm is also influenced by the intensity and duration of the light. Higher intensity and longer durations of exposure produce greater phase change.[37–41] Several studies have assessed phase shifts of the circadian rhythm after exposure to light of varying wavelengths. These studies have shown that shorter-wavelength light (blue-green light) between 470 and 525 nm is more effective than longer-wavelength light in phase delaying,[42] phase advancing,[43] and suppressing melatonin secretion.[42–45]

Evidence of Morning Bright Light Therapy for Sleep-Onset Insomnia

Several studies have assessed the efficacy of morning bright light for individuals with a delayed circadian rhythm. Rosenthal and colleagues[46] exposed participants to 2 hours of either bright light (2500 lux) or dim light (300 lux) between 6:00 and 9:00 AM for 2 weeks. Participants exposed to morning bright light produced significantly advanced core body temperature minimum and sleep-onset times when compared with those exposed to dim light. In a similar study, Watanabe and colleagues[47] exposed participants to 3 hours of bright light timed 1.5 hours after their core body temperature minimum for 5 consecutive mornings. Core body temperature, sleep-onset time, and wake-up time all significantly advanced after the light exposure. Similar benefits have also been reported after the use of a bright light mask in the morning for 26 days.[48,49]

In a more recent pilot study, short-wavelength blue light was used to phase-advance the circadian rhythm and sleep/wake pattern of individuals with a delayed circadian rhythm.[50] Bright light was administered using portable light glasses comprising blue light–emitting diodes. Over a 1-week period, participants initially wore the glasses for 2 hours immediately after waking and then continued to wear them 30 minutes earlier each day until wake-up time occurred at 6:00 AM. The circadian phase of participants was compared with a control group who followed the same procedure but without blue light exposure. Participants in the blue-light group showed a significant phase advance of 2.5 hours, whereas the control group experienced no change in the timing of their circadian phase.

Although the efficacy of morning bright light has been well established to advance the circadian phase, few studies have investigated its efficacy for the treatment of sleep-onset insomnia

associated with a delayed circadian phase. Lack and colleagues[51] selected individuals with sleep-onset insomnia who also had a delayed circadian phase (mean DLMO occurring at 12:28 AM) and exposed them to either bright light (2500 lux) or dim red light (<100 lux) for an hour, timed at 1.5 hours before their habitual wake-up time over 1 week. Participants exposed to bright light had a significant advance of melatonin onset by 1 hour and 21 minutes, a significant mean reduction in sleep latency of 34 minutes, an advance of sleep-onset time, and an increase in total sleep time. The control group showed no change in circadian phase or sleep variables.

Clinical recommendations for the use of morning bright light for sleep-onset insomnia

It is recommended that bright light be administered for 1 hour immediately after the habitual wake-up time initially.[51] After the initial exposure, both wake-up time and bright light exposure should be advanced by 15 minutes each morning until the desired wake-up time is achieved. In the example described earlier (see **Fig. 2**), exposure to bright light would commence at 9:00 AM initially, and then advance by 15 minutes each day to the target wake-up time of 7:15 AM. Once the target wake-up time is achieved, exposure to bright light should continue for 2 weeks to allow time for sleep-onset time to advance and to ensure adequate total sleep time is obtained. After morning bright light therapy, continued adherence to a consistent wake-up time and early light exposure is recommended. In addition, a regimen of dim light exposure and quiet activities in the evening will help avoid the possible phase-delaying effects of ambient bright light and behavioral activation before bedtime.

Cases of chronic insomnia are often multifactorial, as is most probably the case with many who experience sleep-onset insomnia. The authors suggest that a phase-delay of the circadian rhythm is commonly associated with this type of insomnia. It is also common for a learned insomnia to be present. This component of the insomnia disorder should be addressed using behavioral therapies, such as stimulus control therapy. Thus, a combination of this therapy and morning bright light therapy is indicated for many with sleep-onset insomnia.

Evening Bright Light Therapy for Early Morning Awakening Insomnia

To date, 2 studies have successfully used evening bright light to phase-delay the circadian rhythm and improve the sleep of individuals with early-morning-awakening insomnia. In a pilot study,

Lack and Wright[31] administered bright white light (2500 lux) to 9 participants with early-morning-awakening insomnia over 2 consecutive evenings. Participants were exposed to the light for 4 hours from 8:00 PM to 12:00 AM hours. The light pulse was timed to end before the mean core body temperature minimum of the group (2:00 AM hours). The temperature rhythm delayed by 2 to 4 hours, whereas the melatonin rhythm delayed by 1 to 2 hours. The final wake-up time of participants was also significantly delayed, from 4:59 AM to 6:00 AM hours, which resulted in an increase in total sleep time of more than an hour.

In a similar study, 24 adults with early-morning-awakening insomnia were assigned to a bright light exposure (2500 lux of white light) or control (dim red light) condition[32] for 2 consecutive evenings. Participants were again exposed to light over a 4-hour period from 9:00 PM to 1:00 AM hours. Exposure to the bright white light resulted in a significant 2-hour delay of the circadian temperature and melatonin rhythms. This finding was accompanied by a significant delay in wake-up time, a reduction in wake time after sleep onset, and an increase in total sleep time of more than 1 hour. Participants also reported a decrease in negative daytime symptoms, such as depressed mood. The improvements to sleep were durable, with significant improvements still evident 4 weeks after treatment.

Clinical recommendations for the use of evening bright light for early-morning-awakening insomnia

We suggest that clients stay up for approximately 1 hour after their habitual bedtime while maximizing their exposure to ambient light. Use of an artificial bright light source (eg, portable light glasses) is recommended, if available, to achieve a faster phase-delay of the circadian rhythm. In the example described earlier (see **Fig. 3**), the client should remain awake until approximately 11:00 PM. Individuals should be encouraged to keep active in the evening to minimize the likelihood of unintentional napping. Those with a pattern of early morning awakenings should avoid morning bright light using measures such as wearing dark glasses when going outside in the first hours after waking.

Chronic insomnia from any cause is likely to be exacerbated by sleep-disruptive habits and conditioned arousal, which are best addressed with cognitive/behavior therapy. The behavior therapy in the case of early-morning-awakening insomnia would most appropriately be bedtime (or sleep) restriction therapy. This therapy could be administered compatibly with evening bright light therapy that extends beyond the individual's normal bedtime, at least for the first 2 weeks of therapy.

In summary, 2 types of insomnia, sleep-onset insomnia and early-morning-awakening insomnia, have been associated with delayed and advanced circadian rhythms, respectively. These circadian rhythm anomalies can be treated with the use of morning bright light in the case of sleep-onset insomnia, and evening bright light in the case of early-morning-awakening insomnia. Although robust evidence shows that appropriately timed light therapy can retime the body clock, evidence of the therapeutic value of bright light therapy for these types of insomnia needs further development. Large randomized controlled trials of bright light and behavior therapies, alone and in combination, are needed to improve the treatment of these debilitating disorders.

REFERENCES

1. American Psychiatric Association. Diagnostic and statistical manual of mental disorders test revision. 4th edition. Washington, DC: American Psychiatric Association; 2001.
2. American Academy of Sleep Medicine. The international classification of sleep disorders: diagnostic and coding manual. 2nd edition 2005. Westchester (IL).
3. Blackwell T, Yaffe K, Ancoli-Israel S, et al. Poor sleep is associated with impaired cognitive function in older women: the study of osteoporotic fractures. J Gerontol A Biol Sci Med Sci 2006;61(4):405–10.
4. Morin C. Insomnia: psychological assessment and management. New York: The Guilford Pres; 1993.
5. Jansson-Frojmark M, Lindblom K. A bidirectional relationship between anxiety and depression, and insomnia? A prospective study in the general population. J Psychosom Res 2008;64(4):443–9.
6. Ohayon MM, Roth T. Place of chronic insomnia in the course of depressive and anxiety disorders. J Psychiatr Res 2003;37(1):9–15.
7. Borbely A. A two process model of sleep regulation. Hum Neurobiol 1982;1:195–204.
8. Åkerstedt T, Folkard S. Validation of the S and C components of the three-process model of alertness regulation. Sleep 1995;18(1):1–6.
9. Lack L, Wright H. Circadian rhythms and insomnia. In: Attarian HP, Schuman C, editors. Clinical handbook of insomnia. Springer Science + Business Media; 2010. p. 243–53.
10. Arendt J. Melatonin, circadian rhythms, and sleep. N Engl J Med 2000;343(15):1114–6.
11. Arendt J. Melatonin and the mammalian pineal gland. In: Arendt J, editor. Melatonin and the mammalian pineal gland. London: Chapman & Hall; 1995. p. 1–246.

12. Sack R, Lewy A, Hughes R. Use of melatonin for sleep and circadian rhythm disorders. Ann Med 1998;30:115–21.

13. Czeisler CA, Duffy JF, Shanahan TL, et al. Stability, precision, and near-24-hour period of the human circadian pacemaker. Science 1999;284(5423): 2177–81.

14. Voultsios A, Kennaway DJ, Dawson D. Salivary melatonin as a circadian phase marker: validation and comparison to plasma melatonin. J Biol Rhythms 1997;12(5):457–65.

15. Rahman SA, Kayumov L, Tchmoutina EA, et al. Clinical efficacy of dim light melatonin onset testing in diagnosing delayed sleep phase syndrome. Sleep Med 2009;10(5):549–55.

16. Campbell SS. Intrinsic disruption of normal sleep and circadian patterns. In: Turek FW, Zee PC, editors. Regulation of sleep and circadian rhythms, vol. 133. New York: Marcel Dekker; 1999. p. 465–86.

17. Dijk DJ, Edgar DE. Circadian and homeostatic control of wakefulness and sleep. In: Turek FW, Zee PC, editors. Regulation of sleep and circadian rhythms, vol. 133. New York: Marcel Dekker; 1999. p. 111–48.

18. Monk TH, Buysse DJ, Reynolds CF, et al. Circadian rhythms in human performance and mood under constant conditions. J Sleep Res 1997;6:9–18.

19. Strogatz SH, Kronauer RE. Circadian wake maintenance zones and insomnia in man. Sleep Research 1985;14:219.

20. Strogatz SH, Kronauer RE, Czeisler CA. Circadian pacemaker interferes with sleep onset at specific times each day: role in insomnia. Am J Physiol 1987;253(1 Pt 2):R172–178.

21. Morris M, Lack L, Dawson D. Sleep-onset insomniacs have delayed temperature rhythms. Sleep 1990;13(1):1–14.

22. Wright H, Lack L, Bootzin R. Relationship between dim light melatonin onset and the timing of sleep in sleep onset insomniacs. Sleep Biol Rhythm 2006;4: 78–80.

23. Van Veen MM, Kooij S, Boonstra A, et al. Delayed circadian rhythms in adults with attention-deficit/hyperactivity disorder and chronic sleep-onset insomnia. Biol Psychiatry 2010;67:1091–6.

24. Lewy A, Sack R, Fredrickson R, et al. The use of bright light in the treatment of chronobiologic sleep and mood disorders: the phase-response curve. Psychopharmacol Bull 1983;19(3):523–5.

25. Taylor A, Wright H, Lack L. Sleeping-in on the weekend delays circadian phase and increases sleepiness the following week. Sleep Biol Rhythm 2008;6:172–9.

26. Yang C, Spielman AJ. The effect of a delayed weekend sleep pattern on sleep and morning functioning. Psychol Health 2001;16:715–25.

27. Strogatz SH, Kronauer RE, Czeisler CA. Circadian regulation dominates homeostatic control of sleep length and prior wake length in humans. Sleep 1986;9(2):353–64.

28. Duffy JF, Dijk DJ, Klerman EB, et al. Later endogenous circadian temperature nadir relative to an earlier wake time in older people. Am J Physiol 1998;275(5 Pt 2):R1478–1487.

29. Miles LE, Dement WC. Sleep and aging. Sleep 1980;3(2):1–220.

30. Lack L, Mercer J, Wright H. Circadian rhythms of early morning awakening insomniacs. J Sleep Res 1996;5(4):211–9.

31. Lack L, Wright H. The effect of evening bright light in delaying the circadian rhythms and lengthening the sleep of early morning awakening insomniacs. Sleep 1993;16(3):436–43.

32. Lack L, Wright H, Kemp K, et al. The treatment of early-morning awakening insomnia with 2 evenings of bright light. Sleep 2005;28(5):616–23.

33. Khalsa SB, Jewett ME, Cajochen C, et al. A phase response curve to single bright light pulses in human subjects. J Physiol 2003;549(Pt 3):945–52.

34. Czeisler C, Kronauer R, Allan J, et al. Bright light induction of strong (type 0) resetting of the human circadian pacemaker. Science 1989;244:1328–33.

35. Dawson D, Lack L, Morris M. Phase resetting of the human circadian pacemaker with use of a single pulse of bright light. Chronobiol Int 1993;10(2): 94–102.

36. Minors DS, Waterhouse JM, Wirz-Justice A. A human phase-response curve to light. Neurosci Lett 1991;133:36–40.

37. Boivin DD, Brown EN, Yuan A, et al. The onset and offset of melatonin secretion is equally sensitive to the intensity-dependent resetting effect of light in humans. Sleep 1999;22(Suppl):S138.

38. Boivin DB, Duffy JF, Kronauer RE, et al. Sensitivity of the human circadian pacemaker to moderately bright light. J Biol Rhythms 1994;9:315–31.

39. Boivin DB, Duffy JF, Kronauer RE, et al. Dose-response relationships for resetting of human circadian clock by light. Nature 1996;379(6565): 540–2.

40. Kennaway D, Earl C, Shaw P, et al. Phase delay of the rhythm of 6-sulphatoxy melatonin excretion by artificial light. J Pineal Res 1987;4(3):315–20.

41. Van Cauter E, Sturis J, Byrne MM, et al. Demonstration of rapid light-induced advances and delays of the human circadian clock using hormonal phase markers. Am J Physiol 1994;266:E953–963.

42. Wright H, Lack L. Effect of light wavelength on suppression and phase delay of the melatonin rhythm. Chronobiol Int 2001;18(5):801–8.

43. Wright HR, Lack LC, Kennaway DJ. Differential effects of light wavelength in phase advancing the melatonin rhythm. J Pineal Res 2004;36:140–4.

44. Brainard GC, Hanifin JP, Greeson JM, et al. Action spectrum for melatonin regulation in humans: evidence for a novel circadian photoreceptor. J Neurosci 2001;21(16):6405–12.

45. Thapan K, Arendt J, Skene DJ. An action spectrum for melatonin suppression: evidence for a novel non- rod, non-cone photoreceptor system in humans. J Physiol 2001;535(Pt 1):261–7.

46. Rosenthal NE, Joseph-Vanderpool JR, Levendosky AA, et al. Phase-shifting effects of bright morning light as treatment for delayed sleep phase syndrome. Sleep 1990;13(4):354–61.

47. Watanabe T, Kajimura N, Kato M, et al. Effects of phototherapy in patients with delayed sleep phase syndrome. Psychiatry Clin Neurosci 1999;53:231–3.

48. Cole RJ, Smith JS, Alcala YC, et al. Bright light mask treatment of delayed sleep phase syndrome. J Biol Rhythms 2002;17(1):89–101.

49. Czeisler CA, Dijk DJ. Human circadian physiology and sleep-wake regulation. In: Takahashi JS, Turek FW, Moore RY, editors. Handbook of behavioral neurobiology: circadian clocks, vol. 12. New York: Kluwer Academic/Plenum; 2001. p. 531–68.

50. Lack L, Bramwell T, Wright H, et al. Morning bright light can advance the melatonin rhythm in mild delayed sleep phase syndrome. Sleep Biol Rhythm 2007;5:78–90.

51. Lack L, Wright H, Paynter D. The treatment of sleep onset insomnia with bright morning light. Sleep Biol Rhythm 2007;5:173–9.

Insomnia Comorbid to Severe Psychiatric Illness

Adriane M. Soehner, MA, Katherine A. Kaplan, MA,
Allison G. Harvey, PhD*

KEYWORDS

- Insomnia • Bipolar disorder • Schizophrenia • CBT-I

KEY POINTS

- Insomnia, as well as hypersomnia and circadian rhythm disturbances, are common in schizophrenia and bipolar disorder.
- Poor sleep continuity and abnormal sleep architecture are associated with disease-specific symptoms, poor quality of life, and greater impairment in schizophrenia and bipolar disorder.
- Cognitive Behavioral Therapy for insomnia and melatonin agonists may be useful sleep treatments in severe mental illness.
- Preliminary evidence indicates that treatment of sleep can improve psychiatric symptoms in severe mental illness.

INTRODUCTION: NATURE OF THE PROBLEM

There is robust evidence that insomnia frequently co-occurs with a wide range of psychiatric disorders. Indeed, it is estimated that 20% to 40% of individuals with mental illness experience insomnia.[1–3] Because insomnia can be associated with a variety of psychiatric disorders and/or medical illnesses, diagnostic classification systems, such as the DSM-IV-TR[4] and ICSD-2,[5] distinguish between "primary" and "secondary" insomnia. Primary insomnia is considered a freestanding condition, whereas secondary insomnia is diagnosed when the insomnia is considered subordinate to a primary condition, such as a psychiatric disorder; yet, the relationship between insomnia and a co-occurring psychiatric disorder can vary considerably across patients. Indeed, the distinction between primary and secondary insomnia has been blurred by epidemiologic research, suggesting that insomnia may predate, and predict, psychiatric illness.[2,6] As a result, a recent National Institutes of Health State-of-the-Science Conference[7] concluded that the term "secondary" should be replaced with "comorbid" on the basis of evidence that insomnia that is comorbid with another disorder likely contributes to the maintenance of the disorder.[8,9]

In cases of comorbid insomnia, additional empirical and clinical attention is especially important, as there appears to be a cyclical relationship between sleep disturbance and medical or psychiatric illness. For example, worsening sleep problems can lead to exacerbated psychiatric symptoms and daytime distress, with psychiatric symptoms and daytime distress then worsening the sleep problems.[9–11] Fortunately, there is a growing body of evidence suggesting that insomnia responds to Cognitive Behavioral Therapy for Insomnia (CBT-I), even if the psychiatric or medical disorder is not under control.[12] Smith and colleagues[9] concluded that treatment effects are generally moderate to large for CBT-I administered in medical and psychiatric illnesses, and are comparable to treatment effects in primary insomnia.

The goal of the present review was to summarize the role of insomnia and disturbed sleep

Department of Psychology, Berkley University of California, 3210 Tolman Hall, Berkeley, CA 97420-1650, USA
* Corresponding author.
E-mail address: aharvey@berkeley.edu

Sleep Med Clin 8 (2013) 361–371
http://dx.doi.org/10.1016/j.jsmc.2013.04.007
1556-407X/13/$ – see front matter © 2013 Elsevier Inc. All rights reserved.

architecture in 2 severe mental illnesses: bipolar disorder (BD) and schizophrenia. Although the research we review largely examines the importance of insomnia as a mechanism in severe psychiatric illness, it is noteworthy that there is increasing interest in the possibility that hypersomnia, delayed sleep phase, and reduced sleep need may also be mechanisms.[13,14] Current knowledge regarding pharmacologic and psychological treatment approaches for insomnia in these populations are briefly reviewed, as well as challenges clinicians may encounter adapting CBT-I procedures in severe mental illness.

BD

Overview of sleep disturbance across the phases of BD

Sleep disturbance is a core feature of mood episodes in BD. During periods of mania, most patients (69%–99%) experience reduced need for sleep, which has been corroborated by both self-report and polysomnographic (PSG) investigations (see Harvey[15] for review). Additionally, several small studies have shown that, relative to healthy nonpatients, individuals with mania tend to exhibit shortened rapid eye-movement (REM) sleep latency and increased REM density.[16,17]

The rates of insomnia in bipolar depression vary considerably across studies, with one study reporting that 100% of depressed patients with BD experienced insomnia (see Harvey[15] for review). The rates of hypersomnia during the depressive phase of bipolar illness vary between 23% and 78%.[13] Similar to unipolar depression, patients with bipolar depression tend to experience shortened REM latency relative to healthy adults,[18,19] although there have been nonreplications.[20] REM density in a bipolar depressed sample was elevated compared with healthy adults and not significantly different from a unipolar depressed group.[19] Reduced non-REM (NREM) stage 3 (N3), or slow-wave sleep (SWS), has been observed in small samples of depressed patients with BD relative to healthy adults[21] and at a level equivalent to unipolar depressed patients.[22] However, one study found no differences in N3 relative to healthy adults.[20] Finally, in depressed patients with BD, one investigation reported reduced stage N1 sleep,[20] but most reports have not.[19,21]

During the interepisode period, clinically significant sleep disturbance persists in up to 70% of patients with BD.[23,24] Estimates of insomnia prevalence between episodes vary. A recent study in a sample of 14 participants with BD reported that only 2 (14%) met criteria for insomnia,[25] whereas an earlier investigation in a larger sample found

that 50% of patients with BD experienced interepisode insomnia.[23] Another study reported that 25% of patients with BD experienced interepisode hypersomnia.[26] With regard to specific sleep characteristics, studies have shown that during the interepisode period, patients with BD had longer sleep-onset latency,[9,27,28] longer and more variable periods of wakefulness during the night,[29] more nighttime awakenings,[28,30] increased sleep duration,[27] poorer sleep efficiency,[23,28] and more night-to-night variability of sleep patterns[27] relative to healthy adults. During the interepisode period, 2 studies found evidence for increased REM density in both unmedicated[31] and medicated bipolar samples.[32] However, one study found no differences between sleep architecture in healthy adults and participants with BD in the interepisode period.[30] In all 3 studies, there were no observed differences in NREM sleep in the bipolar samples relative to healthy adults.[30–32]

Even among patients with BD treated with "best practice" mood stabilizers in a systematic treatment enhancement program for BD,[33] 66% experienced significant sleep disturbance.[34,35] Furthermore, sleep disturbance is characteristic across the bipolar spectrum. In a recent investigation of a sample of 116 euthymic outpatients with BD, 27.1% of those with BD type 1 reported ongoing sleep disturbance, as well as 21.7% of those with BD type 2, and 16.6% of those with BD not otherwise specified (NOS).[24] Although, the investigators note that these percentages may underestimate patients with underlying sleep disturbance who were receiving treatment with hypnotics and/or sedating antipsychotics.[24] Another study found that total sleep time is shortest in BD NOS, relative to BD type 1 and BD type 2, but the 3 subtypes are equally impaired in night-to-night variability in sleep duration.[34]

Significance of insomnia in BD

Sleep disturbance is an early marker for BD. In a study of early-onset BD, sleep disturbance was retrospectively reported to be one of the earliest symptoms observed by parents.[36] In another study, sleep disturbance was identified as an antecedent to the first onset of BD in a subset of high-risk youth.[37] A thorough review of early symptoms of mania and depression by Jackson and colleagues,[38] identified sleep disturbance as the most common prodrome of manic relapse and the sixth most common prodrome of depressive relapse in BD. In response to experimental sleep deprivation, a substantial proportion of individuals with BD depression show a rapid alleviation of depressed mood, but a subset of participants experienced an onset of hypomania or mania.[39–41]

Furthermore, a recent cross-sectional study found that patients with BD who habitually slept fewer than 6 hours a night exhibited both greater manic and depressive symptoms relative to patients with BD that slept between 6.5 and 8.5 hours.[34] In the same study, participants with BD sleeping more than 9.0 hours also exhibited more depressive symptomatology than did the group with BD that slept between 6.5 and 8.5 hours.

Prospective investigations have reported similar findings. Shortened sleep duration has been found to predict increased daily manic symptoms[42,43] and depressive symptoms at a 6-month follow-up.[44] Lengthened sleep duration also predicted heightened daily depressive symptoms[43] and depressive symptoms at a 6-month follow-up.[26] Lower and more variable sleep efficiency and variability of sleep-onset latency in interepisode BD were related to more lifetime depressive episodes and more current depressive symptoms.[45] There is also evidence to suggest that disturbed sleep in interepisode BD has considerable functional consequences. Disturbed sleep and short habitual sleep duration (<6 hours) were associated with impaired psychosocial functioning and poorer quality of life in patients with BD during the interepisode period.[34,46]

Few investigations have examined the relationship among sleep architecture, mood, and outcome in BD. In one study of interepisode BD, sleep architecture was not correlated with concurrent mood symptoms.[32] However, greater REM density was correlated with more severe depressive symptoms and greater functional impairment at 3 months, whereas prolonged duration of the first REM period and a greater amount of SWS were positively correlated with manic symptoms and impairment at 3 months. Additionally, the amount of N2 sleep was negatively correlated with manic symptoms and impairment at 3 months. Hudson and colleagues[47] found that time spent asleep and REM percentage inversely correlated with mania severity in currently manic patients.

Treating insomnia in BD
Taken together, these data have highlighted the complexity and multiple sleep disturbances that are characteristic of BD (insomnia, hypersomnia, delayed sleep phase, irregular sleep-wake schedule, reduced sleep need) and the importance of an intervention to treat sleep problems as a pathway for improving mood and reducing impairment. However, few studies have explored treatment options for sleep disturbance in BD. A chart review in a private clinic showed that non-benzodiazapine hypnotics appear safe, and 46% of patients with BD prescribed hypnotics were using these medications chronically.[48] In a case report, gabapentin was found to be helpful for treatment-resistant insomnia in BD.[49,50] However, case reports on benzodiazepines for insomnia in BD have not been encouraging.[50]

Open trials of medications targeting the circadian system, such as melatonin[51] and agomelatine,[52] are promising, but preliminary. Two small clinical trials recently evaluated ramelteon for sleep disturbance in BD. One study evaluated the efficacy and tolerability of ramelteon in BD type 1 with manic symptoms and insomnia.[53] Twenty-one outpatients were randomized to receive either 8 mg per day of ramelteon (n = 10) or placebo (n = 11) in an 8-week double-blind treatment design. Although ramelteon did not significantly differ from placebo in reducing symptoms of insomnia, mania, and global severity of illness, it was tolerable and associated with improvement in a global rating of depressive symptoms. Another recent study of ramelteon focused on treating sleep disturbance in euthymic patients with BD.[54] Participants were randomized to receive 8 mg per day of ramelteon (n = 42) or placebo (n = 41) for up to 24 weeks. Relative to the placebo group, participants receiving ramelteon had marginally better subjective sleep quality, and overall risk for depression and mania relapse was cut nearly in half during the 24-week treatment period.

Although these preliminary results using pharmacologic interventions for sleep in BD are encouraging, it is important to develop and test nonpharmacologic approaches to treat sleep in BD because (1) there are fewer side effects or interactions with other treatments for the BD and other conditions; (2) concerns remain about treatment durability, daytime residual effects, tolerance, dependence, and rebound insomnia with pharmacotherapy; (3) certain classes of insomnia medications (most important, the benzodiazepine receptor agonists approved by the Food and Drug Administration) pose a risk of abuse given the comorbidity between BD and substance use disorders.[55]

CBT-I may be a particularly useful intervention to stabilize sleep and circadian rhythms in BD. As described previously, individuals with BD display night-to-night variability in total sleep time,[34] along with reduced sleep efficiency and increased nighttime wakefulness[23,32] that may respond well to sleep restriction and stimulus control. However, in adapting CBT-I for BD it may be important to modify certain components that could lead to sleep deprivation, because of the strong link between sleep loss and relapse.[15] For example, the stimulus control instruction to get out of bed may lead some patients to engage in rewarding and arousing activities that prevent sleep. Also, to avoid changes in mood related to short-term sleep deprivation, minimum time in bed during sleep restriction should likely be no lower than 6.5 hours. Throughout treatment, it is particularly important to monitor depression and/or mania symptoms at the start of each session and negotiate a safety plan with the patient before the start of therapy, should mood grow unstable during treatment. If symptoms of depression or mania emerge, changes in total sleep time that may be contributing to these symptoms should be evaluated, and consideration should be given to modifying or temporarily suspending sleep restriction or stimulus control if necessary. Notwithstanding such concerns, we recently reported preliminary findings suggesting the safety of regularizing bed and wake times using stimulus control and sleep-restriction strategies with patients with BD.[56]

Summary and future directions

Thus far, research evidence consistently supports a link among sleep, mood, impairment, and quality of life in BD. However, several important gaps in knowledge remain. At a foundational level, more research is needed to understand the prevalence of sleep disturbances (insomnia, hypersomnia, delayed sleep phase, reduced sleep need) across the BD subtypes and during mixed mood episodes (ie, when diagnostic criteria are met for *both* a manic episode and an episode of depression). Additionally, the nature and role of sleep architecture in the course of BD remains understudied, with most polysomnographic investigations in BD having been conducted approximately 2 to 3 decades ago.

It will also be crucial to identify causal, and potentially bidirectional, pathways between sleep disturbance and mood in BD. There is robust behavioral and neuroimaging evidence among healthy nonpatient samples that sleep deprivation undermines emotion regulation the following day.[57] Additionally, an interesting study of medical residents by Zohar and colleagues[58] suggests that the context in which the emotion is experienced is important for determining the direction of the effect of sleep disturbance on affective functioning. Specifically, sleep loss increased negative affect following a goal-thwarting event and diminished positive emotions following a goal-enhancing event. Individuals with mood disorders, who already have a vulnerable emotion regulation system, would likely experience even more adverse effects from sleep disturbances. However, this assumption has yet to be tested in a BD sample.

Given the high rates of sleep disturbance in BD, it is surprising that few controlled trials of medication or psychological interventions for sleep have been conducted in this population. There is exciting preliminary evidence that treating sleep or circadian disturbance with ramelteon can reduce the risk of manic and depressive relapse, supporting the idea that treating sleep can improve the course of illness.[54] Furthermore, a recent report has provided encouraging initial support for the efficacy and safety of CBT-I in BD. However, certain treatment complexities in BD need to be better understood, such as the following: Should a clinician approach treating sleep disturbance differently at distinctive phases of the BD illness? During manic or mixed episodes, a pharmacologic approach for sleep may be most appropriate to aid in fully stabilizing a patient. Yet, during bipolar depression or the interepisode period, psychological approaches may be preferable because of the reduced risk of negative side effects. In unipolar depression, CBT-I improves sleep and depressive symptoms when administered in combination with antidepressants[59] or as a stand-alone treatment.[60] Larger controlled trials testing psychological and pharmacologic therapies in BD hold promise for not only improving sleep, but also for stabilizing mood stability and enhancing quality of life.

Schizophrenia and Psychotic Disorders

Overview of sleep in schizophrenia

Sleep disturbance is prevalent in schizophrenia, during both psychosis and remission. An early investigation conducted in psychiatric inpatients found that 83% of 12 acutely ill patients with schizophrenia and 47% of 17 patients with chronic psychosis had at least one type of sleep complaint, such as difficulty falling asleep, early morning awakening, awakening during the night, not sleeping soundly, and having increased time in bed.[61] A later report found that, of 93 stable outpatients with schizophrenia, early insomnia was endorsed by 26% of the patients, middle insomnia by 23%, and early morning awakening by 16% of the patients.[62] Within the Clinical Antipsychotic Trials of Intervention Effectiveness study, 16% to 30% of patients across treatment arms reported insomnia and 24% to 31% reported hypersomnia despite management of symptoms with antipsychotic medication.[63] In a sample of 44 adults with schizophrenia, another study reported poor sleep quality at a rate of 52% using the Pittsburgh Sleep Quality Index.[64] More recently, a study conducted with 175 clinically stable outpatients suffering from schizophrenia or schizoaffective disorder found that 44% met criteria for clinical insomnia using the Insomnia Severity Index.[65]

Consistent with the sleep complaints described previously, self-report and PSG investigations of medicated patients with schizophrenia report prolonged sleep latency, low sleep efficiency, poor sleep quality, and shortened sleep duration.[66–70] These patterns are also observed in drug-free or medication naïve patients with schizophrenia. A meta-analysis of PSG studies in 321 patients and 331 controls reported that the schizophrenia group experienced increased sleep latency, decreased total sleep time, increased wake after sleep onset, and reduced sleep efficiency compared with healthy controls.[71]

Prospective studies involving actigraphy have also provided interesting insights. In a study of 28 older patients with schizophrenia and age-matched controls, monitoring of sleep–wake function with actigraphy showed greater wake time at night, longer time in bed, more sleep during the day, and less robust circadian rhythmicity in the schizophrenia group.[72] Similarly, a sample of 20 middle-aged outpatients with schizophrenia took longer to fall asleep and slept longer than those in the control group regardless of sleep-onset time. Furthermore, 50% of the individuals in the schizophrenia group showed markedly delayed and/or free-running sleep-wake cycles.[73] Thus, in addition to sleep-continuity problems, disrupted circadian rhythmicity is also evident in individuals with treated schizophrenia.

There is also a growing body of evidence demonstrating altered sleep architecture in schizophrenia.[14,74,75] Most studies indicate that SWS, NREM delta activity, and REM latency are reduced in schizophrenia, whether the patients are drug-naïve, acutely psychotic, or medicated and clinically stable.[55,70,76–83] Some studies have found elevated REM density,[16,84] but previously treated and drug-naïve patients with schizophrenia typically exhibit normal REM density.[77,79,82,83,85,86] More recently, reduced spindle activity has been observed in schizophrenia relative to healthy adults.[87]

Significance of insomnia in schizophrenia

Sleep disturbances have also been associated with exacerbated symptoms in schizophrenia, particularly positive symptoms. Positive symptoms include delusions, hallucinations, disorganized thinking, and behavior. For example, a recent actigraphic investigation found that, relative to patients with schizophrenia experiencing predominantly negative symptoms on the Positive and Negative Syndrome Scale (PANSS), those with predominantly positive symptoms experienced more sleep-wake disturbances.[88] Similarly, prolonged sleep latency in inpatients with

schizophrenia was associated with greater "Thinking Disturbance" on the Brief Psychiatric Rating Scale (BPRS).[89] In another study, moderate or severe insomnia symptoms were present in more than 50% of a medicated sample experiencing persecutory delusions.[90] Patients with schizophrenia that exhibited insomnia symptoms, low total sleep time, and poor sleep efficiency were also at a greater risk for worsening of positive symptoms after antipsychotic discontinuation.[91,92] Interestingly, studies have generally found that negative symptoms (ie, anhedonia, social withdrawal, loss of motivation, poor self-care) were unrelated to insomnia symptoms. Finally, a substantial number of studies have reported that sleep continuity disturbances and poor sleep quality detrimentally affect quality of life in patients with schizophrenia, even while on stable medication regimens.[1,62,65,66,69,71,93,94]

PSG investigations have demonstrated relationships between sleep architecture and symptom severity in schizophrenia (for review see Refs.[14,75,95]). Overall illness severity, as assessed by the BPRS or PANSS, has generally been associated with altered REM sleep, such as increased REM percentage, shorter REM latency, and decreased REM density (ie, Refs.[77,82,96,97]). Greater positive symptom severity is typically associated with lower REM density or shortened REM latency in medicated, unmedicated, and drug-naïve patients.[77,82,86,96,97] REM density was also found to correlate specifically with hallucinatory behavior, as assessed by the BPRS.[85] A more recent study reported that spindle activity and spindle number were inversely related to both positive and negative symptoms on the PANSS, namely the stereotyped thinking, conceptual disorganization and hallucination subscales.[87] With regard to negative symptoms, studies have largely reported an association between increased negative symptoms and reduced SWS duration, SWS percentage, or delta activity,[79,98–102] although there have been some nonreplications.[77,82,87] Some investigations have also found REM latency[77,96,98] and REM density[103] to be inversely correlated with negative symptoms.

In addition to the relationship between acute symptomatology and sleep parameters, SWS and REM latency have been found to predict clinical outcome. Keshavan and colleagues[104] reported that lower percentage of delta sleep at baseline predicted poorer functional outcomes at 1-year and 2-year follow-up. Another investigation found that shorter REM latency in medication-free inpatients with schizophrenia predicted poorer global functioning 1 year after hospital discharge.[105] Similarly, relative to 6 inpatients with schizophrenia with sleep-onset REM episodes, 30 inpatients with schizophrenia without this sleep abnormality had better global functioning 1 year after assessment.[106]

Treating insomnia in schizophrenia

As is the case for BD, minimal work has been done to explore treatment options for sleep disturbance associated with schizophrenia despite the high prevalence, persistence, and clinical consequences of sleep disturbance in this mental disorder. In the case of insomnia linked with schizophrenia, treatment most frequently involves antipsychotics and sedative hypnotics.[95] Most first-generation and second-generation antipsychotics, except for risperidone, appear to facilitate an increase in total sleep time and/or sleep efficiency in patients with schizophrenia (for review, see Refs.[10,75]). However, as previously noted, a large proportion of patients continue to experience insomnia and hypersomnia despite treatment with atypical antipsychotics.[63]

Much less is known about the safety and efficacy of hypnotic medications in the context of schizophrenia. Generally, these medications do not have long-term efficacy and are associated with residual sedation during the daytime.[95] In a survey of 93 clinically stable medicated outpatients with schizophrenia, 33 reported using hypnotic medication, but 14 (35.5%) of those patients still considered their sleep to be disturbed.[62] Another study of 6 male outpatients with schizophrenia treated with benzodiazepine hypnotics in combination with antipsychotics found that substituting zopiclone for the benzodiazepine hypnotic improved subjective soundness of sleep and delta activity.[107] However, a recent review of the literature highlighted that no controlled trials of nonbenzodiazepine hypnotics or benzodiazepine hypnotics have been conducted in schizophrenia.[108]

Preliminary findings from treatment trials testing melatonin in schizophrenia have been promising. In outpatients with chronic schizophrenia, Shamir and colleagues[109] used a randomized, blinded, crossover study design to examine the effects of melatonin replacement (2 mg, controlled release) on their sleep. Melatonin improved sleep efficiency measured via actigraphy, particularly for low-efficiency sleepers. A second study reported that melatonin improved the subjective quality of sleep in a randomized, double-blinded, placebo-controlled trial in 40 stable outpatients with schizophrenia with sleep-onset insomnia.[110] Patients were randomly assigned to augment their current medication regimen with either flexibly dosed melatonin (3–12 mg per night; n = 20) or placebo (n = 20). Relative to placebo, melatonin significantly improved sleep quality, reduced the number of nighttime awakenings, increased the duration of sleep, and improved mood. Importantly, melatonin was not associated with self-reported "hangover" symptoms, such as headache, early morning dullness, or head heaviness, which can be associated with conventional hypnotic medications. No concurrent changes in positive and negative symptoms were noted in these melatonin treatment trials.

With regard to psychological approaches, a recent open trial tested CBT-I in patients with persecutory delusions.[111] Participants included outpatients with persecutory delusions that had persisted for at least 6 months (n = 15), including individuals with a diagnosis of schizophrenia (n = 10), psychotic disorder (n = 2), delusional disorder (n = 1), and psychosis (n = 1). A 4-session CBT-I intervention resulted in clinically significant reductions in insomnia severity and improved sleep quality. Furthermore, there was a significant reduction in paranoid thinking, depressive symptoms, and anxiety symptoms following CBT-I. These improvements were maintained though a 1-month follow-up assessment, indicating short-term durability of this intervention. In this case, the adapted CBT-I intervention included sleep psycho-education, sleep hygiene recommendations, and a stimulus control intervention. Cognitive approaches for insomnia and sleep restriction were not used in the 4-session protocol. Although these preliminary results are promising and support the notion that improving sleep is beneficial in a variety psychological domains, the small sample size and lack of a control condition prevent definitive conclusions from being drawn about the efficacy of CBT-I in psychotic disorders. Additionally, as demonstrated by Myers and colleagues,[111] in adapting CBT-I for schizophrenia, it may be important to eliminate certain traditional CBT-I components, such as sleep restriction, which could lead to reduced sleep time and exacerbation of psychotic symptoms.[92] It may also be particularly important to monitor positive symptoms at the start of each session throughout treatment and negotiate a safety plan with the patient before the start of therapy, should psychotic symptoms emerge during treatment.

Summary and future directions

Overall, the literature suggests that sleep problems, namely insomnia and circadian disturbances, are frequent in schizophrenia. Moreover, these sleep disturbances are generally associated with greater symptom severity, impaired quality of life, and the course of schizophrenia. Although there is a growing body of work investigating sleep architecture in schizophrenia, more research examining the rates of sleep disorders using gold-standard diagnostic methods[112] are needed. Facets of both REM and NREM sleep architecture appear altered in schizophrenia, although findings regarding these components of sleep have not been consistent. This is perhaps because of small sample sizes and heterogeneities in the patient populations (ie, not subdividing into paranoid, catatonic, and undifferentiated patient groups), issues that should be addressed in future studies. Additionally, although there is considerable evidence supporting an association between sleep (primarily poor sleep continuity and altered sleep architecture) with symptoms and outcome, much work is still needed to disentangle causal relationships. Future research involving prospective and experimental designs could shed light on the important causal links between sleep disturbance and disease severity.

Two sleep treatment studies in outpatient schizophrenia populations, one testing melatonin[110] and the other testing adapted CBT-I,[111] have provided the best preliminary evidence that normalization of sleep is related to improved clinical outcome. These interventions demonstrated that treating sleep led to improvements in residual positive symptoms and/or mood, and lay the groundwork for future sleep interventions in schizophrenia. Further investigations testing sleep interventions in larger-scale controlled trials would help more rigorously clarify the clinical utility of treating sleep disturbances in schizophrenia. Finally, the timing and selection of sleep treatments requires examination. For instance, certain insomnia interventions may be more effective at different phases of illness (acute vs stable) or based on schizophrenia subtype. Although many gaps remain in the literature, the findings available highlight the importance of developing and testing sleep interventions for schizophrenia, with the aim of reducing symptom burden and improving functional outcomes.

SUMMARY

In both BD and schizophrenia, sleep disturbance is a prominent feature regardless of medication status and phase of the disorder. Insomnia is the most frequent sleep problem in each of these patient populations, yet hypersomnia and circadian rhythm disturbances are also common. These sleep problems, as well as altered sleep architecture, are associated with exacerbated disease-specific symptoms, reduced quality of life, impaired daily functioning, and poor clinical outcome. Although gaps in knowledge remain,

these observations suggest a need for more research focusing on treatment of insomnia in severe psychiatric illness. A few small sleep-focused treatment studies in BD and schizophrenia have provided preliminary evidence that treatment of sleep disturbance may have clinical utility, reducing residual symptoms and risk of acute relapse. Future intervention trials would benefit from use of PSG and sample sizes large enough to assess whether improvements in these psychiatric conditions are driven by the improvement in sleep.

CBT-I appears to be a particularly promising avenue for reducing sleep disturbance, given its effectiveness in other psychiatric disorders and its low side-effect profile. That said, at least one study has documented that greater symptom severity in major depression is associated with poorer adherence to CBT-I,[113] and symptom severity or fluctuation in BD or schizophrenia may present similar challenges to treatment adherence. Some have raised concerns over residual positive, negative, and cognitive symptoms in schizophrenia that may also hinder adherence to CBT-I.[114] It is clear that both pharmacologic and psychological treatments for insomnia, as separate or interwoven interventions, require further testing in BD and schizophrenia. However, the evidence reviewed here suggests an encouraging possibility that treatment of sleep disturbance, in conjunction with the management of severe psychiatric illness, could lead to a more successful outcome and improved quality of life.

REFERENCES

1. Benca RM, Obermeyer WH, Thisted RA, et al. Sleep and psychiatric disorders. A meta-analysis. Arch Gen Psychiatry 1992;49:651–68 [discussion: 69–70].
2. Ford DE, Kamerow DB. Epidemiologic study of sleep disturbances and psychiatric disorders. An opportunity for prevention? J Am Med Assoc 1989;262:1479–84.
3. Ohayon MM. Epidemiology of insomnia: what we know and what we still need to learn. Sleep Med Rev 2002;6:97–111.
4. American Psychiatric Association. Diagnostic and statistical manual of mental disorders. 4th edition. Washington, DC: American Psychiatric Association; 2000. Text revision.
5. American Academy of Sleep Medicine. International classification of sleep disorders: diagnostic and coding manual. 2nd edition. Westchester (IL): American Academy of Sleep Medicine; 2005.
6. Breslau N, Roth T, Rosenthal L, et al. Sleep disturbance and psychiatric disorders: a longitudinal

epidemiological study of young adults. Biol Psychiatry 1996;39(6):411–8.

7. NIH. National Institutes of Health State of the Science Conference Statement: manifestations and management of chronic insomnia in adults. June 13-15, 2005. Sleep 2005;28:1049–57.

8. Harvey AG. Insomnia: symptom or diagnosis? Clin Psychol Rev 2001;21:1037–59.

9. Smith MT, Huang MI, Manber R. Cognitive Behavior Therapy for chronic insomnia occurring within the context of medical and psychiatric disorders. Clin Psychol Rev 2005;25:559–92.

10. Krystal AD, Thakur M, Roth T. Sleep disturbance in psychiatric disorders: effects on function and quality of life in mood disorders, alcoholism, and schizophrenia. Ann Clin Psychiatry 2008;20(1):39–46.

11. Harvey AG. Insomnia, psychiatric disorders, and the transdiagnostic perspective. Curr Dir Psychol Sci 2008;17:299–303.

12. Rybarczyk B, Lopez M, Schelble K, et al. Home-based video CBT for comorbid geriatric insomnia: a pilot study using secondary data analyses. Behav Sleep Med 2005;3:158–75.

13. Kaplan KA, Harvey AG. Hypersomnia across mood disorders: a review and synthesis. Sleep Med Rev 2009;13:275–85.

14. Monti JM, Bahammam AS, Pandi-Perumal SR, et al. Sleep and circadian rhythm dysregulation in schizophrenia. Prog Neuropsychopharmacol Biol Psychiatry 2013;43C:209–16.

15. Harvey AG. Sleep and circadian rhythms in bipolar disorder: seeking synchrony, harmony, and regulation. Am J Psychiatry 2008;165:820–9.

16. Hudson JI, Lipinski JF, Keck PE Jr, et al. Polysomnographic characteristics of schizophrenia in comparison with mania and depression. Biol Psychiatry 1993;34(3):191–3.

17. Linkowski P, Kerkhofs M, Rielaert C, et al. Sleep during mania in manic-depressive males. Eur Arch Psychiatry Neurol Sci 1986;235(6):339–41.

18. Jernajczyk W. Latency of eye movement and other REM sleep parameters in bipolar depression. Biol Psychiatry 1986;21(5–6):465–72.

19. Lauer CJ, Wiegand M, Krieg JC. All-night electroencephalographic sleep and cranial computed tomography in depression. A study of unipolar and bipolar patients. Eur Arch Psychiatry Clin Neurosci 1992;242(2–3):59–68.

20. Thase ME, Himmelhoch JM, Mallinger AG, et al. Sleep EEG and DST findings in anergic bipolar depression. Am J Psychiatry 1989;146:329–33.

21. Jovanovic UJ. The sleep profile in manic-depressive patients in the depressive phase. Waking Sleeping 1977;1:199–210.

22. Fossion P, Staner L, Dramaix M, et al. Does sleep EEG data distinguish between UP, BPI or BPII major depressions? An age and gender controlled study. J Affect Disord 1998;49(3):181–7.

23. Harvey AG, Schmidt DA, Scarna A, et al. Sleep-related functioning in euthymic patients with bipolar disorder, patients with insomnia, and subjects without sleep problems. Am J Psychiatry 2005;162:50–7.

24. Brill S, Penagaluri P, Roberts RJ, et al. Sleep disturbances in euthymic bipolar patients. Ann Clin Psychiatry 2011;23(2):113–6.

25. St-Amand J, Provencher MD, Belanger L, et al. Sleep disturbances in bipolar disorder during remission. J Affect Disord 2013;146(1):112–9.

26. Kaplan KA, Gruber J, Eidelman P, et al. Hypersomnia in inter-episode bipolar disorder: does it have prognostic significance? J Affect Disord 2011;132(3):438–44.

27. Millar A, Espie CA, Scott J. The sleep of remitted bipolar outpatients: a controlled naturalistic study using actigraphy. J Affect Disord 2004;80:145–53.

28. Talbot LS, Stone S, Gruber J, et al. A test of the bidirectional association between sleep and mood in bipolar disorder and insomnia. J Abnorm Psychol 2012;121(1):39–50.

29. Gershon A, Thompson WK, Eidelman P, et al. Restless pillow, ruffled mind: sleep and affect coupling in interepisode bipolar disorder. J Abnorm Psychol 2012;121(4):863–73.

30. Knowles JB, Cairns J, MacLean AW, et al. The sleep of remitted bipolar depressives: comparison with sex and age-matched controls. Can J Psychiatry 1986;31(4):295–8.

31. Sitaram N, Nurnberger JI Jr, Gershon ES, et al. Cholinergic regulation of mood and REM sleep: potential model and marker of vulnerability to affective disorder. Am J Psychiatry 1982;139(5):571–6.

32. Eidelman P, Talbot LS, Gruber J, et al. Sleep architecture as correlate and predictor of symptoms and impairment in inter-episode bipolar disorder: taking on the challenge of medication effects. J Sleep Res 2010;19(4):516–24.

33. Sachs GS, Thase ME, Otto MW, et al. Rationale, design, and methods of the systematic treatment enhancement program for bipolar disorder (STEP-BD). Biol Psychiatry 2003;53(11):1028–42.

34. Gruber J, Harvey AG, Wang PW, et al. Sleep functioning in relation to mood, function, and quality of life at entry to the Systematic Treatment Enhancement Program for Bipolar Disorder (STEP-BD). J Affect Disord 2009;114(1–3):41–9.

35. Gruber J, Miklowitz DJ, Harvey AG, et al. Sleep matters: sleep functioning and course of illness in bipolar disorder. J Affect Disord 2011;134(1–3):416–20.

36. Faedda GL, Baldessarini RJ, Glovinsky IP, et al. Pediatric bipolar disorder: phenomenology and course of illness. Bipolar Disord 2004;6:305–13.

37. Duffy A, Alda M, Crawford L, et al. The early manifestations of bipolar disorder: a longitudinal prospective study of the offspring of bipolar parents. Bipolar Disord 2007;9:828–38.

38. Jackson A, Cavanagh J, Scott J. A systematic review of manic and depressive prodromes. J Affect Disord 2003;74:209–17.

39. Colombo C, Benedetti F, Barbini B, et al. Rate of switch from depression into mania after therapeutic sleep deprivation in bipolar depression. Psychiatry Res 1999;86:267–70.

40. Szuba MP, Baxter LR Jr, Fairbanks LA, et al. Effects of partial sleep deprivation on the diurnal variation of mood and motor activity in major depression. Biol Psychiatry 1991;30(8):817–29.

41. Wehr TA, Sack DA, Rosenthal NE. Sleep reduction as a final common pathway in the genesis of mania. Am J Psychiatry 1987;144:201–4.

42. Barbini B, Bertelli S, Colombo C, et al. Sleep loss, a possible factor in augmenting manic episode. Psychiatry Res 1996;65:121–5.

43. Bauer M, Grof P, Rasgon N, et al. Temporal relation between sleep and mood in patients with bipolar disorder. Bipolar Disord 2006;8:160–7.

44. Perlman CA, Johnson SL, Mellman TA. The prospective impact of sleep duration on depression and mania. Bipolar Disord 2006;8(3):271–4.

45. Eidelman P, Talbot LS, Gruber J, et al. Sleep, illness course, and concurrent symptoms in inter-episode bipolar disorder. J Behav Ther Exp Psychiatry 2010;41(2):145–9.

46. Giglio LM, Andreazza AC, Andersen M, et al. Sleep in bipolar patients. Sleep Breath 2009;13(2):169–73.

47. Hudson JI, Lipinski JF, Frankenburg FR, et al. Electroencephalographic sleep in mania. Arch Gen Psychiatry 1988;45(3):267–73.

48. Schaffer CB, Schaffer LC, Miller AR, et al. Efficacy and safety of nonbenzodiazepine hypnotics for chronic insomnia in patients with bipolar disorder. J Affect Disord 2011;128:305–8.

49. Egashira T, Inoue T, Shirai Y, et al. Adjunctive gabapentin for treatment-resistant insomnia of bipolar disorder: a case report. Clin Neuropharmacol 2011;34:129–30.

50. Weilburg JB, Sachs G, Falk WE. Triazolam-induced brief episodes of secondary mania in a depressed patient. J Clin Psychiatry 1987;48:492–3.

51. Bersani G, Garavini A. Melatonin add-on in manic patients with treatment resistant insomnia. Prog Neuropsychopharmacol Biol Psychiatry 2000;24:185–91.

52. Calabrese JR, Guelfi JD, Perdrizet-Chevallier C. Agomelatine adjunctive therapy for acute bipolar depression: preliminary open data. Bipolar Disord 2007;9(6):628–35.

53. McElroy SL, Winstanley EL, Martens B, et al. A randomized, placebo-controlled study of adjunctive ramelteon in ambulatory bipolar I disorder with manic symptoms and sleep disturbance. Int Clin Psychopharmacol 2011;26(1):48–53.

54. Norris ER, Karen B, Correll JR, et al. A double-blind, randomized, placebo-controlled trial of adjunctive ramelteon for the treatment of insomnia and mood stability in patients with euthymic bipolar disorder. J Affect Disord 2013;144(1–2):141–7.

55. Levin FR, Hennessy G. Bipolar disorder and substance abuse. Biol Psychiatry 2004;56:738–48.

56. Kaplan KA, Harvey AG. Behavioral treatment of insomnia in bipolar disorder. Am J Psychiatry, in press.

57. Yoo SS, Gujar N, Hu P, et al. The human emotional brain without sleep—a prefrontal amygdala disconnect. Curr Biol 2007;17:R877–8.

58. Zohar D, Tzischinsky O, Epsten R, et al. The effects of sleep loss on medical residents' emotional reactions to work events: a cognitive-energy model. Sleep 2005;28:47–54.

59. Manber R, Edinger JD, Gress JL, et al. Cognitive behavioral therapy for insomnia enhances depression outcome in patients with comorbid major depressive disorder and insomnia. Sleep 2008; 31:489–95.

60. Taylor DJ, Lichstein KL, Weinstock J, et al. A pilot study of cognitive-behavioral therapy of insomnia in people with mild depression. Behav Ther 2007; 38:49–57.

61. Detre T. Sleep disorder and psychosis. Can Psychiatr Assoc J 1966;11(Suppl):169–77.

62. Haffmans PM, Hoencamp E, Knegtering HJ, et al. Sleep disturbance in schizophrenia. Br J Psychiatry 1994;165(5):697–8.

63. Lieberman JA, Stroup TS, McEvoy JP, et al. Effectiveness of antipsychotic drugs in patients with chronic schizophrenia. N Engl J Med 2005; 353(12):1209–23.

64. Royuela AMJ, Gil-Verona JA. Sleep in schizophrenia: a preliminary study using the Pittsburgh Sleep Quality Index. Neurobiol Sleep Wakefulness Cycle 2002;2(2):37–9.

65. Palmese LB, DeGeorge PC, Ratliff JC, et al. Insomnia is frequent in schizophrenia and associated with night eating and obesity. Schizophr Res 2011;133(1–3):238–43.

66. Afonso P, Figueira ML, Paiva T. Sleep-wake patterns in schizophrenia patients compared to healthy controls. World J Biol Psychiatry 2013. [Epub ahead of print].

67. Poulin J, Chouinard S, Pampoulova T, et al. Sleep habits in middle-aged, non-hospitalized men and women with schizophrenia: a comparison with healthy controls. Psychiatry Res 2010;179(3):274–8.

68. Doi Y, Minowa M, Uchiyama M, et al. Psychometric assessment of subjective sleep quality using the Japanese version of the Pittsburgh Sleep Quality

Index (PSQI-J) in psychiatric disordered and control subjects. Psychiatry Res 2000;97(2–3):165–72.

69. Xiang YT, Weng YZ, Leung CM, et al. Prevalence and correlates of insomnia and its impact on quality of life in Chinese schizophrenia patients. Sleep 2009;32(1):105–9.

70. Monti JM, Monti D. Sleep disturbance in schizophrenia. Int Rev Psychiatry 2005;17(4):247–53.

71. Chouinard S, Poulin J, Stip E, et al. Sleep in untreated patients with schizophrenia: a meta-analysis. Schizophr Bull 2004;30(4):957–67.

72. Martin JL, Jeste DV, Ancoli-Israel S. Older schizophrenia patients have more disrupted sleep and circadian rhythms than age-matched comparison subjects. J Psychiatr Res 2005;39(3):251–9.

73. Wulff K, Dijk DJ, Middleton B, et al. Sleep and circadian rhythm disruption in schizophrenia. Br J Psychiatry 2012;200(4):308–16.

74. Benson KL. Sleep in schizophrenia: impairments, correlates, and treatment. Psychiatr Clin North Am 2006;29(4):1033–45 [abstract ix-x].

75. Cohrs S. Sleep disturbances in patients with schizophrenia: impact and effect of antipsychotics. CNS Drugs 2008;22(11):939–62.

76. Keshavan MS, Reynolds CF 3rd, Miewald JM, et al. A longitudinal study of EEG sleep in schizophrenia. Psychiatry Res 1996;59(3):203–11.

77. Tandon R, Shipley JE, Taylor S, et al. Electroencephalographic sleep abnormalities in schizophrenia. Relationship to positive/negative symptoms and prior neuroleptic treatment. Arch Gen Psychiatry 1992;49(3):185–94.

78. Ganguli R, Rabin BS, Kelly RH, et al. Clinical and laboratory evidence of autoimmunity in acute schizophrenia. Ann N Y Acad Sci 1987;496:676–85.

79. Ganguli R, Reynolds CF 3rd, Kupfer DJ. Electroencephalographic sleep in young, never-medicated schizophrenics. A comparison with delusional and nondelusional depressives and with healthy controls. Arch Gen Psychiatry 1987;44(1):36–44.

80. Stern M, Fram DH, Wyatt R, et al. All-night sleep studies of acute schizophrenics. Arch Gen Psychiatry 1969;20(4):470–7.

81. Hiatt JF, Floyd TC, Katz PH, et al. Further evidence of abnormal non-rapid-eye-movement sleep in schizophrenia. Arch Gen Psychiatry 1985;42(8):797–802.

82. Poulin J, Daoust AM, Forest G, et al. Sleep architecture and its clinical correlates in first episode and neuroleptic-naive patients with schizophrenia. Schizophr Res 2003;62(1–2):147–53.

83. Kempenaers C, Kerkhofs M, Linkowski P, et al. Sleep EEG variables in young schizophrenic and depressive patients. Biol Psychiatry 1988;24(7):833–8.

84. Keshavan MS, Reynolds CF, Kupfer DJ. Electroencephalographic sleep in schizophrenia: a critical review. Compr Psychiatry 1990;31(1):34–47.

85. Benson KL, Zarcone VP Jr. Rapid eye movement sleep eye movements in schizophrenia and depression. Arch Gen Psychiatry 1993;50(6):474–82.

86. Lauer CJ, Schreiber W, Pollmacher T, et al. Sleep in schizophrenia: a polysomnographic study on drug-naive patients. Neuropsychopharmacology 1997;16(1):51–60.

87. Ferrarelli F, Peterson MJ, Sarasso S, et al. Thalamic dysfunction in schizophrenia suggested by whole-night deficits in slow and fast spindles. Am J Psychiatry 2010;167(11):1339–48.

88. Afonso P, Brissos S, Figueira ML, et al. Schizophrenia patients with predominantly positive symptoms have more disturbed sleep-wake cycles measured by actigraphy. Psychiatry Res 2011;189(1):62–6.

89. Zarcone VP, Benson KL. BPRS symptom factors and sleep variables in schizophrenia. Psychiatry Res 1997;66(2–3):111–20.

90. Freeman D, Pugh K, Vorontsova N, et al. Insomnia and paranoia. Schizophr Res 2009;108(1–3):280–4.

91. Chemerinski E, Ho BC, Flaum M, et al. Insomnia as a predictor for symptom worsening following antipsychotic withdrawal in schizophrenia. Compr Psychiatry 2002;43(5):393–6.

92. Neylan TC, van Kammen DP, Kelley ME, et al. Sleep in schizophrenic patients on and off haloperidol therapy. Clinically stable vs relapsed patients. Arch Gen Psychiatry 1992;49(8):643–9.

93. Ritsner M, Kurs R, Ponizovsky A, et al. Perceived quality of life in schizophrenia: relationships to sleep quality. Qual Life Res 2004;13(4):783–91.

94. Hofstetter JR, Lysaker PH, Mayeda AR. Quality of sleep in patients with schizophrenia is associated with quality of life and coping. BMC Psychiatry 2005;5:13.

95. Kantrowitz J, Citrome L, Javitt D. GABA(B) receptors, schizophrenia and sleep dysfunction: a review of the relationship and its potential clinical and therapeutic implications. CNS Drugs 2009;23(8):681–91.

96. Taylor SF, Tandon R, Shipley JE, et al. Effect of neuroleptic treatment on polysomnographic measures in schizophrenia. Biol Psychiatry 1991;30(9):904–12.

97. Yang C, Winkelman JW. Clinical significance of sleep EEG abnormalities in chronic schizophrenia. Schizophr Res 2006;82(2–3):251–60.

98. Tandon R, DeQuardo JR, Taylor SF, et al. Phasic and enduring negative symptoms in schizophrenia: biological markers and relationship to outcome. Schizophr Res 2000;45(3):191–201.

99. Keshavan MS, Miewald J, Haas G, et al. Slow-wave sleep and symptomatology in schizophrenia and related psychotic disorders. J Psychiatr Res 1995;29(4):303–14.

100. Keshavan MS, Pettegrew JW, Reynolds CF 3rd, et al. Biological correlates of slow wave sleep

deficits in functional psychoses: 31P-magnetic resonance spectroscopy. Psychiatry Res 1995; 57(2):91–100.

101. Kato M, Kajimura N, Okuma T, et al. Association between delta waves during sleep and negative symptoms in schizophrenia. Pharmaco-EEG studies by using structurally different hypnotics. Neuropsychobiology 1999;39(3):165–72.

102. Kajimura N, Kato M, Okuma T, et al. Relationship between delta activity during all-night sleep and negative symptoms in schizophrenia: a preliminary study. Biol Psychiatry 1996;39(6):451–4.

103. Riemann D, Hohagen F, Krieger S, et al. Cholinergic REM induction test: muscarinic supersensitivity underlies polysomnographic findings in both depression and schizophrenia. J Psychiatr Res 1994;28(3):195–210.

104. Keshavan MS, Reynolds CF 3rd, Miewald J, et al. Slow-wave sleep deficits and outcome in schizophrenia and schizoaffective disorder. Acta Psychiatr Scand 1995;91(5):289–92.

105. Goldman M, Tandon R, DeQuardo JR, et al. Biological predictors of 1-year outcome in schizophrenia in males and females. Schizophr Res 1996;21(2):65–73.

106. Taylor SF, Tandon R, Shipley JE, et al. Sleep onset REM periods in schizophrenic patients. Biol Psychiatry 1991;30(2):205–9.

107. Kajimura N, Kato M, Okuma T, et al. A quantitative sleep-EEG study on the effects of benzodiazepine and zopiclone in schizophrenic patients. Schizophr Res 1995;15(3):303–12.

108. Baandrup L, Jennum P, Lublin H, et al. Treatment options for residual insomnia in schizophrenia. Acta Psychiatr Scand 2013;127(1):81–2.

109. Shamir E, Laudon M, Barak Y, et al. Melatonin improves sleep quality of patients with chronic schizophrenia. J Clin Psychiatry 2000;61(5):373–7.

110. Suresh Kumar PA, Andrade C, Bhakta SG, et al. Melatonin in schizophrenic outpatients with insomnia: a double-blind, placebo-controlled study. J Clin Psychiatry 2007;68(2):237–41.

111. Myers E, Startup H, Freeman D. Cognitive behavioural treatment of insomnia in individuals with persistent persecutory delusions: a pilot trial. J Behav Ther Exp Psychiatry 2011;42(3):330–6.

112. Buysse D, Ancoli-Israel S, Edinger JD, et al. Recommendations for a standard research assessment of insomnia. Sleep 2006;29:1155–73.

113. Manber R, Bernert RA, Suh S, et al. CBT for insomnia in patients with high and low depressive symptom severity: adherence and clinical outcomes. J Clin Sleep Med 2011;7(6):645–52.

114. Andrade C, Suresh Kumar PN. Treating residual insomnia in schizophrenia: examining the options. Acta Psychiatr Scand 2013;127(1):11.

Insomnia and Cancer
Prevalence, Nature, and Nonpharmacologic Treatment

Josée Savard, PhD[a,b,*], Marie-Hélène Savard, PhD[b]

KEYWORDS

- Insomnia • Cancer • Prevalence • Risk factors • Nonpharmacologic treatment
- Cognitive-behavioral therapy • Self-help treatment • Stepped-care model

KEY POINTS

- Insomnia is very common in patients with cancer, especially in those with breast or gynecologic cancer.
- Several cancer-specific factors may trigger the onset of sleep disturbances, including surgery and hospitalization, adjuvant treatments, nocturnal hot flashes, fatigue, and pain.
- Cognitive-behavioral therapy (CBT) is increasingly recognized as the treatment of choice for insomnia comorbid with cancer.
- More research is warranted on patients' acceptability and efficacy of CBT for insomnia during the active phase of cancer treatment and in patients with advanced disease. It is also important to determine whether it would be appropriate to concurrently treat other cancer-related symptoms that are associated with the occurrence of insomnia (eg, hot flashes, fatigue, pain) to increase treatment efficacy.
- The accessibility of CBT for insomnia, which is currently highly limited in oncology settings, could be improved through the use of more minimal interventions (eg, self-administered) and a stepped-care approach, but their efficacy and cost-effectiveness need to be assessed using large, randomized controlled trials.

PREVALENCE AND EVOLUTION OF INSOMNIA IN PATIENTS WITH CANCER

Sleep disturbances are amongst the most common symptoms reported by patients with cancer. Early cross-sectional studies, mainly conducted in the posttreatment phase, revealed that between 30% and 50% of patients with cancer report insomnia symptoms. More recent epidemiologic evidence from large-scale longitudinal studies suggests that these rates may even be higher in patients undergoing cancer treatments, at least in certain subgroups of patients. Overall, rates of insomnia symptoms and syndrome found in patients with cancer appear to be at least 2 to 3 times higher than in the general population. Various definitions have been used, although typically the insomnia syndrome has been defined by a combination of criteria on frequency (eg, ≥ 3 nights), severity (eg, sleep-onset latency or wake after sleep onset >30 minutes), duration (eg, >1 month), and consequences on daytime functioning. Insomnia symptoms have mostly been defined as a subjective complaint of sleep difficulties not meeting full criteria for an insomnia syndrome.

[a] School of Psychology, Laval University, 2325, rue des Bibliothèques, Québec, Québec, G1V 0A6, Canada;
[b] Centre de Recherche du CHU de Québec, Laval University Cancer Research Center, 11, Côte du Palais, Québec, Québec G1R 2J6, Canada
* Corresponding author.
E-mail address: josee.savard@psy.ulaval.ca

Sleep Med Clin 8 (2013) 373–387
http://dx.doi.org/10.1016/j.jsmc.2013.04.006
1556-407X/13/$ – see front matter © 2013 Elsevier Inc. All rights reserved.

Cross-Sectional Studies

The numerous cross-sectional studies that have assessed the presence of sleep impairments in patients with cancer have been reviewed extensively.[1–8] Overall, these studies suggest that 30% to 50% of patients with cancer complain of sleep difficulties and that nearly 20% meet the diagnostic criteria for an insomnia syndrome (or disorder), although this last issue has received much less attention. However, these studies were characterized by several limitations, including the use of small convenience samples and by use of sleep measures composed of single or a small number of items, as well as sleep often being assessed in the posttreatment phase, in many cases several years later. Moreover, because of their cross-sectional nature these studies did not provide any information on the natural course of sleep impairments (incidence, remission, persistence) throughout the cancer care trajectory and beyond.

Longitudinal Studies

Nonmetastatic cancer

Two large-scale longitudinal studies have been conducted in nonmetastatic patients with heterogeneous cancer sites to better assess the differential prevalence of sleep impairments across cancer sites and their evolution over time. The authors' research team followed 991 patients awaiting surgery for mixed cancer sites.[9,10] Patients were assessed at baseline (ie, during the perioperative phase) and 2, 6, 10, 14, and 18 months later. At baseline, 59% had insomnia symptoms, including the 28% with an insomnia syndrome, as assessed using a telephone diagnostic interview and the algorithm developed by LeBlanc and colleagues.[11] Accordingly, patients were considered to have an insomnia syndrome when they met the following criteria: sleep-onset latency (SOL) or wake after sleep onset (WASO) more than 30 minutes, at least 3 nights per week; sleep efficiency (SE) less than 85%, for at least 1 month; impaired daytime functioning or marked distress, or using a hypnotic medication 3 nights per week or more for at least 1 month. Although these rates steadily decreased over time, 36% of the sample still suffered from insomnia symptoms, whereas 21% met the criteria for an insomnia syndrome 18 months later, which remains much higher than in the general population. Rates of insomnia were especially high in patients with breast (42%–69%) and gynecologic (33%–68%) cancer, and lower in men with prostate cancer (25%–39%) throughout the study. Moreover, the general persistence rate (ie, insomnia present at 2 consecutive time points on 2–4-month intervals) was

51%, and 35% of patients had insomnia persisting for at least 3 consecutive time points. Insomnia syndrome was a particularly enduring condition, with persistence rates ranging from 69% to 80%.

In another large-scale prospective study, Palesh and colleagues[12] assessed the presence of insomnia in 823 patients scheduled to receive at least 4 cycles of chemotherapy for various types of cancer (all stages). Sleep difficulties were assessed on day 7 of cycles 1 and 2 of chemotherapy using the 6 sleep-related questions from the Hamilton Depression Inventory. The insomnia syndrome was defined by the presence of difficulty falling asleep, difficulty staying asleep, and/or early morning awakenings (at least 30 minutes each) for at least 3 nights a week for 2 weeks. This more liberal definition (not taking into account SE and insomnia-related functioning impairments), coupled with the fact that the information was derived from a questionnaire rather than from a diagnostic interview, yielded greater prevalence rates. At cycle 1, 80% of the patients displayed insomnia symptoms, including the 43% meeting the criteria for an insomnia syndrome; these rates decreased to 68% and 35%, respectively, at cycle 2. Among good sleepers at cycle 1, 35% developed insomnia symptoms at cycle 2 (of whom 10% developed an insomnia syndrome). When comparing cancer sites (ie, breast, gynecologic, hematologic, lung, gastrointestinal), the prevalence of insomnia symptoms (including those with a syndrome) was the highest in patients with breast cancer (85%), followed closely by those with gynecologic cancer (83%). The prevalence of the insomnia syndrome was highest in patients with lung cancer (51%) and lowest in those with a gastrointestinal malignancy (24%).

Advanced cancer

Very little research has assessed the prevalence of sleep disturbances in patients with advanced cancer. Data from our longitudinal study described above included 194 patients with advanced cancer (ie, stages III–IV; various cancer sites) who received surgery.[13] During the perioperative period, 20% to 46% reported insomnia symptoms, whereas an additional 14% to 27% met criteria for an insomnia syndrome (total 35%–73%). Again, higher rates were found in patients with breast cancer than in those with prostate cancer. The prevalence of insomnia syndrome was fairly stable or increased over time depending on the cancer type, which suggests that it is often a chronic condition in these patients. However, in this study patients with distant metastasis were excluded, and surgery had to have curative intent. Hence it is unclear whether the results are generalizable to patients with more advanced disease.

Another longitudinal study conducted in 209 terminally ill patients with cancer in Japan showed that 15% of them had sleep disturbance and 29% had subthreshold disturbance at the moment of registration to a palliative care unit.[14] The presence of sleep disturbance was determined using the insomnia/hypersomnia item of the major depressive episode module of the Structured Clinical Interview for DSM-III-R. These rates increased to 26% and 37%, respectively, at the time of admission to the unit (follow-up assessment). There was a change in sleep status in 67% of the patients between the two time points; sleep deteriorated (46%) more frequently than it improved (21%). Given that hypersomnia is common in this population, future efforts should be devoted to distinguish this condition from insomnia. In addition, more studies are needed to identify medical, psychological, and environmental factors associated with sleep impairment among patients with advanced cancer.

Risk Factors of Insomnia in the Context of Cancer

According to the model devised by Spielman and Glovinsky,[15] there are 3 categories of etiologic factors involved in the development of insomnia: (1) predisposing factors, or enduring traits that increase the individual's general vulnerability to develop insomnia; (2) precipitating factors, or situational conditions that trigger the onset of insomnia; and (3) perpetuating factors, or variables contributing to the maintenance of insomnia over time. A particular focus herein is on factors more specific to cancer.

Predisposing factors

Contrary to what has been found in primary insomnia, insomnia comorbid with cancer is more prevalent in younger patients,[16–18] perhaps because this subgroup also generally displays the highest levels of psychological distress. This difference can also be attributable to the fact that, in women, a younger age is associated with an increased susceptibility to experience menopausal transition during cancer treatments, which may lead to poor sleep (see Precipitating Factors section). Other predisposing factors are the same as those in primary insomnia (**Box 1**). Female gender and the presence of a hyperarousability trait have been found to increase the risk for developing insomnia symptoms in cancer.[9] Available evidence on the comorbidity of insomnia with depression and anxiety disorders has revealed that, although these disorders often co-occur, insomnia frequently develops independently of mood disturbances.[19,20]

Box 1
Predisposing factors for insomnia comorbid with cancer

Younger age

Female gender

Hyperarousability trait

Personal and family history of insomnia

Antecedents of a psychiatric disorder (eg, depressive or anxiety disorders)

Precipitating factors

In the general population, insomnia is generally precipitated by stressful life events such as job loss/work stress, separation/divorce, death of a loved one, and medical conditions.[21] Illnesses such as cancer represent a potentially potent precipitating factor for insomnia. In fact, cancer does not represent a single event; it is rather characterized by a succession of severe stressors, each of which can serve as a precipitating factor for insomnia. Insomnia can be triggered at any point during the cancer process: at the initial diagnosis, at the time of surgery, during treatment, at the time of diagnosis and treatment of a recurrence, and during the palliative and terminal stages of the disease (**Box 2**).[1]

The period surrounding the cancer surgery, generally occurring soon after cancer diagnosis, is associated with particularly high levels of sleep disturbances. Longitudinal studies following patients during the cancer care trajectory indicated that the prevalence of insomnia was the highest at this point.[10,22] A study conducted among 96 patients with colorectal or gastrointestinal cancer showed a significant aggravation of sleep difficulties 6 weeks following the surgery in comparison with the presurgical evaluation.[23] It is important to note that hospitalization, in itself, can trigger sleep disturbances,[24] because of environmental factors (eg, noise, bed discomfort, administration of medications during sleeping periods), as well as psychological and behavioral factors (eg, anxiety, modification of sleep routine). Surgery-related pain and nocturia (eg, following radical prostatectomy) can also play a role.

All adjuvant treatments may increase the risk of developing insomnia, because of their emotional impact, direct physiologic effects, or side effects. Chemotherapy is thought to be particularly harmful.[25,26] Patients report more subjective sleep disturbance (sleep quality and duration, total sleep time) during the active phases of chemotherapy compared with nontreatment periods.[27] Longitudinal studies using subjective measures have also

Box 2
Precipitating factors for insomnia comorbid with cancer

Psychological reaction (eg, depressive/anxiety symptoms) to:

    Initial diagnosis

    Recurrence diagnosis

    Progression

Cancer treatments

    Surgery

        Psychological reaction

        Hospitalization (eg, environment, changes in sleep routine)

        Side effects (eg, pain, nocturia)

    Chemotherapy

        Side effects (eg, nausea/vomiting, fatigue) and medications used (eg, antiemetics)

        Deficiency in sexual hormones (eg, nocturnal hot flashes)

        Changes in circadian rhythms

        Inflammation

    Hormone therapy

        Deficiency in sexual hormones (eg, nocturnal hot flashes)

    Radiation therapy

        Side effects (eg, fatigue, nocturia, pain)

        Changes in circadian rhythms

Cancer symptoms (eg, pain, dyspnea)

Delirium

shown increased sleep impairment with this treatment,[22] as well as persistence of elevated insomnia rates across chemotherapy cycles.[12]

Reasons for this deleterious effect of chemotherapy have yet to be established, but are likely to involve both behavioral and physiologic mechanisms. On the behavioral side, patients receiving chemotherapy are likely to nap more during the day and spend less time outside, thus limiting their exposure to natural daylight. Together, these behavioral changes may alter patients' circadian rhythms. Consistent with this hypothesis, the repeated administration of chemotherapy for breast cancer has been found to be associated with an increased perturbation of sleep/wake rhythms assessed with actigraphy.[28] Chemotherapy also induces inflammation (ie, increased secretion of proinflammatory cytokines), which

may have a deleterious effect on sleep.[17] Side effects of chemotherapy (nausea/vomiting) and medications that are used to prevent them can also contribute to the development of sleep disturbances. For instance, insomnia is a well-known side effect of dexamethasone, a corticosteroid commonly used for that purpose.[29,30]

Hormone therapy for cancer, in both women and men, appears to be another important risk factor for insomnia. Among patients with prostate cancer, androgen deprivation therapy was associated with an increased risk of insomnia compared with radiotherapy in a recent study by the authors.[31] This effect was significantly mediated by increased hot flashes and night sweats. Although specific evidence is lacking on the effect of hormone therapy for cancer on sleep in women, it is likely to be the same.

Indeed, the deficiency in sexual hormones (estrogen in women, testosterone in men) caused by hormone therapy (eg, tamoxifen, arimidex, goserelin) but also by chemotherapy, surgery (eg, bilateral orchiectomy), and the abrupt cessation of hormone replacement therapy in women may induce or exacerbate nocturnal hot flashes, which can interfere with sleep. Increasing evidence from the breast cancer literature supports the relationship between hot flashes and sleep disturbances. In one of the authors' studies, changes occurring in self-reported vasomotor symptoms between the end of initial adjuvant treatments and a 3-month follow-up were significantly associated with parallel changes in insomnia complaints.[32] Using objective measures of nocturnal hot flashes and sleep, the study by Savard and colleagues[33] of 24 survivors of breast cancer showed that the 10-minute periods around hot flashes had more wake time and more stage changes to lighter sleep than other 10-minute periods during the night. In addition, nights with hot flashes had a significantly higher percentage of wake time, a lower percentage of Stage 2 sleep, and a longer rapid eye movement (REM) sleep latency compared with nights without hot flashes. A more recent investigation by this team conducted in 56 women treated for breast cancer revealed that slower and longer hot flashes, but not increased hot-flash frequency, were associated with several sleep impairments including greater total wake time, poorer SE, and a higher number of awakenings.[34]

There is also some evidence suggesting that cancer-related fatigue, another highly common symptom, is a risk factor for the development or increase of insomnia symptoms in patients with cancer. As much as 75% of patients undergoing chemotherapy or radiotherapy report symptoms of weakness and tiredness.[3] Being the most common complaint of insomnia sufferers, fatigue is often perceived as a consequence of poor sleep. However, additional analyses of our aforementioned longitudinal study using structural equation modeling showed that greater fatigue significantly predicted a subsequent increase in insomnia symptoms during the cancer care trajectory, whereas insomnia was not found to predict subsequent fatigue.[35] Empirical evidence is lacking on the mechanisms through which fatigue could lead to insomnia, but it could be the consequence of impaired circadian rhythms caused by increased napping and rest and reduced light exposure, as already explained, or may be due to a common pathophysiologic mechanism (eg, inflammation[36,37]).

Insomnia can also be triggered by cancer pain. It has been estimated that 30% to 50% of ambulatory patients with cancer or patients undergoing antineoplastic treatment, and 60% to 80% of patients with advanced cancer, experience pain.[38–41] In a sample of 2862 cancer outpatients, the risk of reporting insomnia symptoms was 2.7 times higher for those having pain.[42] In a longitudinal study of 93 women with metastatic breast cancer, increases in pain levels over 12 months significantly predicted more difficulties in falling asleep and nocturnal awakenings.[43] There are also data showing increased objectively assessed sleep disturbances and circadian-rhythm impairments (with actigraphy) among men (but not women) with pain, compared with cancer patients without pain.[41]

Dyspnea and nocturia are other somatic symptoms that may affect sleep negatively,[19,44–46] although their impact has been less studied in cancer. Finally, sleep disturbances represent a typical clinical feature of delirium, a condition occurring mostly in terminal cancer. In this context, sleep difficulties are most frequently characterized by daytime sleepiness, nighttime agitation, difficulty falling asleep, and in some cases complete reversal of the sleep-wake cycle.[47,48]

Perpetuating factors

Although some precipitating factors of insomnia may be chronic in nature and can perpetuate sleep impairment, such as cancer-related pain, the individual responses to the sleep problem determine in large part whether the sleep disturbance will cease or become chronic. According to a cognitive-behavioral conceptualization of insomnia,[21] the most salient conditions maintaining insomnia are maladaptive sleep habits and dysfunctional cognitions about sleep (**Box 3**). Both types of factors are believed to exert their negative effects by increasing arousal (ie, physiologic, cognitive, and

> **Box 3**
> **Perpetuating factors for insomnia comorbid with cancer**
>
> Maladaptive sleep behaviors
>
> > Excessive amount of time spent in bed
> >
> > Irregular sleep-wake schedule
> >
> > Napping
> >
> > Engaging in sleep-interfering activities in the bedroom
>
> Faulty beliefs and attitudes about sleep
>
> > Unrealistic sleep requirement expectations
> >
> > Faulty causal attributions
> >
> > Misattribution/amplification of perceived consequences of insomnia
> >
> > Decreased perception of control/predictability of sleep
> >
> > Faulty beliefs about sleep-promoting practices

emotional) and performance anxiety, which are in direct opposition to the relaxation state required for sleep. Results from the authors' longitudinal study[9] support this model in the context of cancer; that is, the persistence of insomnia from baseline to the 2-month evaluation was significantly predicted by higher baseline levels and increases from T1 to T2 in dysfunctional beliefs about sleep, cognitive monitoring of sleep-related threat (eg, calculating the number of hours that one hopes to get), and maladaptive sleep behaviors.

Maladaptive sleep behaviors, such as napping and spending too much time in bed, are particularly frequent in patients with cancer who are encouraged to get rest and sleep to recuperate from their cancer treatments.[49–51] In part, this may explain why patients with cancer appear to be at higher risk for developing chronic insomnia. Also, in addition to typical faulty beliefs and attitudes about sleep encountered in individuals with chronic insomnia, patients with cancer entertain specific erroneous beliefs including "If I don't sleep well, my cancer will come back," which may induce great levels of arousal and performance anxiety ("I really need to sleep tonight") as bedtime approaches.

NONPHARMACOLOGIC TREATMENT: COGNITIVE-BEHAVIORAL THERAPY

Because maladaptive sleep habits and dysfunctional cognitions about sleep are amenable to change, cognitive-behavioral therapy (CBT), which directly addresses these perpetuating factors, is particularly relevant for the treatment of insomnia, including the insomnia experienced by patients with cancer. CBT is increasingly recognized as the treatment of choice for cancer-related insomnia.[52] In this section, evidence for the efficacy of CBT specifically in the context of cancer is reviewed, and areas for future research and issues regarding its accessibility are discussed.

Efficacy of CBT in Patients with Cancer

Description of the evidence

There is accumulating evidence supporting the efficacy of CBT in patients with cancer. **Table 1** presents the methodological characteristics of studies that have been published thus far. Most sleep-intervention studies have been conducted after the year 2000.[53] Overall, findings indicate that CBT for insomnia is associated with improvements in subjective measures of sleep (eg, sleep diary parameters, scores on the Insomnia Severity Index [ISI] and the Pittsburgh Sleep Quality Index [PSQI]), decreased psychological distress (eg, anxiety, depression), and increased quality of life. Some studies have also included objective measures of sleep (polysomnographic and actigraphic recording) but results have been more equivocal,[54–56] as in studies of primary insomnia.

The strongest evidence supporting the efficacy of CBT for insomnia in the context of cancer is provided by randomized controlled trials (RCTs). In the first RCT conducted, 57 survivors of breast cancer meeting criteria for a chronic insomnia syndrome were randomized to CBT for insomnia (8 weekly sessions administered in small groups) or a waiting-list control condition.[54] Results indicated larger improvements in subjective sleep parameters (ISI score; SOL, WASO, SE, total wake time), decreases in psychological distress (depression and anxiety), and increases in quality of life, as well as a lower frequency of medicated nights in women treated with CBT (**Fig. 1**). These positive effects were well sustained up to 12 months after the intervention. An interesting finding of this study is that control patients slightly improved during their waiting period, most likely because of the effect of the passage of time, but it was only when they finally received CBT that they achieved the same level of improvement as CBT patients after treatment. This finding could indicate that the specific therapeutic ingredients of CBT are needed to obtain clinically significant benefits.

More recently, Espie and colleagues[55] randomized 150 patients who had completed their cancer treatment to either CBT for insomnia, composed of

5 group sessions administered by trained nurses, or treatment as usual (TAU). CBT was associated with a reduction of wake time (SOL + WASO) of nearly 1 hour and an increase of 10% in SE, whereas no change was observed in TAU patients posttreatment. Moreover, these beneficial effects were maintained at the 6-month follow-up.

Avenues for future research

Despite the increasing body of literature supporting the efficacy of CBT for insomnia in patients with cancer, many issues still need to be better documented (**Box 4**). For instance, given that previous work has mostly been conducted in the posttreatment phase,[54,55,57–59] sometimes years after the termination of oncologic treatment, it is unclear whether CBT is as beneficial when administered during cancer care. Although intervening in insomnia patients earlier in the cancer care trajectory seems appealing to prevent symptoms from becoming chronic, the patients' acceptability and the efficacy of this approach are not guaranteed. Indeed, patients undergoing treatment may not be as willing to receive an insomnia intervention while they are occupied with their radiation therapy and chemotherapy sessions, and have to deal with their side effects (eg, nausea, fatigue) that are often severe and incapacitating. In addition, still receiving treatments that have potential sleep-altering side effects (eg, corticosteroids used for nausea and vomiting during chemotherapy) could negatively affect the efficacy of CBT for insomnia.

A series of studies conducted by Berger and colleagues[60,61] has looked at the efficacy of the Individualized Sleep Promotion Plan (ISPP), an adaptation of CBT for insomnia (see later discussion), in patients with breast cancer undergoing chemotherapy. Results of their recent RCT of 219 participants indicated that sleep quality, as assessed with the PSQI, and the number of awakenings, WASO, and SE from a sleep diary, significantly improved immediately after the ISPP intervention.[61] However, at the 1-year assessment, PSQI scores were significantly more improved in the ISPP group when compared with a healthy-eating control condition, but no between-groups differences were found on any sleep diary (and actigraphic) parameter.[56] Although these findings could suggest that CBT for insomnia leads to less enduring effects during cancer treatment, they may be due to a floor effect. In fact, patients were not selected on the basis of clinical insomnia at baseline in that study, and the intent of the intervention was mostly preventive (to prevent insomnia symptoms from developing/aggravating during chemotherapy).

Clearly more prevention and intervention studies on the effect of CBT for insomnia during cancer care are needed.

Moreover, a large proportion of clinical trials on the efficacy of CBT for insomnia have focused on women, particularly those with breast cancer. Although this fact reflects the higher prevalence of insomnia in this specific population, research is needed to assess whether CBT for insomnia may be as effective in males and patients with other cancer types. The efficacy of nonpharmacologic interventions for sleep impairments also needs to be investigated in patients with advanced cancer. Although patients who are still ambulatory despite their illness progression are likely to benefit from the same treatment strategies, the treatment protocol probably needs to be adapted for patients with more functional disabilities and who are approaching death. In this population sleep impairments may take the form of insomnia symptoms, but excessive daytime sleepiness and hypersomnia are also common,[62,63] and may constitute an adverse effect of medication for cancer pain such as morphine.[64] A greater recourse to environmental strategies (eg, increased exposure to natural or artificial light during the day and reduced exposure during nighttime; augmented activity during the day) to resynchronize the sleep/wake cycle appears to be especially relevant in such cases. Although such approaches have been used successfully in patients with dementia[65,66] and in nursing home residents,[67] their feasibility and usefulness need to be explored in patients with advanced cancer.

The specific strategies that need to be included in the treatment protocol also need to be better defined. Thus far, the majority of clinical trials have used the standard CBT protocol for insomnia, with remission rates comparable with those found in primary insomnia; this includes behavioral strategies such as stimulus control and sleep restriction, cognitive restructuring, and basic sleep hygiene principles.[54,55,57–59] Several investigators have included relaxation,[57,58,60,61,68] but not all. The possible additional benefit of relaxation has yet to be demonstrated, in the context of both cancer and primary insomnia.

Nonetheless, adaptations of the standard CBT for insomnia protocol have been tested in a few trials. For instance, Berger and colleagues[60,61] developed and tested the efficacy of the ISPP in patients with breast cancer undergoing chemotherapy. The ISPP was administered in very brief sessions (15–30 minutes), and was developed collaboratively with the patients and tailored to their specific needs. While it aimed at including 4 standard components (ie, stimulus control,

modified sleep restriction, relaxation therapy, and sleep hygiene), patients had the freedom to design their own plan and could therefore select the strategies they wished to try. Such adaptation could have affected the treatment efficacy and may explain, at least partly, why beneficial effects were obtained on sleep quality ratings (ie, PSQI scores) but not on sleep diary data at the 1-year follow-up as described earlier.[56]

More specific to the cancer context is the question as to whether targeting more directly other cancer-related symptoms that are associated with the occurrence of insomnia would increase treatment efficacy. As already discussed, symptoms such as hot flashes, fatigue, and pain often contribute to triggering the onset of insomnia and its persistence in this population, and specific CBT strategies targeting these symptoms have been found to be efficacious in noncancer individuals (eg, CBT for pain offered to patients with chronic pain). Savard and colleagues[54] added a brief fatigue management strategy, targeting physical deconditioning and promoting physical activity, to the standard CBT for insomnia protocol, but it was impossible in this study to delineate the potential additional benefit of this component. In a recent RCT (N = 96) of survivors of breast cancer, the efficacy of a group CBT targeting hot flashes/night sweats (paced breathing and relaxation, decatastrophizing), sleep (behavioral and cognitive strategies administered in 2 sessions), and stress and anxiety was compared with TAU.[69] Results indicated that the intervention was associated with reduced problematic hot flashes, but also improved sleep as assessed using the 4 items of the Women's Health Questionnaire. Hence, adding CBT strategies targeting other cancer-related symptoms that are often associated with sleep disturbances (eg, hot flashes, fatigue, pain) to standard CBT for insomnia is a promising approach to increase intervention efficacy and the scope of treatment effects. However, this hypothesis needs further verification.

Accessibility of CBT in Patients with Cancer

Although CBT for insomnia appears to be efficacious in patients with cancer, its accessibility is extremely limited in this population. There are several reasons for this. Insomnia remains a largely underdiagnosed and undertreated condition. Sleep difficulties and their impact are trivialized, and there is a common perception that they will fade away by themselves or be improved through the beneficial effect of more general psychological interventions. Also, when a treatment

Table 1
Methodological aspects of studies having assessed the efficacy of CBT for insomnia among patients with cancer

Authors,[Ref,] Year	N[a]	Study Design	Patients	Inclusion Criteria for Clinical Insomnia	Treatment Duration	Treatment Components (SC, SR, SH, CR, Re)	Therapists	Main Sleep Measures	Time Assessments
RCT									
Berger et al,[56,61] 2009	219	Individual BT-I (n = 113) Healthy eating (n = 106)	Breast cancer Undergoing tx	No	8–12 sessions of 15–90 min Total of 5.5 h of clinical contact in 6.3 sessions on average, over 3 mo	SC, SR, SH, Re	Research nurse	*Subjective:* sleep diary, PSQI *Objective:* Actigraphy	Pre-CTX; After each CTX; 1, 2, 3, and 12-mo FU (after last CTX)
Epstein & Dirksen,[87] 2007	81	Group CBT-I (n = 40) Group sleep education and hygiene (n = 41)	Breast cancer 3 mo to 31 y post-dx	Yes	4 sessions of 1–2 h plus 2 telephone sessions of 0.5–1 h over 6 wk	SC, SR, SH	Clinical nurse	*Subjective:* Sleep diary; 4 items assessing sleep improvement *Objective:* Actigraphy	Pre-tx; Post-tx
Espie et al,[55] 2008	150	Group CBT-I (n = 100) Treatment as usual (n = 50)	Breast, prostate, bowel, or gynecologic cancer ≥1 mo post-tx (median = 23.5–33.5 mo)	Yes	5 weekly sessions of 50 min	SC, SR, SH, CR, Re	Cancer nurse	*Subjective:* Sleep diary *Objective:* Actigraphy	Pre-tx; Post-tx; 6-mo FU
Fiorentino et al,[58] 2009	21 (5 patients excluded postrandomization)	*Crossover design* Individual CBT-I (n = 8) Waiting list, 6 wk (n = 8)	Breast cancer 5 mo to 24 y post-tx	Yes	6 weekly 1-h sessions	SC, SR, SH, CR, Re	Not provided	*Subjective:* Sleep diary; ISI; PSQI *Other:* sleep medication form *Objective:* Actigraphy	Pre-tx/pre-waiting; Weekly during tx/waiting; Post-tx/Post-waiting; 6-wk FU
Savard et al,[54] 2005	58	Group CBT-I (n = 28) Waiting list (n = 30)	Breast cancer ≥1 mo post-tx (mean = 30.7 mo)	Yes	8 weekly sessions of 90 min plus 1 optional booster session	SC, SR, SH, CR	Master's level psychologist	*Subjective:* Sleep diary, ISI *Objective:* Laboratory PSG	Pre-tx/pre-waiting; Post-tx/Post-waiting; 3, 6, and 12-mo FU
Non-RTC									
Berger et al,[60] 2002	25	Feasibility study; single group design with repeated measurement Individual BT-I	Breast cancer Undergoing tx	(patients with chronic insomnia were excluded)	8 sessions (no duration provided) over 4 cycles of chemotherapy	SC, SR, SH, Re	Research assistant	*Subjective:* Sleep diary, PSQI *Objective:* Actigraphy	Days -2 to +7 of each 4 cycles of CTX

Study	Sample size	Design	Cancer type	RCT	Session format	Components	Therapist	Measures	Assessment
Davidson et al,[57] 2001	14	Single group design with repeated measurement Group CBT-I (n = 14)	Various types of cancer ≥1 mo post-tx (median = 20.8 mo)	Yes	6 sessions of 1–1.5 h over 8 wk	SC, SH, CR, Re	Two doctoral students in clinical psychology	*Subjective*: Sleep diary, ISI	Pre-tx; Week 4 (during tx); Week 8 (last tx session)
Quesnel et al,[59] 2003	10	Multiple baseline A-B experimental design Group CBT-I (n = 10)	Breast cancer ≥1 mo post-tx (mean = 52.3 mo)	Yes	8 weekly sessions of 90 min plus 1 optional booster session	SC, SR, SH, CR	Master's level psychologist	*Subjective*: Sleep diary, ISI *Objective*: Laboratory PSG	Baseline (3–10 wk); Post-tx; 3 and 6 mo FU
Simeit et al,[68] 2004	229	Three nonrandomized groups with repeated measurement Progressive muscle relaxation + BT (n = 80) Autogenic training + BT (n = 71) Treatment as usual (n = 78)	Various types of cancer 10.7 mo post-dx on average	Yes	3 1-h sessions	SC, SH, Re	Not provided	*Subjective*: PSQI	Pre-tx; Post-tx; 6-wk FU; 6-mo FU
Self-Help Treatment									
Ritterband et al,[73] 2012	28	RCT Online CBT-I (n = 14) Control (n = 14)	Various types of cancer ≥1 mo post-tx (mean = 3.9 y)	Yes	6 interactive cores (45–60 min each) over 6–9 wk	SC, SR, SH, CR	N/A	*Subjective*: Online sleep diary; ISI	Pre-tx; Post-tx
Savard et al,[72] 2011	11	Single group design with repeated measurement Self-administered CBT-I (n = 11)	Breast cancer From 21 d after radiotherapy initiation to 60 d post-tx	Yes	60-min video plus 6 short booklets over 6–8 wk	SC, SR, SH, CR	N/A	*Subjective*: Sleep diary; ISI	Pre-tx; Post-tx; 3-mo FU

Abbreviations: BT-I, behavioral therapy for insomnia; CBT-I, cognitive-behavioral therapy for insomnia; CR, cognitive restructuring; CTX, chemotherapy; dx, diagnostic; FU, follow-up; ISI, Insomnia Severity Index; N/A, not available; PSG, polysomnography; PSQI, Pittsburgh Sleep Quality Index; RCT, randomized controlled trial; Re, relaxation; SC, stimulus control; SH, sleep hygiene; SR, sleep restriction; tx, treatment.

a The sample size reported here is the total number at randomization; the final sample size used for the statistical analyses may vary.

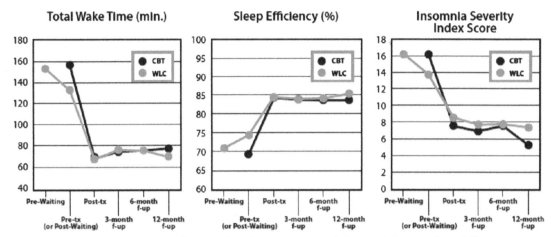

Fig. 1. Findings from Savard and colleagues (2005). CBT, cognitive-behavioral therapy; f-up, follow-up; post-tx, posttreatment; pre-tx, pretreatment; WLC, waiting-list control condition. (*Adapted from* Savard J, Simard S, Hervouet S, et al. Insomnia in men treated with radical prostatectomy for prostate cancer. Psychooncology 2005;14:147–56.)

is initiated it is often a pharmacologic one that is chosen,[70] despite the well-known limitations of such an approach. Cancer care providers are commonly unaware of the existence of effective nonpharmacologic options for insomnia, and these alternatives are rarely available in their clinical setting. Indeed, there are very few psychosocial oncology professionals who have the necessary training to administer CBT for insomnia. Even when such resources are available they are habitually insufficient to meet all needs, given the high prevalence of insomnia symptoms in this population.

One obvious solution would be to train more mental health care providers in the administration

of CBT for insomnia. Clinical workshops given in psychosocial oncology meetings may be a way to achieve this goal. However, offering professional training is not a panacea. Many patients with cancer do not have any access to mental health professionals because they live too far away from cancer centers or have limited financial resources. In addition, the significant number of sessions that usually comprise CBT for insomnia, and costs associated with it, preclude its implementation as part of routine cancer care. Finally, some patients are reluctant to meet with a mental health cancer care provider to treat a sleep problem.

Efficacy of self-help CBT for insomnia

For all aforementioned reasons, it is imperative to develop alternatives to face-to-face sessions for the treatment of insomnia in patients with cancer. Self-help interventions for primary insomnia have received increased empirical support in recent years, with effects that have been found to be similar to those associated with professionally administered treatments.[71] Whereas early studies investigated more traditional forms of self-help treatments (ie, bibliotherapy), more recent ones have evaluated the feasibility and efficacy of interventions using new technologies (see **Table 1**).

In the context of cancer, 2 such studies have been published. The first was conducted by the authors' group, and evaluated the feasibility of a video-based CBT for insomnia in 11 patients with breast cancer who had completed their radiation therapy.[72] All patients received the intervention, which comprised a 60-minute animated video and 6 short booklets covering stimulus control,

---

Box 4
Avenues for future research on cancer-related insomnia

- Evaluate the efficacy of CBT for insomnia:

  ○ In patients undergoing treatment

  ○ In males and patients with cancer types other than breast

  ○ In patients with advanced cancer

- Assess the possible added value of integrating treatment components targeting symptoms potentially involved in insomnia etiology (eg, hot flashes, pain, fatigue)

- Investigate the effectiveness of minimal CBT for insomnia and stepped-care models

- Compare the efficacy of alternative interventions (exercise, yoga) with that of CBT for insomnia

sleep restriction, cognitive restructuring, and sleep hygiene. Overall, results indicated that patients were highly satisfied with the treatment they received, its content, and the sleep improvements that stemmed from it. Preliminary efficacy data also indicated the presence of statistically and clinically significant improvements after treatment on sleep diary parameters, which were maintained at a 3-month follow-up. More recently, Ritterband and colleagues[73] conducted a small-scale RCT in 28 patients with mixed cancer sites. Half of the patients were randomized to an Internet-based CBT for insomnia (called Sleep Healthy Using the Internet, or SHUTi) while the other 14 were assigned to a waiting-list control condition. The intervention was composed of 6 interactive cores (45–60 minutes each) combining stimulus control, sleep restriction, cognitive restructuring, and sleep hygiene strategies. Significantly larger sleep improvements, as assessed with a sleep diary and the ISI, were found in the CBT group when compared with the control group after treatment. A greater reduction in fatigue scores was also observed.

Together, these preliminary findings suggest that CBT for insomnia can be delivered efficaciously to patients with cancer through the use of new technologies. However, these encouraging results need to be confirmed in larger RCTs. Comparisons with more traditional, professionally administered forms of CBT for insomnia are especially warranted. In addition, it would be important to investigate whether there are individuals for whom such self-help interventions are not as beneficial. Indeed, although self-administered CBT for insomnia appears to be efficacious in general, this treatment modality may not be appropriate or optimal for all patients. A recently completed RCT by the authors randomized 242 patients with breast cancer who had just completed their radiation therapy to 1 of 3 groups: (1) 6 weekly sessions of professionally administered CBT for insomnia; (2) video-based CBT for insomnia as described above; (3) no treatment. Preliminary findings of this trial, of which analysis is still ongoing, suggest that patients with more severe insomnia (ISI score ≥ 15) at baseline were much less likely to become good sleepers (ISI score <8) following a video-based CBT for insomnia than when receiving face-to-face sessions (21% vs 50%).[74] Many other variables could negatively affect the response to a self-help intervention, and need to be studied. These factors include some demographic characteristics (eg, age, education), health literacy (ie, the basic set of skills to seek, understand, and use health information), self-efficacy, and the level of comfort with new technologies. More information on the effect of such variables is critical to be able to target specific subgroups of patients more likely to benefit from a self-help approach.

Stepped-care model: the ultimate approach to make CBT for insomnia more accessible

As more information becomes available on variables that have some impact on treatment response associated with self-help CBT for insomnia, it will undoubtedly become clear that such minimal interventions should not be considered a complete substitute for a professionally administered treatment. A stepped-care approach has recently been proposed as an ideal delivery model for making CBT for insomnia more accessible.[75] Typically the entry level is a minimal intervention (eg, self-administered). Patients who go into remission following such minimal treatment receive no further treatment, whereas others "step up" to a more intense form (eg, professionally administered sessions). Thus, more intensive treatments are reserved for people who do not benefit from simpler first-line treatments, or for those not expected to benefit right away from such treatments.[76] Consequently, treatment costs are significantly reduced and resource allocation in therapy is maximized.[77] Although a stepped-care model seems feasible and cost-effective for the administration of CBT for insomnia in the context of cancer, its efficacy and cost-effectiveness need to be established before it is integrated in routine care.

OTHER NONPHARMACOLOGIC OPTIONS

A few other nonpharmacologic options have been tested for improving the sleep of patients with cancer, among which exercise interventions have received the greatest attention. This alternative is an interesting one, given all the other positive effects regular exercising can have on the health of cancer patients (eg, body-weight reduction, increased physical fitness and functioning, decreased psychological distress, improved quality of life). Nevertheless, RCTs on the effect of exercise on sleep quality in patients with cancer have revealed mixed findings, with some studies showing benefits[78–80] while others did not.[81,82] Yoga and mindfulness-based stress reduction (MBSR) interventions have also received some support,[83–85] although effects on sleep have been considered to be small and nonsignificant in a recent meta-analysis.[86]

Most of these studies were conducted in patients with subclinical sleep disturbances at baseline, so it is unknown whether these interventions are potent enough to treat clinical insomnia. In the study by Courneya and colleagues,[81] an aerobic exercise intervention was not associated with greater sleep improvements on the PSQI in comparison with a usual care condition when analyzing the total sample of patients with lymphoma, of whom approximately 50% were good sleepers at baseline. However, a subgroup analysis showed a between-group difference on sleep improvements in patients who were poor sleepers at baseline. Although these findings appear to suggest that exercise programs are effective in patients who have clinical insomnia, there is other evidence indicating that exercise may not be sufficient. In a study investigating a walking exercise intervention that selected exclusively patients with poor sleep at baseline,[79] a significantly greater reduction of PSQI scores at 1-month and 2-month assessments was found in comparison with usual care, but the mean PSQI remained in the clinical range at both time points (at 1 month 10.7 and at 2 months 9.8, compared with 13.4 at baseline).

Moreover, no study has yet been published comparing the efficacy of exercise and yoga/MBSR interventions with that of more established treatments such as CBT for insomnia. This aspect is important because these less specific approaches may lead to some improvements in sleep quality in comparison with a no-treatment condition, but the gains achieved may remain lower than what is obtained with CBT for insomnia.

SUMMARY

Research on insomnia comorbid with cancer has flourished in the past decade. The high prevalence and persistence of the insomnia problem has been well established and, although more work is certainly needed, available findings have provided a better understanding of the factors that are associated with its incidence and persistence in the context of cancer. CBT has been found to be efficacious in RCTs, and is increasingly recognized as the treatment of choice for insomnia therapy in oncology. However, some subgroups of patients have been understudied (eg, males, patients with cancer types other than breast cancer, patients with advanced cancer), and should be the focus of future work. Moreover, the accessibility to CBT for insomnia is extremely limited. This problem may be resolved through the use of self-help treatments and stepped-care models, but the effectiveness of these approaches needs to be ascertained before they are integrated into routine care.

REFERENCES

1. Savard J, Morin CM. Insomnia in the context of cancer: a review of a neglected problem. J Clin Oncol 2001;19:895–908.
2. Fiorentino L, Ancoli-Israel S. Sleep dysfunction in patients with cancer. Curr Treat Options Neurol 2007;9:337–46.
3. Savard J, Ancoli-Israel S. Sleep and fatigue in cancer patients. In: Kryger MH, Roth T, Dement WC, editors. Principles and practice of sleep medicine. 5th edition. St Louis (MO): Elsevier Saunders; 2011. p. 1416–21.
4. Fiorentino L, Ancoli-Israel S. Insomnia and its treatment in women with breast cancer. Sleep Med Rev 2006;10:419–29.
5. Kvale EA, Shuster JL. Sleep disturbance in supportive care of cancer: a review. J Palliat Med 2006;9:437–50.
6. Parish JM. Sleep-related problems in common medical conditions. Chest 2009;135:563–72.
7. Berger AM. Update on the state of the science: sleep-wake disturbances in adult patients with cancer. Oncol Nurs Forum 2009;36:E165–77.
8. Ancoli-Israel S, Moores R, Moores J. Recognition and treatment of sleep disturbances in cancer. J Clin Oncol 2009;27:5864–6.
9. Savard J, Villa J, Ivers H, et al. Prevalence, natural course, and risk factors of insomnia comorbid with cancer over a 2-month period. J Clin Oncol 2009; 27:5233–9.
10. Savard J, Ivers H, Villa J, et al. Natural course of insomnia comorbid with cancer: an 18-month longitudinal study. J Clin Oncol 2011;29:3580–6.
11. LeBlanc M, Merette C, Savard J, et al. Incidence and risk factors of insomnia in a population-based sample. Sleep 2009;32:1027–37.
12. Palesh OG, Roscoe JA, Mustian KM, et al. Prevalence, demographics, and psychological associations of sleep disruption in patients with cancer: University of Rochester Cancer Center-Community Clinical Oncology Program. J Clin Oncol 2010;28:292–8.
13. Bernatchez MS, Savard J, Ivers H. Prevalence and evolution of insomnia among advanced cancer patients. 26th Annual Conference of the Canadian Association of Psychosocial Oncology. Toronto, May 2013.
14. Akechi T, Okuyama T, Akizuki N, et al. Associated and predictive factors of sleep disturbance in advanced cancer patients. Psychooncology 2007; 16:888–94.
15. Spielman AJ, Glovinsky P. Case studies in insomnia. In: Hauri PJ, editor. The varied nature of insomnia. New York: Plenum Press; 1991. p. 1–15.
16. Davidson JR, MacLean AW, Brundage MD, et al. Sleep disturbance in cancer patients. Soc Sci Med 2002;54:1309–21.

17. Palesh OG, Peppone L, Innominato P, et al. Prevalence, putative mechanisms and management of sleep problems during chemotherapy for cancer. Nat Sci Sleep 2012;4:151–62.

18. Desai K, Mao JJ, Su I, et al. Prevalence and risk factors for insomnia among breast cancer patients on aromatase inhibitors. Support Care Cancer 2013;21:43–51.

19. Savard J, Simard S, Hervouet S, et al. Insomnia in men treated with radical prostatectomy for prostate cancer. Psychooncology 2005;14:147–56.

20. Ginsburg ML, Quirt C, Ginsburg AD, et al. Psychiatric illness and psychosocial concerns of patients with newly diagnosed lung cancer. CMAJ 1995; 152:701–9.

21. Morin CM. Insomnia: psychological assessment and management. New York: The Guilford Press; 1993.

22. Van Onselen C, Paul SM, Lee K, et al. Trajectories of sleep disturbance and daytime sleepiness in women before and after surgery for breast cancer. J Pain Symptom Manage 2013;45:244–60.

23. Forsberg C, Bjorvell H, Cedermark B. Well-being and its relation to coping ability in patients with colo-rectal and gastric cancer before and after surgery. Scand J Caring Sci 1996;10:35–44.

24. Sheely LC. Sleep disturbances in hospitalized patients with cancer. Oncol Nurs Forum 1996;23: 109–11.

25. Enderlin CA, Coleman EA, Cole C, et al. Sleep across chemotherapy treatment: a growing concern for women older than 50 with breast cancer. Oncol Nurs Forum 2010;37:461–A3.

26. Beck SL, Berger AM, Barsevick AM, et al. Sleep quality after initial chemotherapy for breast cancer. Support Care Cancer 2010;18:679–89.

27. Chen ML, Yu CT, Yang CH. Sleep disturbances and quality of life in lung cancer patients undergoing chemotherapy. Lung Cancer 2008;62:391–400.

28. Savard J, Liu L, Natarajan L, et al. Breast cancer patients have progressively impaired sleep-wake activity rhythms during chemotherapy. Sleep 2009;32:1155–60.

29. Cassileth PA, Lusk EJ, Torri S, et al. Antiemetic efficacy of dexamethasone therapy in patients receiving cancer chemotherapy. Arch Intern Med 1983;143:1347–9.

30. Ling MH, Perry PJ, Tsuang MT. Side effects of corticosteroid therapy: psychiatric aspects. Arch Gen Psychiatry 1981;38:471–7.

31. Savard J, Hervouet S, Ivers H. Prostate cancer treatments and their side effects are associated with increased insomnia. Psychooncology 2012 Aug 8. http://dx.doi.org/10.1002/pon.3150. [Epub ahead of print].

32. Savard MH, Savard J, Trudel-Fitzgerald C, et al. Changes in hot flashes are associated with concurrent changes in insomnia symptoms among breast cancer patients. Menopause 2011;18:985–93.

33. Savard J, Davidson JR, Ivers H, et al. The association between nocturnal hot flashes and sleep in breast cancer survivors. J Pain Symptom Manage 2004;27:513–22.

34. Savard MH, Savard J, Caplette-Gingras A, et al. Relationship between objectively recorded hot flashes and sleep disturbances among breast cancer patients: investigating hot flash characteristics other than frequency. Menopause 2013 Apr 29. [Epub ahead of print].

35. Trudel-Fitzgerald C, Savard J, Ivers H. Which symptoms come first? Exploration of temporal relationships between cancer-related symptoms over an 18-month period. Ann Behav Med 2013 Jun; 45(3):329–37.

36. Kamath J. Cancer-related fatigue, inflammation and thyrotropin-releasing hormone. Curr Aging Sci 2012;5:195–202.

37. Wood LJ, Weymann K. Inflammation and neural signaling: etiologic mechanisms of the cancer treatment-related symptom cluster. Curr Opin Support Palliat Care 2013;7:54–9.

38. Belgrade MJ. Control of pain in cancer patients. Postgrad Med 1989;85:319–29.

39. Portenoy RK, Miransky J, Thaler HT, et al. Pain in ambulatory patients with lung or colon cancer. Cancer 1992;70:1616–24.

40. Taddeini L, Rotschafer JC. Pain syndromes associated with cancer. Postgrad Med 1984;75:101–8.

41. Buffum D, Koetters T, Cho M, et al. The effects of pain, gender, and age on sleep/wake and circadian rhythm parameters in oncology patients at the initiation of radiation therapy. J Pain 2011;12:390–400.

42. Sharma N, Hansen CH, O'Connor M, et al. Sleep problems in cancer patients: prevalence and association with distress and pain. Psychooncology 2013;21:1003–9.

43. Palesh OG, Collie K, Batiuchok D, et al. A longitudinal study of depression, pain, and stress as predictors of sleep disturbance among women with metastatic breast cancer. Biol Psychol 2007; 75:37–44.

44. Zeitzer JM, Bliwise DL, Hernandez B, et al. Nocturia compounds nocturnal wakefulness in older individuals with insomnia. J Clin Sleep Med 2013;9: 259–62.

45. Hanisch LJ, Gooneratne NS, Soin K, et al. Sleep and daily functioning during androgen deprivation therapy for prostate cancer. Eur J Cancer Care 2011;20:549–54.

46. Ozturk A, Sarihan S, Ercan I, et al. Evaluating quality of life and pulmonary function of long-term survivors of non-small cell lung cancer treated with radical or postoperative radiotherapy. Am J Clin Oncol 2009;32:65–72.

47. American Psychiatric Association. Diagnostic and statistical manual of mental disorders, text revision. 4th edition. Washington, DC: American Psychiatric Association; 2000.

48. Breitbart W, Cohen KR. Delirium. In: Holland JC, editor. Psycho-oncology. New York: Oxford University Press; 1998. p. 564–75.

49. Graydon JE, Bubela N, Irvine D, et al. Fatigue-reducing strategies used by patients receiving treatment for cancer. Cancer Nurs 1995;18:23–8.

50. Irvine DM, Vincent L, Graydon JE, et al. Fatigue in women with breast cancer receiving radiation therapy. Cancer Nurs 1998;21:127–35.

51. Richardson A, Ream EK. Self-care behaviours initiated by chemotherapy patients in response to fatigue. Int J Nurs Stud 1997;34:35–43.

52. Howell D, Oliver TK, Keller-Olaman S, et al. A Pan-Canadian practice guideline: Prevention, screening, assessment, and treatment of sleep disturbances in adults with cancer. Supportive Care in Cancer 2013 May 25. [Epub ahead of print].

53. Langford DJ, Lee K, Miaskowski C. Sleep disturbance interventions in oncology patients and family caregivers: a comprehensive review and meta-analysis. Sleep Med Rev 2012;16:397–414.

54. Savard J, Simard S, Ivers H, et al. Randomized study on the efficacy of cognitive-behavioral therapy for insomnia secondary to breast cancer, part I: sleep and psychological effects. J Clin Oncol 2005;23:6083–95.

55. Espie CA, Fleming L, Cassidy J, et al. Randomized controlled clinical effectiveness trial of cognitive behavior therapy compared with treatment as usual for persistent insomnia in patients with cancer. J Clin Oncol 2008;26:4651–8.

56. Berger AM, Kuhn BR, Farr LA, et al. One-year outcomes of a behavioral therapy intervention trial on sleep quality and cancer-related fatigue. J Clin Oncol 2009;27:6033–40.

57. Davidson JR, Waisberg JL, Brundage MD, et al. Nonpharmacologic group treatment of insomnia: a preliminary study with cancer survivors. Psychooncology 2001;10:389–97.

58. Fiorentino L, McQuaid JR, Liu L, et al. Individual cognitive behavioral therapy for insomnia in breast cancer survivors: a randomized controlled cross-over pilot study. Nat Sci Sleep 2009;2010:1–8.

59. Quesnel C, Savard J, Simard S, et al. Efficacy of cognitive-behavioral therapy for insomnia in women treated for nonmetastatic breast cancer. J Consult Clin Psychol 2003;71:189–200.

60. Berger AM, VonEssen S, Khun BR, et al. Feasibility of a sleep intervention during adjuvant breast cancer chemotherapy. Oncol Nurs Forum 2002;29:1431–41.

61. Berger AM, Kuhn BR, Farr LA, et al. Behavioral therapy intervention trial to improve sleep quality and cancer-related fatigue. Psychooncology 2009;18:634–46.

62. Parker KP, Bliwise DL, Ribeiro M, et al. Sleep/wake patterns of individuals with advanced cancer measured by ambulatory polysomnography. J Clin Oncol 2008;26:2464–72.

63. Vena C, Parker K, Allen R, et al. Sleep-wake disturbances and quality of life in patients with advanced lung cancer. Oncol Nurs Forum 2006;33:761–9.

64. Glare P, Walsh D, Sheehan D. The adverse effects of morphine: a prospective survey of common symptoms during repeated dosing for chronic cancer pain. Am J Hosp Palliat Care 2006;23:229–35.

65. McCurry SM, Pike KC, Vitiello MV, et al. Increasing walking and bright light exposure to improve sleep in community-dwelling persons with Alzheimer's disease: results of a randomized, controlled trial. J Am Geriatr Soc 2011;59:1393–402.

66. McCurry SM, Gibbons LE, Logsdon RG, et al. Nighttime insomnia treatment and education for Alzheimer's disease: a randomized, controlled trial. J Am Geriatr Soc 2005;53:793–802.

67. Alessi CA, Martin JL, Webber AP, et al. Randomized, controlled trial of a nonpharmacological intervention to improve abnormal sleep/wake patterns in nursing home residents. J Am Geriatr Soc 2005;53:803–10.

68. Simeit R, Deck R, Conta-Marx B. Sleep management training for cancer patients with insomnia. Support Care Cancer 2004;12:176–83.

69. Mann E, Smith MJ, Hellier J, et al. Cognitive behavioural treatment for women who have menopausal symptoms after breast cancer treatment (MENOS 1): a randomised controlled trial. Lancet Oncol 2012;13:309–18.

70. Casault L, Savard J, Ivers H, et al. Utilization of hypnotic medication in the context of cancer: predictors and frequency of use. Support Care Cancer 2012;20:1203–10.

71. van Straten A, Cuijpers P. Self-help therapy for insomnia: a meta-analysis. Sleep Med Rev 2009;13:61–71.

72. Savard J, Villa J, Simard S, et al. Feasibility of a self-help treatment for insomnia comorbid with cancer. Psychooncology 2011;20:1013–9.

73. Ritterband LM, Bailey ET, Thorndike FP, et al. Initial evaluation of an internet intervention to improve the sleep of cancer survivors with insomnia. Psychooncology 2012;21:695–705.

74. Savard J, Ivers H, Savard MH, et al. Is a video-based cognitive-behavioral therapy as efficacious as a professionally-administered treatment for insomnia comorbid with cancer? Preliminary results of a randomized controlled trial, 10th conference of the American Psychosocial Oncology Society. Huntington Beach (CA): 2013.

75. Espie CA. Stepped care: a health technology solution for delivering cognitive behavioral therapy as a first line insomnia treatment. Sleep 2009;32: 1549–58.

76. Newman MG. Recommendations for a cost-offset model of psychotherapy allocation using generalized anxiety disorder as an example. J Consult Clin Psychol 2000;68:549–55.

77. Haaga DA. Introduction to the special section on stepped care models in psychotherapy. J Consult Clin Psychol 2000;68:547–8.

78. Payne JK, Held J, Thorpe J, et al. Effect of exercise on biomarkers, fatigue, sleep disturbances, and depressive symptoms in older women with breast cancer receiving hormonal therapy. Oncol Nurs Forum 2008;35:635–42.

79. Tang MF, Liou TH, Lin CC. Improving sleep quality for cancer patients: benefits of a home-based exercise intervention. Support Care Cancer 2010;18: 1329–39.

80. Wang YJ, Boehmke M, Wu YW, et al. Effects of a 6-week walking program on Taiwanese women newly diagnosed with early-stage breast cancer. Cancer Nurs 2011;34:E1–13.

81. Courneya KS, Sellar CM, Trinh L, et al. A randomized trial of aerobic exercise and sleep quality in lymphoma patients receiving chemotherapy or no treatments. Cancer Epidemiol Biomarkers Prev 2012;21:887–94.

82. Dodd MJ, Cho MH, Miaskowski C, et al. A randomized controlled trial of home-based exercise for cancer-related fatigue in women during and after chemotherapy with or without radiation therapy. Cancer Nurs 2010;33:245–57.

83. Andersen SR, Wurtzen H, Steding-Jessen M, et al. Effect of mindfulness-based stress reduction on sleep quality: results of a randomized trial among Danish breast cancer patients. Acta Oncol 2013; 52:336–44.

84. Carson JW, Carson KM, Porter LS, et al. Yoga of Awareness program for menopausal symptoms in breast cancer survivors: results from a randomized trial. Support Care Cancer 2009;17: 1301–9.

85. Cohen L, Warneke C, Fouladi RT, et al. Psychological adjustment and sleep quality in a randomized trial of the effects of a Tibetan yoga intervention in patients with lymphoma. Cancer 2004;100: 2253–60.

86. Buffart LM, van Uffelen JG, Riphagen II, et al. Physical and psychosocial benefits of yoga in cancer patients and survivors, a systematic review and meta-analysis of randomized controlled trials. BMC Cancer 2012;12:559–80.

87. Esptein DR, Dirksen SR. Randomized trial of a cognitive-behavioral intervention for insomnia in breast cancer survivors. Oncology Nursing Forum 2007;34:E51–9.

Insomnia and Obstructive Sleep Apnea

Jason C. Ong, PhD*, Megan R. Crawford, PhD

KEYWORDS

- Obstructive sleep apnea • Insomnia • Comorbidity

KEY POINTS

- The comorbidity between insomnia and obstructive sleep apnea (OSA) is highly prevalent in patients presenting to sleep clinics and is associated with significant morbidity.
- Sleep clinicians should conduct comprehensive evaluations for both OSA and insomnia regardless of the presenting complaint.
- Patient management should include considerations to both OSA and insomnia treatments.

INTRODUCTION

With more than 80 distinct sleep disorders classified in the International Classification of Sleep Disorders (ICSD-2[1]), comorbidity of sleep disorders has emerged as an important topic with clinical and research significance. In particular, obstructive sleep apnea (OSA) and insomnia are 2 sleep disorders that co-occur frequently, involve clinical features and associations that are distinct from the separate conditions, and are treatable. OSA, which affects about 10% to 20% of middle to older aged adults,[2] is characterized by the repeated obstruction of the upper airway during sleep that leads to complete cessation (apnea) or reduction (hyperpnea) of airflow, occurring irrespective of continued ventilatory effort. Before termination, these events lead to a decrease in blood oxygen saturation and an associated increase in carbon dioxide levels during longer events. The termination of the apnea is often preceded by an arousal, which leads to sleep fragmentation and activation of the sympathetic nervous system. The former is hypothesized to be involved in the neurocognitive sequelae, whereas the latter leads to cardiovascular dysregulation. This process is identified as the possible cause for the daytime sleepiness and cardiovascular health and functioning problems witnessed in these individuals.[3–7] Severe OSA has been linked to a 4- to 6-fold increased risk of mortality, irrespective of factors such as age, diabetes, or high cholesterol.[8,9]

Symptoms of insomnia include difficulty initiating and/or maintaining sleep, waking too early, and/or nonrestorative sleep. When the nocturnal symptoms are associated with significant distress or daytime dysfunction and last for at least 3 months, the condition is considered an insomnia disorder.[10] As a result of evolving diagnostic criteria for insomnia, there are large variations in the cited prevalence rates of these types of sleep difficulties, ranging from around 6% to 30%.[11–13] The pathophysiology of insomnia is thought to involve hyperarousal in the form of cognitive arousal (eg, increased cognitive activity or negative tone of cognitions) and physiologic arousal (eg, elevations in core body temperature, muscle tension, and sympathetic activation).[14] The most frequently cited consequences of insomnia are the reduction in quality of life and productivity, and increased risk of accidents, and absenteeism.[13,15] Insomnia may also be a risk factor for various psychiatric

Preparation of this article was supported in part by a research grant from the National Heart, Lung, Blood Institute (NHLBI) awarded to the first author (R01HL114529).
Department of Behavioral Science, Rush University Medical Center, 710 South Paulina Street, Suite 600, Chicago, IL 60612, USA
* Corresponding author.
E-mail address: jason_ong@rush.edu

conditions[16,17] and health problems such as hypertension,[18] type 2 diabetes,[19] and even mortality after controlling for hypertension and diabetes.[20]

The co-occurrence of both conditions was first described in 1973 by Guilleminault and colleagues,[21] who reported on 3 individual cases who presented to the sleep laboratory for evaluation of insomnia and were subsequently investigated for sleep-disordered breathing. More recently, the comorbidity between sleep apnea and insomnia has garnered increased research and clinical interest, likely resulting from a paradigm shift in how insomnia is conceptualized. Whereas insomnia was previously considered secondary to a primary condition, a consensus statement released by the US National Institutes of Health[22] regards insomnia as a distinct disorder that can also be comorbid to another condition. This conceptualization challenges the traditional assumption that insomnia is merely a symptom of another condition, and allows for a separate diagnosis of "comorbid insomnia" even in the context of another sleep disorder such as sleep apnea.

Diagnosing comorbid insomnia in the context of another sleep disorder can be challenging, as there can be overlap in the complaint of sleep disturbance (eg, difficulty maintaining sleep) and daytime dysfunction (eg, daytime fatigue). Moreover, our understanding of the mechanisms involved in the comorbid relationship remains very limited. Even well-trained clinicians cannot make reliable distinctions with regard to the attribution of insomnia symptoms.[23] As a response, recent recommendations[10,24] enable a diagnosis of an insomnia disorder without attributing the causal relationship between the symptoms and the co-occurring disorder. In the *Diagnostic and Statistical Manual of Mental Disorders*, fifth edition (DSM-V), specifiers are used with an insomnia disorder to note the comorbid condition rather than attempting to assign causal attributions, as was the case in previous classification systems such as DSM-IV (ie, primary vs secondary insomnia). With these shifts in conceptualization and nosology, several research studies focusing on the insomnia/OSA comorbidity have emerged. This growing body of literature is shaping our understanding of the relationship, consequences, and treatment implications of comorbid insomnia and sleep apnea.

This review of the literature is organized on the basis of the progression of research on the comorbidity between insomnia and sleep apnea. First, clinical features and associations with this comorbidity are discussed, much of which has been informed by cross-sectional studies. Second, the authors discuss models of pathogenesis that have been proposed in the literature. Here, emerging data from longitudinal studies and relevant retrospective studies that are capable of examining the time course of the two disorders are highlighted. Finally, the clinical implications of this review are discussed, and suggestions are made regarding future research.

CLINICAL FEATURES AND ASSOCIATIONS

Given that most patients are not aware of the classification of sleep disorders or possible comorbidity, the rates of comorbidity can depend on the chief complaint (**Table 1**). Among individuals with a presenting complaint related to sleep apnea (eg, snoring, excessive daytime sleepiness, nocturnal breathing issues), the co-occurrence of insomnia varies between 6% and 84%.[25–30,33,35,36,40,42,43] By contrast, in those seeking evaluation for insomnia, rates of co-occurring sleep apnea ranged from 7% to 69%.[31,32,34,37–39,41] Of note, these reports may underestimate the true rates of comorbidity. These prevalence rates have emerged largely from samples that were excluded from the primary study because of the comorbid sleep apnea as determined through polysomnography. These rates often do not include those who present with clinical symptoms of sleep apnea who are excluded during previous screenings. For example, in one such study 17% of the recruited sample were excluded because of witness apneas and snoring or sleepiness during telephone/hospital interviews.[37] The variability in rates is likely affected by several other factors. First, the criteria for insomnia vary across studies. When insomnia is defined as the presence of at least 1 nocturnal symptom (onset, maintenance difficulties, or early morning awakening), rates are higher (6%–84%)[25–27,29,33,35,42,43] than if insomnia is classified as nighttime symptoms with concomitant daytime dysfunction that would justify a diagnosis of insomnia disorder (21%–39%).[28,40] The discrepancy might also vary according to insomnia subtypes (ie, difficulty falling asleep vs difficulty maintaining sleep). In a group of 157 individuals referred to a sleep clinic for suspected OSA, more individuals reported problems with sleep maintenance or waking too early (26% and 19%, respectively) relative to difficulties falling asleep (6%).[29] Subsequent studies (eg, Refs.[26,27,33]) have found similar differences across subtypes, suggesting different etiologic pathways. Finally, rates of insomnia vary as a function of OSA severity. However, results are in conflict with some that have shown a strong positive relationship between severity and prevalence of insomnia,[33] whereas others have not.[27,36]

Several cross-sectional studies also shed light on some of the clinical features of these comorbid conditions. As with the prevalence rates, the features differ as a function of the "primary" condition. Individuals with a primary complaint of OSA were more likely female,[26,36,42–45] had more dysfunctional beliefs about sleep,[40,46] were more likely to present with restless legs syndrome,[26,35,36] and reported less alcohol use[36] compared with OSA-only individuals. In individuals with a primary complaint of insomnia, patients were more likely than those without OSA to be male,[37,39] have a higher body mass index,[31,32,34,37,39] be older,[31,39] and have more daytime and nighttime nocturnal symptoms consistent with OSA.[32,34] These findings suggest that the patient's chief complaint (OSA or insomnia) might yield different clinical considerations, and that secondary complaints should be fully explored.

In addition to clinical features, comorbidity of insomnia and sleep apnea is associated with increased morbidity and impairment. In this regard the literature suggests that concurrent insomnia and OSA increase risks for depression or other comorbid psychiatric conditions,[35,36,40,43] medical conditions such as chronic pain,[36] cardiovascular disease (hypertension and congestive heart failure),[43] reduced quality of life,[26] functional impairment,[32] sleepiness (only found in sleep maintenance insomnia),[26,29] and absenteeism from work.[47] Because the majority of these findings are from cross-sectional data, it is unclear as to whether the increased morbidity is a cause or a consequence of the comorbidity of insomnia and OSA.

The presence of both OSA and insomnia can also have a negative impact on the treatment process and outcomes. Specifically, the presence of insomnia can negatively affect treatment outcomes of OSA. In 20 OSA patients who were unsuccessfully treated with a mandibular advancement device, Machado and colleagues[48] reported 'that the presence of insomnia was the only significant predictor of nonimprovement. Other studies have examined the impact of insomnia on adherence to continuous positive airway pressure (CPAP). Wickwire and colleagues[49] conducted a retrospective chart review of 232 OSA patients who had been prescribed CPAP and had provided information on possible insomnia symptoms. After controlling for age and gender, sleep maintenance symptoms were associated with worse objective CPAP adherence at clinical follow-up, assessed 4 months after titration. Similarly, a recent longitudinal study of 705 OSA individuals treated with positive airway pressure (PAP) revealed that insomnia symptoms (both initial and maintenance) at baseline were

predictive of reduced PAP use at the 2-year follow-up.[27] Other studies have found similar evidence for the negative impact of insomnia before initiating CPAP, on CPAP use during the first 7 days of use as well as the first 6 months of use.[50,51] However, one study did not find a relationship between insomnia (as measured by the Insomnia Severity Index) and CPAP adherence at 6 months.[52]

In contrast to the impact of insomnia on OSA, much less is known about the potential impact of OSA on insomnia treatment outcome. One preliminary report found that the presence of OSA did not negatively affect the outcomes of cognitive-behavioral therapy (CBT) for insomnia.[53] In another study, Nguyen and colleagues[54] reported the improvement of insomnia symptoms after 24 months of auto-PAP treatment in 80 individuals with sleep apnea. Of the 39 subjects who had insomnia, baseline sleepiness and disease severity were associated with insomnia improvement after 24 months. Taken together, the available literature suggests that the coexistence of insomnia and OSA is likely to have a negative impact on OSA treatment, but if or how it might affect insomnia treatment is unclear. Indeed, further research is needed to clarify the potential impact of comorbidity on treatment, as this has very important implications for patient management.

MODELS OF PATHOGENESIS

The pathophysiology and developmental course of comorbid OSA and insomnia is not clearly understood. A few theoretical models outlining possible pathways have been proposed and discussed in the literature.[55,56] One pathway is that OSA is a precursor and putative risk factor for an insomnia disorder. This notion has intuitive appeal, given that respiratory events could lead to nocturnal awakenings and repeated awakenings could lead to chronic insomnia.[55,57] Krakow and colleagues[58] found that nocturnal awakenings reported by patients with insomnia were frequently due to respiratory events. This conceptualization would also fit the diathesis stress-response model of insomnia proposed by Spielman and colleagues[59] whereby the onset of OSA is a precipitating factor for insomnia. Another hypothesis supporting this pathway is that respiratory events can also lead to sympathetic activation thereby increasing hyperarousal, which is a key feature of insomnia.[29,58] A third hypothesis is that treatment of OSA can precipitate insomnia. One study examining retrospective data of patients treated at a sleep clinic reported that 21.4% (12 of 56) of patients who did not report insomnia at baseline developed

Table 1
Prevalence rates of comorbid sleep apnea and insomnia

Authors,[Ref.] Year	Sample Size	Criteria for Sleep Apnea	Criteria for Insomnia	Prevalence of Comorbid Insomnia	Prevalence of Comorbid Sleep Apnea
Billings et al,[25] 2013	191	OSA (AHI ≥15)	DIS frequent or always	24%	
Bjornsdottir et al,[26] 2012	826[a]	Untreated OSA patients referred for CPAP	DIS, DMS nearly every day	DIS: 12.6% men and 27.3% women; DMS: 51.6% men and 62.4% women	
Bjornsdottir et al,[27] in press	705	OSA (AHI ≥15)	DIS, DMS or EMA ≥3 nights/wk	DIS = 15.5%, DMS = 59.3%, EMA = 27.7%	
Caetano Mota et al,[28] 2012	80	OSA (AHI ≥5)	Self-reported present and new onset (self-report questionnaires)	30% present, 21.4% new onset	
Chung,[29] 2005	157	OSA meeting ICSD criteria and AHI ≥5	Insomnia symptoms (DIS, EMA and DMS [difficulty returning back to sleep and multiple wakenings])	42% at least 1 symptom; DIS = 6%, DMS = 26% (multiple wakenings) and 12% (difficulty returning to sleep), and EMA = 19%	
Chung,[30] 2003	119[a]	OSA (AHI ≥5)	Insomnia symptoms (DIS, EMA and DMS [difficulty returning back to sleep and multiple wakenings])	DMS = 33% (multiple wakenings) and 16% (difficulty returning to sleep), EMA = 21%, and DIS = 9%	
Cronlein et al,[31] 2012	93	SAS (AHI ≥10)	Meet ICSD-2 criteria for psychophysiological insomnia		23%
Gooneratne et al,[32] 2006	99[a]	SRBD (AHI ≥15)	Insomnia symptoms ≥3 nights/wk for ≥3 wk		29.3%
Johansson et al,[33] 2009	183[a]	OSA (AHI ≥5)	Some or more problems with DIS, DMS, EMA reported	DIS = 44%, DMS = 63%, EMA = 37%	
Kinugawa et al,[34] 2012	64	SAS (AHI ≥15)	ICSD-2 criteria for insomnia		68.7%

Study	n	Criteria	Insomnia definition	Prevalence
Krakow et al,[35] 2001	231	SDB (UARS or OSA: clinical criteria and AHI ≥5)	Clinically apparent insomnia symptoms (2 or more insomnia symptoms)	50%
Krell and Kapur,[36] 2005	228[a]	SDB (AHI ≥10)	At least DIS, DMS, or EMA often/almost always	54.9% (DIS = 33.4%, DMS = 38.8%, EMA = 31.4%)
Lichstein et al,[37] 1999	80	AHI >15	ICSD criteria for insomnia	29% (43% with AHI >5)
McCall et al,[38] 2009	73	AHI ≥15	SOL >30 min and SE <85% or RDC for ≥4 nights/wk	7%
Ong et al,[39] 2009	51	ICSD-2 criteria and AHI ≥15	DSM-IV-TR criteria for insomnia	39%
Smith et al,[40] 2004	105	OSAHS (unclear)	Presenting with insomnia disorder	39%
Stone et al,[41] 1994	45	OSA (RDI ≥10)	TST <6 h, SOL/WASO >30 min for minimum 6 mo	40%
Subramanian et al,[42] 2001	300	OSA (AHI >10)	Insomnia (unclear), DIS, DMS, EMA, PPI	Insomnia = 84%, DIS = 57%, DMS = 68%, EMA = 48%, PPI = 49%
Vozoris,[43] 2012	546[a]	Self-reported health professional diagnosis of sleep apnea	DIS, DMS, EMA often or almost always	Any symptom 43.3% DIS = 25.9%, DMS = 28.8%, EMA = 20.8%

Abbreviations: AHI, apnea-hypopnea index; CPAP, continuous positive airway pressure; DIS, difficulty initiating sleep; DMS, difficulty maintaining sleep; DSM-IV-TR, *Diagnostic and Statistical Manual of Mental Disorders*, 4th edition, text revised; EMA, early morning awakenings; ICSD, International Classification of Sleep Disorders; OSA, obstructive sleep apnea; OSAHS, obstructive sleep apnea and hypopnea syndrome; PPI, psychophysiologic insomnia; RDC, research diagnostic criteria; RDI, respiratory disturbance index; SDB, sleep-disordered breathing; SOL, sleep-onset latency; TST, total sleep time; UARS, upper airway resistance syndrome; WASO, wake after sleep onset.
[a] Sample size is not identical to the overall sample size recruited.

insomnia after 3 months or more of receiving PAP (primarily auto-PAP).[28] The investigators speculated that this type of pressure delivery, with changing pressure levels, can actually lead to more sleep fragmentation, and could be a possible contributor to the development of insomnia resulting from PAP treatment. Thus, insomnia might emerge from poor tolerance to OSA therapy. However, another viable explanation of these data is that the auto-PAP effectively treated the OSA, and insomnia emerged once the sleep debt was resolved and the homeostatic sleep drive was regulated. In other words, effective treatment of OSA could unmask an underlying insomnia disorder.

Despite the intuitive appeal of this pathway, recent longitudinal data dispute this temporal relationship. In one report OSA at baseline, defined as an apnea-hypopnea index score of 5 or greater, was not a significant predictor of patients' responses to the question, "Do you feel you have insomnia?" posed at a 7.5-year follow-up.[60] Another report from the same dataset found that moderate to severe sleep apnea, defined as an AHI of 15 or greater, is a risk factor for the development of poor sleep (moderate to severe ratings on nocturnal symptoms of insomnia) but not chronic insomnia as defined earlier.[61] The investigators propose that respiratory events in the context of OSA can lead to acute sleep disruption but do not evolve into an insomnia disorder over time, as earlier hypotheses have posited.

A second pathway is suggested whereby the insomnia disorder develops first and is a precursor to OSA. This pathway has less intuitive appeal in that prolonged awakenings or hyperarousal from insomnia do not have obvious causal connections with respiratory mechanisms. It has been hypothesized that the sleep deprivation resulting from chronic insomnia might compromise the upper airway (eg, pharyngeal) muscle tone.[35,57] Unfortunately, no empirical studies have been found to support or dispute this pathway.

A third potential pathway involves an underlying mechanism that links the two sleep disorders. Theoretical models have focused on the potential role of the hypothalamic-pituitary-adrenal axis (HPA) pathway and metabolic factors.[55,62] It is hypothesized that stress increases HPA activity, leading to sleep fragmentation associated with insomnia. In addition, repeated respiratory events in the context of OSA can lead to autonomic activation, triggering HPA activation.[62] Furthermore, the increased HPA activity might disrupt metabolic activity associated with metabolic syndrome (eg, glucose imbalance). To the authors' knowledge, there is no published evidence directly testing these theoretical models or the possibility that a third variable, such as depression, is a mediator between the onset of sleep apnea and the development of insomnia.

CLINICAL IMPLICATIONS FOR SLEEP MEDICINE
Assessment

Given the literature showing that insomnia symptoms can predict OSA and can also have a negative impact on treatment, effective assessment of both OSA and insomnia is advised to provide comprehensive care. First, the chief complaint (insomnia or sleep-related breathing issues) should give rise to more specific considerations regarding the comorbid (or "secondary") condition. For example, women might appear to fit a profile for an insomnia disorder (eg, complain of sleep disturbance, hold dysfunctional sleep-related cognitions), but a comprehensive assessment for sleep-related breathing disorder should still be considered. Appropriate assessment can give rise to considerations regarding the timing of treatment sequences (see later discussion) or whether the patient might be aided by use of a hypnotic during the overnight polysomnography. Indeed, there is evidence that higher sleep efficiency on the night of the CPAP titration predicts future compliance with CPAP.[63] Lettieri and colleagues[64,65] have found that administration of eszopiclone (3 mg) on the titration night improved the quality of the titration study and improved CPAP adherence when compared with placebo. This finding can serve as an example of how comprehensive baseline assessment can improve patient management of these comorbid sleep disorders.

Treatment Strategies

Effective treatments are available when insomnia and sleep apnea occur separately. Pharmacologic therapy using hypnotic medication is the most common treatment option for insomnia. However, some hypnotics, such as benzodiazepines, can have adverse effects on nocturnal respiration, thus exacerbating the OSA.[66,67] Therefore, these should be used with caution for the patient with both OSA and insomnia. The newer nonbenzodiazepine agents, such as zolpidem and eszopiclone, seem to have less effect on the airway.[68,69] CBT has become the first-line nonpharmacologic treatment for insomnia. Although CBT is generally regarded as safe and effective across a variety of comorbid conditions, it remains unclear as to whether there are specific counterindications when insomnia and OSA are comorbid. For example, sleep restriction could exacerbate daytime sleepiness because of the OSA. As noted earlier, only one study has documented that the presence of OSA did not negatively affect the outcomes of CBT for insomnia.[53] This finding would suggest that CBT is a potential treatment for those with comorbid insomnia and OSA. Components such as sleep restriction and stimulus control, aimed at eliminating the extended periods of wakefulness spent in bed, might also potentially improve poor sleeping habits in individuals with comorbid insomnia and OSA (eg, napping and extended time in bed).

The first-line treatment for moderate to severe OSA is CPAP.[70–72] Although treatment of OSA using CPAP provides many health benefits, it is currently unclear whether this will also improve insomnia for patients with both OSA and insomnia. Bjornsdottir and colleagues[27] showed that effective use was associated with a 50% reduction in the prevalence of sleep maintenance insomnia, but symptoms of initial insomnia were largely still present at follow-up. Other treatments for OSA include a dental oral appliance, positional training, and surgery. These treatments are typically recommended based on specific features related to the OSA (eg, mild OSA, position-dependent OSA, enlarged tonsils). However, to the authors' knowledge no studies have examined the impact of these procedures on comorbid insomnia.

While there are effective treatments available for insomnia and OSA separately, there are currently no known monotherapies that effectively treat insomnia and sleep apnea simultaneously. Therefore, management of patients with both OSA and insomnia entails the combining of treatments for insomnia with treatments for OSA. One study by Krakow and colleagues[73] examined a sequence of CBT for insomnia followed by treatment for OSA (CPAP, oral appliance, turbinectomy). Of the 17 patients treated, 8 reported clinically significant improvements from insomnia after CBT, with an additional 7 (for a total of 15 of 17) reporting clinically significant improvements in insomnia after receiving both treatments. Guilleminault and colleagues[74] tested sequences of CBT before or after ear/nose/throat surgery for 30 patients with mild OSA and insomnia. Optimal outcomes were achieved for patients who received both treatments, with some evidence that treating OSA first led to resolution of insomnia in some patients before CBT. The retrospective study by Caetano Mota and colleagues[28] found that 45.8% (11 of 24) of patients who reported insomnia and were diagnosed with sleep apnea no longer reported insomnia following PAP treatment. However, 21.4% of patients (12 of 56) who did not have insomnia at baseline developed insomnia during the course of PAP treatment. Thus, insomnia

symptoms might be present at baseline or could appear during treatment, suggesting that insomnia symptoms should be monitored over time and that appropriate treatment should be delivered should it arise during OSA treatment. For patients who initially present with OSA but develop treatment-emergent insomnia after starting OSA therapy, a course of CBT or hypnotic medications should be considered as an adjunct to the OSA therapy. For other patients who initially present with insomnia (particularly sleep maintenance insomnia) but are treatment resistant to CBT or hypnotics, evaluation for OSA should be considered because the insomnia could be masking the symptoms of OSA. Finally, some patients might initially present with both insomnia and OSA symptoms. For these patients it is advisable to treat both disorders, but there currently is no clear guidance as to the order or sequence of treatment. Until a uniform treatment is developed, considerations should be given to combination approaches in treating the patient with OSA and insomnia.

FUTURE RESEARCH AGENDA

As the comorbidity between sleep apnea and insomnia gains more research attention, future studies should be hypothesis driven with an eye toward improving patient care. First, research should examine methods for diagnosing the co-occurrence of insomnia and OSA. Studies examining the reliability and validity of various diagnostic questionnaires, interviews, or objective measures could improve the precision of the prevalence and incidence of this comorbid condition. Second, research should seek to clarify the pathophysiology and time course of these disorders. Prospective studies using longitudinal designs would be particularly useful to examine temporal precedence and the natural course of the co-occurrence of the two disorders. Studies examining the clinical course of treatment-emergent or treatment-resistant insomnia as it relates to OSA could inform clinicians regarding treatment implementation. At the mechanistic level, studies examining the relationship between repeated respiratory events and their associated sequelae with insomnia mechanisms such as hyperarousal or changes in sleep-related thoughts and behaviors could provide further insight into the etiology of the comorbid condition. Finally, treatment studies examining various combinations or sequences of treatment could provide evidence to optimize the care of this population. A more ambitious aim would be to investigate a unified treatment for both sleep apnea and insomnia. For example, preliminary evidence has indicated that cannabimimetic drugs have promise as a drug treatment for OSA.[75] Such treatment could serve as a tool to reduce AHI and improve sleep continuity, thus targeting symptoms of OSA and sleep maintenance insomnia. It could also be a potential tool for the treatment of OSA while preventing treatment-emergent insomnia. Another approach would be to combine behavioral treatments into one treatment package for subtypes of comorbid OSA and insomnia. For example, positional training could be integrated into CBT for patients with positional sleep apnea and comorbid insomnia. Such studies could also provide insights into the causes and consequences of the two disorders. Achieving these research goals would significantly improve our understanding and treatment of these common sleep disorders.

REFERENCES

1. American Academy of Sleep Medicine. International classification of sleep disorders—2: diagnostic and coding manual. Westchester (IL): American Academy of Sleep Medicine; 2005.
2. Balk EM, Moorthy D, Obadan NO, et al. Diagnosis and treatment of obstructive sleep apnea in adults (No. Report number: 11–EHC052). Rockville (MD): Agency for Healthcare Research and Quality; 2011.
3. Marin JM, Agusti A, Villar I, et al. Association between treated and untreated obstructive sleep apnea and risk of hypertension. JAMA 2012; 307(20):2169–76.
4. Nieto FJ, Young TB, Lind BK, et al. Association of sleep-disordered breathing, sleep apnea, and hypertension in a large community-based study. Sleep Heart Health Study. JAMA 2000;283(14): 1829–36.
5. Peppard PE, Young T, Palta M, et al. Prospective study of the association between sleep-disordered breathing and hypertension. N Engl J Med 2000;342(19):1378–84.
6. Weaver TE, George CF. Cognition and performance in patients with obstructive sleep apnea. In: Kryger MH, Roth TI, Dement WC, editors. Principles and practice of sleep medicine. 5th edition. St Louis (MO): Elsevier Saunders; 2011. p. 1194–206.
7. Young T, Palta M, Dempsey J, et al. The occurrence of sleep-disordered breathing among middle-aged adults. N Engl J Med 1993;328(17): 1230–5.
8. Marshall NS, Wong KK, Liu PY, et al. Sleep apnea as an independent risk factor for all-cause mortality: the Busselton Health Study. Sleep 2008;31(8): 1079–85.
9. Young T, Finn L, Peppard PE, et al. Sleep disordered breathing and mortality: eighteen-year follow-up of the Wisconsin sleep cohort. Sleep 2008;31(8):1071–8.
10. American Psychiatric Association. American Psychiatric Association DSM-5 Development. 2012. Available at: http://www.dsm5.org/ProposedRevision/Pages/proposedrevision.aspx?rid=65#. Accessed July 21, 2012.
11. Morin CM, LeBlanc M, Daley M, et al. Epidemiology of insomnia: prevalence, self-help treatments, consultations, and determinants of help-seeking behaviors. Sleep Med 2006;7(2):123–30.
12. Ohayon MM, Reynolds CF 3rd. Epidemiological and clinical relevance of insomnia diagnosis algorithms according to the DSM-IV and the International Classification of Sleep Disorders (ICSD). Sleep Med 2009;10(9):952–60.
13. Roth T. Insomnia: definition, prevalence, etiology, and consequences. J Clin Sleep Med 2007; 3(Suppl 5):S7–10.
14. Riemann D, Spiegelhalder K, Feige B, et al. The hyperarousal model of insomnia: a review of the concept and its evidence. Sleep Med Rev 2010; 14(1):19–31.
15. Kyle SD, Morgan K, Espie CA. Insomnia and health-related quality of life. Sleep Med Rev 2010; 14(1):69–82.
16. Baglioni C, Battagliese G, Feige B, et al. Insomnia as a predictor of depression: a meta-analytic evaluation of longitudinal epidemiological studies. J Affect Disord 2011;135(1–3):10–9.
17. Ford DE, Kamerow DB. Epidemiologic study of sleep disturbances and psychiatric disorders. An opportunity for prevention? JAMA 1989;262(11): 1479–84.
18. Vgontzas AN, Liao D, Bixler EO, et al. Insomnia with objective short sleep duration is associated with a high risk for hypertension. Sleep 2009; 32(4):491–7.
19. Vgontzas AN, Liao D, Pejovic S, et al. Insomnia with objective short sleep duration is associated with type 2 diabetes: a population-based study. Diabetes Care 2009;32(11):1980–5.
20. Vgontzas AN, Liao D, Pejovic S, et al. Insomnia with short sleep duration and mortality: the Penn State cohort. Sleep 2010;33(9):1159–64.
21. Guilleminault C, Eldridge FL, Dement WC. Insomnia with sleep apnea: a new syndrome. Science 1973;181(4102):856–8.
22. National Institutes of Health. National Institutes of Health state of the science conference statement on manifestations and management of chronic insomnia in adults. Sleep 2005;28(9):1049–57.
23. Edinger JD, Wyatt JK, Stepanski EJ, et al. Testing the reliability and validity of DSM-IV-TR and ICSD-2 insomnia diagnoses. Results of a multitrait-multimethod analysis. Arch Gen Psychiatry 2011; 68(10):992–1002.

24. Edinger JD, Bonnet MH, Bootzin RR, et al. Derivation of research diagnostic criteria for insomnia: report of an American Academy of Sleep Medicine Work Group. Sleep 2004;27(8):1567–96.

25. Billings ME, Rosen CL, Wang R, et al. Is the relationship between race and continuous positive airway pressure adherence mediated by sleep duration? Sleep 2013;36(2):221–7.

26. Bjornsdottir E, Janson C, Gislason T, et al. Insomnia in untreated sleep apnea patients compared to controls. J Sleep Res 2012;21(2):131–8.

27. Bjornsdottir E, Janson C, Sigurdsson JF, et al. Symptoms of insomnia among OSA patients before and after 2 years of PAP treatment. Sleep, in press accepted for publication 3/4/2013.

28. Caetano Mota P, Morais Cardoso S, Drummond M, et al. Prevalence of new-onset insomnia in patients with obstructive sleep apnoea syndrome treated with nocturnal ventilatory support. Rev Port Pneumol 2012;18(1):15–21.

29. Chung KF. Insomnia subtypes and their relationships to daytime sleepiness in patients with obstructive sleep apnea. Respiration 2005;72(5):460–5.

30. Chung KF. Relationships between insomnia and sleep-disordered breathing. Chest 2003;123(1):310–1 [author reply: 311–3].

31. Cronlein T, Geisler P, Langguth B, et al. Polysomnography reveals unexpectedly high rates of organic sleep disorders in patients with prediagnosed primary insomnia. Sleep Breath 2012;16(4):1097–103.

32. Gooneratne NS, Gehrman PR, Nkwuo JE, et al. Consequences of comorbid insomnia symptoms and sleep-related breathing disorder in elderly subjects. Arch Intern Med 2006;166(16):1732–8.

33. Johansson P, Alehagen U, Svanborg E, et al. Sleep disordered breathing in an elderly community-living population: relationship to cardiac function, insomnia symptoms and daytime sleepiness. Sleep Med 2009;10(9):1005–11.

34. Kinugawa K, Doulazmi M, Sebban C, et al. Sleep apnea in elderly adults with chronic insomnia. J Am Geriatr Soc 2012;60(12):2366–8.

35. Krakow B, Melendrez D, Ferreira E, et al. Prevalence of insomnia symptoms in patients with sleep-disordered breathing. Chest 2001;120(6):1923–9.

36. Krell SB, Kapur VK. Insomnia complaints in patients evaluated for obstructive sleep apnea. Sleep Breath 2005;9(3):104–10.

37. Lichstein KL, Riedel BW, Lester KW, et al. Occult sleep apnea in a recruited sample of older adults with insomnia. J Consult Clin Psychol 1999;67(3):405–10.

38. McCall WV, Kimball J, Boggs N, et al. Prevalence and prediction of primary sleep disorders in a clinical trial of depressed patients with insomnia. J Clin Sleep Med 2009;5(5):454–8.

39. Ong JC, Gress JL, San Pedro-Salcedo MG, et al. Frequency and predictors of obstructive sleep apnea among individuals with major depressive disorder and insomnia. J Psychosom Res 2009;67(2):135–41.

40. Smith S, Sullivan K, Hopkins W, et al. Frequency of insomnia report in patients with obstructive sleep apnoea hypopnea syndrome (OSAHS). Sleep Med 2004;5(5):449–56.

41. Stone J, Morin CM, Hart RP, et al. Neuropsychological functioning in older insomniacs with or without obstructive sleep apnea. Psychol Aging 1994;9(2):231–6.

42. Subramanian S, Guntupalli B, Murugan T, et al. Gender and ethnic differences in prevalence of self-reported insomnia among patients with obstructive sleep apnea. Sleep Breath 2011;15(4):711–5.

43. Vozoris NT. Sleep apnea-plus: prevalence, risk factors, and association with cardiovascular diseases using United States population-level data. Sleep Med 2012;13(6):637–44.

44. Glidewell RN, Roby EK, Orr WC. Is insomnia an independent predictor of obstructive sleep apnea? J Am Board Fam Med 2012;25(1):104–10.

45. Shepertycky MR, Banno K, Kryger MH. Differences between men and women in the clinical presentation of patients diagnosed with obstructive sleep apnea syndrome. Sleep 2005;28(3):309–14.

46. Yang CM, Liao YS, Lin CM, et al. Psychological and behavioral factors in patients with comorbid obstructive sleep apnea and insomnia. J Psychosom Res 2011;70(4):355–61.

47. Sivertsen B, Bjornsdottir E, Overland S, et al. The joint contribution of insomnia and obstructive sleep apnoea on sickness absence. J Sleep Res 2013;22(2):223–30.

48. Machado MA, de Carvalho LB, Juliano ML, et al. Clinical co-morbidities in obstructive sleep apnea syndrome treated with mandibular repositioning appliance. Respir Med 2006;100(6):988–95.

49. Wickwire EM, Smith MT, Birnbaum S, et al. Sleep maintenance insomnia complaints predict poor CPAP adherence: a clinical case series. Sleep Med 2010;11(8):772–6.

50. Pieh C, Bach M, Popp R, et al. Insomnia symptoms influence CPAP compliance. Sleep Breath 2013;17(1):99–104.

51. Wallace DM, Vargas SS, Schwartz SJ, et al. Determinants of continuous positive airway pressure adherence in a sleep clinic cohort of South Florida Hispanic veterans. Sleep Breath 2013;17(1):351–63.

52. Nguyen XL, Chaskalovic J, Rakotonanahary D, et al. Insomnia symptoms and CPAP compliance in OSAS patients: a descriptive study using data mining methods. Sleep Med 2010;11(8):777–84.

53. Lack LC, Hunter M, Gradisar M, et al. Is the treatment of insomnia impared when OSA is also present? Sleep 2011;34(Abstract Supplement):508.

54. Nguyen XL, Rakotonanahary D, Chaskalovic J, et al. Insomnia related to sleep apnoea: effect of long-term auto-adjusting positive airway pressure treatment. Eur Respir J 2013;41(3): 593–600.

55. Beneto A, Gomez-Siurana E, Rubio-Sanchez P. Comorbidity between sleep apnea and insomnia. Sleep Med Rev 2009;13(4):287–93.

56. Luyster FS, Buysse DJ, Strollo PJ Jr. Comorbid insomnia and obstructive sleep apnea: challenges for clinical practice and research. J Clin Sleep Med 2010;6(2):196–204.

57. Al-Jawder SE, Bahammam AS. Comorbid insomnia in sleep-related breathing disorders: an under-recognized association. Sleep Breath 2012;16(2): 295–304.

58. Krakow B, Romero E, Ulibarri VA, et al. Prospective assessment of nocturnal awakenings in a case series of treatment-seeking chronic insomnia patients: a pilot study of subjective and objective causes. Sleep 2012;35(12):1685–92.

59. Spielman AJ, Caruso LS, Glovinsky PB. A behavioral perspective on insomnia treatment. Psychiatr Clin North Am 1987;10(4):541–53.

60. Singareddy R, Vgontzas AN, Fernandez-Mendoza J, et al. Risk factors for incident chronic insomnia: a general population prospective study. Sleep Med 2012;13(4):346–53.

61. Fernandez-Mendoza J, Vgontzas AN, Bixler EO, et al. Clinical and polysomnographic predictors of the natural history of poor sleep in the general population. Sleep 2012;35(5):689–97.

62. Buckley TM, Schatzberg AF. On the interactions of the hypothalamic-pituitary-adrenal (HPA) axis and sleep: normal HPA axis activity and circadian rhythm, exemplary sleep disorders. J Clin Endocrinol Metab 2005;90(5):3106–14.

63. Drake CL, Day R, Hudgel D, et al. Sleep during titration predicts continuous positive airway pressure compliance. Sleep 2003;26(3):308–11.

64. Lettieri CJ, Collen JF, Eliasson AH, et al. Sedative use during continuous positive airway pressure titration improves subsequent compliance. Chest 2009;136(5):1263–8.

65. Lettieri CJ, Quast TN, Eliasson AH, et al. Eszopiclone improves overnight polysomnography and continuous positive airway pressure titration: a prospective, randomized, placebo-controlled trial. Sleep 2008;31(9):1310–6.

66. Berry RB, Kouchi K, Bower J, et al. Triazolam in patients with obstructive sleep apnea. Am J Respir Crit Care Med 1995;151(2 Pt 1):450–4.

67. Dolly FR, Block AJ. Effect of flurazepam on sleep-disordered breathing and nocturnal oxygen desaturation in asymptomatic subjects. Am J Med 1982;73(2):239–43.

68. Kryger M, Wang-Weigand S, Roth T. Safety of ramelteon in individuals with mild to moderate obstructive sleep apnea. Sleep Breath 2007; 11(3):159–64.

69. Rosenberg R, Roach JM, Scharf M, et al. A pilot study evaluating acute use of eszopiclone in patients with mild to moderate obstructive sleep apnea syndrome. Sleep Med 2007;8(5):464–70.

70. Epstein LJ, Kristo D, Strollo PJ Jr, et al. Clinical guideline for the evaluation, management and long-term care of obstructive sleep apnea in adults. J Clin Sleep Med 2009;5(3):263–76.

71. Kushida CA, Littner MR, Hirshkowitz M, et al. Practice parameters for the use of continuous and bilevel positive airway pressure devices to treat adult patients with sleep-related breathing disorders. Sleep 2006;29(3):375–80.

72. Loube DI, Gay PC, Strohl KP, et al. Indications for positive airway pressure treatment of adult obstructive sleep apnea patients: a consensus statement. Chest 1999;115(3):863–6.

73. Krakow B, Melendrez D, Lee SA, et al. Refractory insomnia and sleep-disordered breathing: a pilot study. Sleep Breath 2004;8(1):15–29.

74. Guilleminault C, Davis K, Huynh NT. Prospective randomized study of patients with insomnia and mild sleep disordered breathing. Sleep 2008; 31(11):1527–33.

75. Prasad B, Radulovacki MG, Carley DW. Proof of concept trial of dronabinol in obstructive sleep apnea. Front Psychiatry 2013;4:1.

Lessons Learned from the National Dissemination of Cognitive Behavioral Therapy for Insomnia in the Veterans Health Administration

Impact of Training on Therapists' Self-Efficacy and Attitudes

Rachel Manber, PhD[a],*, Mickey Trockel, MD, PhD[a],
Wendy Batdorf, PhD[b,c], Allison T. Siebern, PhD[d],
C. Barr Taylor, MD[a], Julia Gimeno, BA[a], Bradley E. Karlin, PhD[b,e]

KEYWORDS

- Cognitive behavioral therapy for insomnia - CBT-I • Insomnia • Dissemination training
- Veterans Health Administration - VHA

KEY POINTS

- Chronic insomnia, common among veterans, is associated with negative physical health, and, if untreated, can impact the severity of comorbid medical and psychiatric conditions.
- Cognitive behavioral therapy for insomnia (CBT-I) is a highly effective and well-established treatment, but patient access is limited because few clinicians are trained to deliver the therapy.
- This article describes the training methods and the impact of training on therapists' use of CBT-I and on their self-efficacy to deliver and attitudes toward CBT-I.

INTRODUCTION

Chronic insomnia is a common sleep disorder,[1–3] particularly among Veterans,[4,5] and it is associated with negative physical health (eg, myocardial infarction, congestive heart failure, diabetes mellitus) and mental health (eg, depression).[6,7] Untreated insomnia can impact the severity of comorbid medical and psychiatric conditions and can hinder treatment of the coexisting disorder.[1,8,9] Insomnia is also associated with increased health care use and economic burden in the workplace, with an estimated annual cost of $100 billion.[10,11] Poor sleep, common among individuals with mental disorders, is often unresolved with general psychotherapy.[12]

---

[a] Psychiatry & Behavioral Sciences, 401 Quarry Road, Stanford, CA 94305, USA; [b] Mental Health Services, U.S. Department of Veterans Affairs Central Office, 810 Vermont Avenue, Northwest Washington, DC 20420, USA; [c] Department of Veterans Affairs, 6200 Aurora Avenue, 636A6/MHM6 Urbandale, IA 50322, USA; [d] The Stanford Center for Sleep Sciences and Medicine, 450 Broadway, Redwood City, California 94063-5730, USA; [e] Department of Mental Health, Bloomberg School of Public Health, Johns Hopkins University, 624 N. Broadway, 8th Floor, Baltimore, MD 21205, USA
* Corresponding author.
E-mail address: rmanber@stanford.edu

Sleep Med Clin 8 (2013) 399–405
http://dx.doi.org/10.1016/j.jsmc.2013.05.003
1556-407X/13/$ – see front matter © 2013 Elsevier Inc. All rights reserved.

Cognitive behavioral therapy for insomnia (CBT-I) is an empirically supported, nonpharmacologic treatment for insomnia. The National Institutes of Health (NIH) Consensus Statement and the British Association of Psychopharmacology have both classified CBT-I as a first-line treatment for insomnia.[3,13] Randomized trials comparing CBT-I with sleep medication (zolpidem, zopiclone, and temazepam) found that CBT-I has comparable efficacy short-term, and better long-term maintenance of gains after treatments are discontinued.[14–16] Moreover, CBT-I is effective, even when insomnia is comorbid with other disorders, such as chronic pain conditions and major depressive disorder.[17,18] However, patient access to CBT-I is not always possible because of the limited number of clinicians trained to deliver this therapy.[19,20] Accordingly, training in and dissemination of CBT-I are greatly needed.

The Veterans Health Administration (VHA) is disseminating CBT-I nationally as part of its efforts to make evidence-based psychotherapies widely available to veterans.[21] Seeking to provide access to CBT-I to veterans with insomnia across the nation, the VHA has implemented a national, competency-based CBT-I Training Program to train licensed mental health clinicians from a variety of disciplines (psychiatrists, psychologists, social workers, nurses, licensed professional mental health counselors, and marriage and family therapists) working in a multitude of settings across the system. In a previous article, the authors described the decisions that have shaped the development of the Department of Veterans Affairs (VA) CBT-I Training Program.[22] Initial program evaluation results indicate that the implementation of CBT-I by newly trained therapists is associated with an overall large reduction in insomnia severity and improvements in depression and quality of life among veterans.[23]

This article describes the training process, including steps taken to support long-term use of CBT-I; reports on therapist outcomes in terms of successful completion of the training program and continued use of CBT-I after completion; and describes the effects of the training on participants' self-efficacy to deliver and attitudes toward CBT-I. The data analysis focused on the following 2 questions: (1) To what extent do therapists continue to provide CBT-I after completing training? (2) Do self-efficacy and attitudes toward providing CBT-I improve during training? Key lessons learned from the initiative are also shared.

THE VA CBT-I TRAINING PROGRAM

Using a competency-based training model, the VA CBT-I training program provides a 4-month case-based consultation period, during which training participants receive corrective feedback on the implementation of CBT-I with veterans from experts in CBI-I. The consultation period complements an education component (experiential workshop and reading materials). Both the workshop and consultation components are described.

Workshop

The training begins with a 3-day workshop designed to provide a foundation for CBT-I. The workshop includes modeling of specific CBT-I skills and opportunities for experiential learning. The workshop is led by a behavioral sleep medicine expert and includes a discussion of sleep regulation (Borbely's 2-process model[24]), provides an overview of sleep architecture, describes the theories of insomnia, and outlines the components of CBT-I (sleep education, stimulus control, sleep restriction therapy, cognitive therapy strategies, and methods for reducing cognitive and somatic arousal). The workshop provides training in comprehensive assessment and case conceptualization and presents a flexible, case-formulation based, 6-session CBT-I protocol. The workshop also addresses adherence challenges and adaptations of the CBT-I protocol for insomnia occurring comorbid to other disorders common in the veteran population, including post-traumatic stress disorder (PTSD) (avoidance of bed because of fear of nightmares or checking behaviors), major depressive disorder (hopelessness of sleep improving, low motivation, and using the bed as an escape from emotional pain), chronic pain (using bed as escape from physical pain), and mild traumatic brain injury (cognitive impairment). Extensive modeling in therapeutic technique delivery takes place with demonstration videos by CBT-I experts, and experiential learning takes place with small and large group discussions and role-play exercises. Immediate corrective feedback from expert CBT-I training consultants is provided and valued by training participants.

Learning is facilitated by materials that support the administration of treatment. These include (1) a comprehensive treatment manual that provides in-depth explanation about what is learned in the workshop and additional reference materials to be used as resources, (2) patient handouts, (3) session-by-session checklists, (4) an intake form, (5) a case conceptualization form, (6) 2 published books,[25,26] and (7) an excel spreadsheet to facilitate calculation of variables, derived from sleep diary data, which are essential for administering sleep restriction therapy.

Consultation Phase

After the training workshop, training participants participate in 4 months of weekly telephone consultation sessions in small groups (4 training participants (consultees) per group), led by CBT-I experts serving as training consultants. During the consultation phase, training participants provide individual CBT-I to veterans who have consented to be a training case and to be audiotaped. Training participants send 6 taped sessions to the CBT-I experts (training consultants) for them to review and rate for competency. A competency rating scale was developed by the CBT-I training program development team.[22] Training consultants (CBT-I experts) listen to full audiotaped sessions and rate the training participant's administration of CBT-I–specific components and more general psychotherapy skills. Minimum competency standards are part of the criteria for successful completion of the training program.[22]

The 90-minute consultation calls are held weekly and provide a forum for constructive feedback, based on tape review. The calls also provide opportunities for questions to be answered, further learning about sleep and sleep disorders, role-play practice of CBT-I skills, and discussions of clinical issues that emerge in the course of treatment implementation.

STEPS TO SUPPORT IMPLEMENTATION OF CBT-I AND SUSTAINABILITY

To support the implementation of CBT-I during and after the training, the training program has developed a Web-based SharePoint site that provides central access to training materials and ongoing access to VA CBT-I consultants via monthly conference calls ("virtual office hours"). Each of these conference calls is moderated by a CBT-I expert and provides training participants who have competed the training program an opportunity to ask questions about issues and challenges that have emerged in the context of delivering CBT-I. This consultation support is designed to promote sustained implementation of CBT-I and help with challenging cases and implementation issues after completion of the training program.

To further promote internal sustainability of training in CBT-I, significant focus has been placed on training new consultants, selected from the pool of participants who completed the training program. Given the limited number of trained CBT-I providers, the initial group of training consultants was a mix of VA-affiliated and external CBT-I experts, many of whom had certification in behavioral sleep medicine. Existing training consultants may recommend consultees to apply to become consultants through a structured recommendation and application process. Accepted applicants then receive training in how to serve as a training consultant, which includes participation in a workshop. A substantial proportion of this workshop is dedicated to education about sleep medicine topics, including sleep-related breathing disorders, restless leg syndrome, periodic limb movement disorder, parasomnias, and circadian rhythm disorders. This aspect of training is designed to help these future training consultants guide their future consultees in selecting cases for CBT-I training and in making appropriate referrals for further assessment and treatment of sleep disorders other than insomnia. The training consultant workshop also provides a review of program logistics and the consultation process, and guidelines about conducting the consultation calls and providing feedback based on review of taped CBT-I sessions. A substantial amount of time during the consultant training workshop is spent on familiarizing the future training consultants with the CBT-I-Competency Rating Scale (CBT-I-CRS), which is used by training consultants to rate consultees' taped sessions. During the consultant training workshop, future training consultants rate taped sessions, discuss their ratings, and receive corrective feedback from the trainer. Ratings are ultimately calibrated across the future training consultants. After this initial training, future training consultants attend a second therapist training workshop. During their 4-month consultation period with their first cohort of training participants, the newly trained training consultants attend weekly group consultation calls with a consultant trainer. These weekly calls provide opportunities for asking questions and discussing emerging sleep and consultation process issues.

PROGRAM EVALUATION

Program evaluation is a central component of the training program and includes evaluation of patient- and therapist-level variables. This article reports on therapist training outcomes, specifically the impact of training on therapist attitudes toward and self-efficacy to deliver CBT-I. The Institutional Review Board at Stanford University determined that using de-identified data obtained in the course of this program evaluation is exempt from further review. At the time of writing, 6-month posttraining de-identified data were available from the first 6 cohorts of training participants.

TRAINING PARTICIPANTS

Training participants come from every region, or Veterans Integrated Service Network, of VHA, including sites in Puerto Rico and Guam, and work in a variety of clinical settings. Treatment settings include outpatient mental health clinics, primary care clinics, and residential treatment programs (including programs for PTSD and substance use disorders) within VA medical centers and in community-based outpatient clinics. Therapists are selected to participate in this training program through a structured application process. To be eligible for the training program, therapists had to (1) be licensed mental health staff in VA; (2) deliver individual psychotherapy services on a regular basis; (3) work in settings where insomnia is a presenting issue and CBT-I can be implemented; (4) have committed to participating in a 4-month consultation period after the workshop; (5) express a commitment to provide CBT-I after completion of the training program; and (6) indicate willingness to recruit at least 1 to 2 patients with insomnia for the consultation process.

MEASURES
CBT-I Self-Efficacy Scale

The 32-item CBT-I Self-Efficacy Scale was developed for this initiative by behavioral sleep medicine experts who were involved in the development of the training program. Similar to the CBT-I-CRS, the scale includes items assessing confidence in using both specific CBT-I skills (eg, "Address cognitions that interfere with sleep") and general psychotherapy skills (eg, "Display a balance of warmth, concern, confidence, genuineness, and professionalism during therapy sessions"). Response options are on a 6-point Likert scale and range from not at all confident to completely confident.

Attitudes Toward CBT-I Scale

The 6-item Attitudes Toward CBT-I Scale includes 3 items assessing positive attitude toward CBT-I (eg, "CBT-I is an effective treatment for patients with insomnia") and 3 items assessing negative attitudes toward CBT-I (eg, "Therapists' adherence to a CBT-I protocol decreases their job satisfaction"). Response options are arranged on a 5-point Likert scale, ranging from strongly disagree to strongly agree.

The CBT-I Self-Efficacy and Attitudes Toward CBT-I Scales were completed at the following 4 time points: before the training workshop, immediately after the training workshop, at the end of the consultation period, and approximately 6 months after the consultation period ended. At the 6-month follow-up assessment, therapists were asked to report the number of patients they treated for insomnia during the prior month and the percent of those treated with individual CBT-I. From this information, the authors derived the number of patients therapists treated with individual CBT-I in the past month.

RESULTS

To date, the VA CBT-I training program provided training to 12 cohorts of clinicians between September 2010 and September 2012. At the time of writing, de-identified data were available from the first 6 cohorts.

Of the 207 therapists in the first 6 training cohorts, 141 were women and 66 were men; 135 were psychologists, 50 were clinical social workers, 11 were nurses, 10 were psychiatrists, and 1 did not indicate discipline. All but 14 of the 207 successfully completed training (8 dropped out of training and 6 did not meet minimum competency criteria for successful completion). Of the 193 who successfully completed the program, 171 also responded to the 6-month follow-up survey consultation. Approximately 74% (136) reported having provided CBT-I during the previous month. Of the 988 patients with insomnia seen during the month before the survey, the mean number of patients therapists reported treating with individual CBT-I was 3.4 (standard deviation [SD], 5.3), with a median of 2 (range, 0–52; interquartile range, 0–4). The most common challenges to continued use of CBT-I identified by training participants were (1) competing professional time demands, cited by 35 training participants, and (2) issues related to patients (eg, no-shows and patients' distance form clinic), cited by 14 training participants.

Principle components analysis with direct oblimin rotation of CBT-I Self-Efficacy Scale items demonstrated 2 components: 1 for CBT-I skills–specific self-efficacy, consisting of 22 items (eigenvalue = 16.7; α = 0.98), and 1 for general psychotherapy skills self-efficacy, consisting of 10 items (eigenvalue = 5.0; α = 0.93). These 2 components explained 68% of baseline variance in the self-efficacy item set. All other possible components had eigenvalues less than 1 and were not retained. Principle components analysis of the Attitudes Toward CBT-I Scale, with direct oblimin rotation, identified a single component, which explained 46% of variance (α = 0.77).

No significant change was seen in general psychotherapy self-efficacy from pre-workshop to post-workshop assessment. However, average item score on therapists' general psychotherapy skills self-efficacy did increase from post-workshop to post-consultation assessment 4 months later (from 4.9 [SD = 0.59] to 5.3 [SD = 0.54]; difference = 0.46 [95% CI, 0.36–0.56]; t_{161} = 9.3; P<.001; Cohen's d = 0.77).

From pre-workshop to post-workshop assessment, average item score on therapists' CBT-I skills–specific self-efficacy subscale increased from 3.6 (SD = 1.1) to 4.3 (SD = 0.67) (difference = 0.70 [95% CI, 0.56–0.85]; t_{186} = 9.5; P<.001; d = 0.65). From post-workshop to post-consultation assessment, CBT-I skills–specific self-efficacy increased further, from 4.3 (SD = 0.65) to 5.1 (SD = 0.66) (difference = 0.82 [95% CI, 0.71–0.93]; t_{160} = 15; P<.001; d = 1.3).

The average item score on the Attitudes Toward CBT-I scale increased from pre-workshop to post-workshop assessment, from 4.0 (SD = 0.54) to 4.4 (SD = 0.50) (difference = 0.45 [95% CI, 0.38–0.52]; t_{188} = 12; P<.001; d = 0.83). No significant change was seen from post-workshop to post-consultation in this scale.

DISCUSSION

Within 2 years of its initiation, the VA CBT-I training program provided training to 12 cohorts of clinicians. The first 6 cohorts involved 207 training participants, with 93% meeting process and competency requirements for completion of training. Approximately three-quarters of these clinicians continued to provide individual CBT-I during the month preceding the 6-month follow-up assessment (6 months after the consultation period ended). With the typical 6 weekly sessions, a therapist who continues to provide CBT-I to the average of 3.4 patients per month for the sample will provide a course of 6 individual CBT-I sessions to at least 27 patients per 48 work weeks per year, which, with 196 therapists, translates to 5292 veterans treated with individual CBT for insomnia each year. Data are not available on the number of patients treated with group CBT-I. The authors anticipate at least comparable uptake among subsequent VA CBT-I training cohorts. As word about the availability and effectiveness of CBT-I with veterans spreads, and an increasing number of therapists are trained in CBT-I, the number of patients receiving CBT-I in the VHA should continue to grow.

The authors found that the CBT-I skills–specific self-efficacy increased from pre-workshop to post-workshop, with further increase from post-workshop to the end of the consultation period (effect sizes of d = 0.65 and 1.3, respectively). This large additional increase in CBT-I skills–specific

self-efficacy between post-workshop and post-consultation provides further support for the important role of consultation in the training of therapists in evidence-based psychotherapies, such as CBT-I.[27] Moreover, Bandura's[28] work on self-efficacy suggests that increasing therapists' self-efficacy in CBT-I will lead to increased initial adoption and long-term implementation of CBT-I.

Although the workshop training alone did not impact self-efficacy in general therapy skills, the experience in providing CBT-I during the 4-month consultation period did lead to improved self-efficacy in general psychotherapy skills. This finding is not surprising given that the process of consultation includes discussion and feedback on general psychotherapy skills that are a part of CBT-I and are rated on the CBT-I-CRS. Thus, the findings indicate that the consultation yields benefits broader than enhanced CBT-I skills and provides greater confidence in more general psychotherapy skills, even among licensed independent mental health professionals. Moreover, it is possible that the additional increase in CBT-I skills–specific self-efficacy from post-workshop to the end of the 4-month consultation period generalized to self-efficacy regarding nonspecific therapeutic skills. Perhaps the experience of successfully improving the sleep of their patients provided the CBT-I trainees positive reinforcement about their skills as therapists in general.

Although the authors found a large effect size for the increase of positive attitudes toward CBT-I from pre-workshop to post-workshop participation, positive attitudes toward CBT-I did not increase significantly from post-workshop to post-consultation, possibly because of a ceiling effect.

The most common obstacle to long-term use of CBT-I has been competing time demands. Group CBT-I may improve therapists' ability to treat more patients. It is effective[29] and increases access to treatment by reaching a greater number of patients simultaneously. However, group administration of CBT-I is more difficult and requires additional skills, particularly in the context of comorbidities. Over time, as therapists gain experience in administering individual CBT-I, they will, with some additional training, be able to increasingly provide group CBT-I effectively. Supplemental training resources are being developed by the CBT-I training program to extend individual CBT-I skills and competencies to groups.

The current data have limitations that should be considered. First, the therapist-level measures (ie, Attitudes Toward CBT-I Scale and CBT-I Self-Efficacy Scale) have not been previously validated. However, as part of the development of the scales, behavioral sleep medicine experts reviewed the items of each and approved their face validity. In addition, results of principle components analyses and Chronbach's α estimates reported herein suggest good convergent validity for items comprising these scales. An additional limitation of this evaluation is the lack of a comparison group. Additional research is needed to confirm the current findings.

SUMMARY

Of the therapists who enrolled in the VA CBT-I training program, 93% successfully completed the process and competency-based requirements of the training, and 6 months after completion, three-quarters continued to deliver individual CBT-I consistent with the training. Training was associated with improved CBT-I skills–specific self-efficacy and attitudes toward CBT-I. The 4-month consultation period was associated with enhanced self-efficacy beyond the improvements post-workshop, which is likely attributable to receiving feedback that is based on observed work sample and improving patients' insomnia. Patients served by clinical care delivery systems outside of the VHA may benefit from similar CBT-I dissemination efforts.

REFERENCES

1. Nowell PD, Buysse DJ, Reynolds CF 3rd, et al. Clinical factors contributing to the differential diagnosis of primary insomnia and insomnia related to mental disorders. Am J Psychiatry 1997;154(10):1412–6.
2. Ford DE, Kamerow DB. Epidemiologic study of sleep disturbances and psychiatric disorders. An opportunity for prevention? JAMA 1989;262(11): 1479–84.
3. National Institutes of Health. National Institutes of Health State of the Science Conference statement on manifestations and management of chronic insomnia in adults, June 13-15, 2005. Sleep 2005; 28(9):1049–57.
4. Mustafa M, Erokwu N, Ebose I, et al. Sleep problems and the risk for sleep disorders in an outpatient veteran population. Sleep Breath 2005;9(2):57–63.
5. Lew HL, Pogoda TK, Hsu PT, et al. Impact of the "polytrauma clinical triad" on sleep disturbance in a department of Veterans Affairs outpatient rehabilitation setting. Am J Phys Med Rehabil 2010;89(6):437–45.
6. Katz DA, McHorney CA. Clinical correlates of insomnia in patients with chronic illness. Arch Intern Med 1998;158(10):1099–107.
7. Katz DA, McHorney CA. The relationship between insomnia and health-related quality of life in patients with chronic illness. J Fam Pract 2002;51(3):229–35.
8. Buysse DJ, Tu XM, Cherry CR, et al. Pretreatment REM sleep and subjective sleep quality distinguish depressed psychotherapy remitters and nonremitters. Biol Psychiatry 1999;45(2):205–13.
9. Thase ME, Simons AD, Reynolds CF 3rd. Abnormal electroencephalographic sleep profiles in major depression: association with response to cognitive behavior therapy. Arch Gen Psychiatry 1996;53(2): 99–108.
10. Ozminkowski RJ, Wang S, Walsh JK. The direct and indirect costs of untreated insomnia in adults in the United States. Sleep 2007;30(3):263–73.
11. Fullerton DS. The economic impact of insomnia in managed care: a clearer picture emerges. Am J Manag Care 2006;12(Suppl 8):S246–52.
12. Kopta SM, Howard KI, Lowry JL, et al. Patterns of symptomatic recovery in psychotherapy. J Consult Clin Psychol 1994;62(5):1009–16.
13. Wilson SJ, Nutt DJ, Alford C, et al. British Association for Psychopharmacology consensus statement on evidence-based treatment of insomnia, parasomnias and circadian rhythm disorders. J Psychopharmacol 2010;24(11):1577–601.
14. Jacobs GD, Pace-Schott EF, Stickgold R, et al. Cognitive behavior therapy and pharmacotherapy for insomnia: a randomized controlled trial and direct comparison. Arch Intern Med 2004;164(17): 1888–96.
15. Sivertsen B, Omvik S, Pallesen S, et al. Cognitive behavioral therapy vs zopiclone for treatment of chronic primary insomnia in older adults: a randomized controlled trial. JAMA 2006;295(24):2851–8.
16. Morin CM, Vallieres A, Guay B, et al. Cognitive behavioral therapy, singly and combined with medication, for persistent insomnia: a randomized controlled trial. JAMA 2009;301(19):2005–15.
17. Lichstein KL, Wilson NM, Johnson CT. Psychological treatment of secondary insomnia. Psychol Aging 2000;15(2):232–40.
18. Manber R, Edinger JD, Gress JL, et al. Cognitive behavioral therapy for insomnia enhances depression outcome in patients with comorbid major depressive disorder and insomnia. Sleep 2008; 31(4):489–95.
19. Lamberg L. Despite effectiveness, behavioral therapy for chronic insomnia still underused. JAMA 2008;300(21):2474–5.
20. Pigeon WR, Crabtree VM, Scherer MR. The future of behavioral sleep medicine. J Clin Sleep Med 2007; 3(1):73–9.
21. Karlin BE, Ruzek JI, Chard KM, et al. Dissemination of evidence-based psychological treatments for posttraumatic stress disorder in the Veterans Health Administration. J Trauma Stress 2010; 23(6):663–73.
22. Manber R, Carney C, Edinger J, et al. Dissemination of CBTI to the non-sleep specialist: protocol

development and training issues. J Clin Sleep Med 2012;8(2):209–18.

23. Karlin BE, Trockel M, Taylor CB, Gimeno J, Manber R. National dissemination of Cognitive Behavioral Therapy for insomnia in Veterans: Clinician and patient-level outcomes. Journal of Consulting and Clinical Psychology 2013. Advance online publication.

24. Borbely AA, Achermann P. Sleep homeostasis and models of sleep regulation. J Biol Rhythms 1999; 14(6):557–68.

25. Carney CE, Manber R. Quiet your mind & get to sleep: solutions for insomnia in those with depression, anxiety, or chronic pain. Oakland (CA): New Harbinger; 2009.

26. Edinger JD, Carney CE. Overcoming insomnia: a cognitive-behavioral therapy approach therapist guide. New York: Oxford University Press; 2008.

27. Karlin B, Brown G, Trockel M, et al. National dissemination of cognitive behavioral therapy for depression in the Department of Veterans Affairs health care system: therapist and patient-level outcomes. J Consult Clin Psychol 2012;80:707–18.

28. Bandura A. Self-efficacy: the exercise of control. New York: W.H. Freeman; 1997.

29. Morin CM, Colecchi C, Stone J, et al. Behavioral and pharmacological therapies for late-life insomnia: a randomized controlled trial. JAMA 1999;281(11): 991–9.

Use of the Internet and Mobile Media for Delivery of Cognitive Behavioral Insomnia Therapy

Colin A. Espie, PhD, FBPsS[a],*, Peter Hames, MA(Oxon)[b],
Brian McKinstry, MD[c]

KEYWORDS

• Insomnia • Sleep disorder • CBT • Intervention • Online • Digital

KEY POINTS

• Web and mobile (digital) technology is increasingly accessible, worldwide.
• Cognitive behavioral therapy (CBT) for insomnia is effective, and it comprises a transferable protocol.
• Digital delivery, using outstanding technology, is likely to enhance insomnia care.
• There is already level 1 evidence for the efficacy of online CBT, but more research is required.
• Effectiveness is important, but so too is choice. The delivery mechanism is in good measure a matter of pragmatics.
• Traditional clinical care and digital resources can be complementary not competitive. There is a need for clear governance guidelines for both.

INTRODUCTION

In the early 1990s, I (CE) was a Clinical Director in the National Health Service (NHS) in Scotland. We served a population base of around 350,000 people. I had budgetary as well as professional responsibilities, and sat on the Executive Board for that NHS region. It was in that management context that I first raised the question about the use of the Internet, although we did not call it that in those days. I remember the response when I suggested we should look into having an electronic mail system for staff to communicate with one another. "It will never catch on" was the general view, and so the idea was shelved-for a while.

How times have changed, and how rapidly they still are changing. Most of us will remember when e-mail first came on the scene. Many were initially skeptical, some were reluctant, and a few were (and perhaps still are) resistant. However, it feels like professional life would be impossible to sustain nowadays using the old way of doing things. Indeed, for some people, using last year's model of laptop, tablet, or smart phone would be a considerable challenge! There can, I am sure, be an element of *de rigeur*, but there is little doubt that it did "catch on," and it is not merely a fashion. The Internet, and the whole new vocabulary that goes with the digital age, is here to stay at least

Disclosure/Conflicts of Interest: Colin Espie is Clinical & Scientific Director of Sleepio Ltd and is a shareholder but does not receive a salary from the company. He has conducted consultancy work or speaking engagements for UCB, Novartis and Boots UK. Peter Hames is CEO, a shareholder and receives a salary from Sleepio Ltd. Brian McKinstry has no conflicts of interest to declare.
[a] Nuffield Department of Clinical Neurosciences, Sleep and Circadian Neuroscience Institute, John Radcliffe Hospital, University of Oxford, Level 6, West Wing, Oxford OX3 9DU, UK; [b] Sleepio Ltd, 2nd Floor, 60-62 Commercial Street, London E1 6LT, United Kingdom; [c] Centre for Population Health Sciences, University of Edinburgh, Edinburgh, United Kingdom
* Corresponding author.
E-mail address: colin.espie@ndcn.ox.ac.uk

Sleep Med Clin 8 (2013) 407–419
http://dx.doi.org/10.1016/j.jsmc.2013.06.001
1556-407X/13/$ – see front matter © 2013 Elsevier Inc. All rights reserved.

until something even more transformational comes along, and it will.

I remember the first piece of data analysis that I conducted on "a computer." Those were heady days in the 1970s. Punching code in "Fortran" and carefully carrying my stack of cards, all in the right order, from one room in the university's computing center to another where I loaded them into a machine linked to the university "mainframe." It felt like some underground bunker from a James Bond movie. The magic was going to happen overnight and I would need to check the next morning that it had "run," and run properly. I recall the excitement when it had all worked and also the frustration when it had failed, usually because of a misplaced comma or space. Need to load that up again tonight then! A few years later, I had an exulted desktop called a "Superbrain." It must have weighed the same as a small adult, but it took floppy disks! I would not labor the historical review, or my point, any further. Suffice to say at each and every time when we believe we are at the peak, they all turn out to be false summits. Things are modern only fleetingly.

Peter Hames studied Experimental Psychology at the University of Oxford and is my cofounder in PocketProf, a company dedicated to creating automated ways of delivering behavioral medicine. Having worked previously developing Internet businesses for Web entrepreneur Martha Lane Fox, and having experienced insomnia first hand, he was perfectly placed to develop our first product Sleepio, a digital sleep improvement program.

Brian McKinstry is Professor of Primary Care eHealth in the Centre for Population Health Studies at the University of Edinburgh, and a practicing general practitioner. His main interest is in remote consulting especially telehealth and telephone consulting. He leads the Telescot program of research into the use of telemetry to manage long-term conditions and is conducting several projects exploring the acceptability, safety and efficacy of telephone consulting and developing new ways of remotely measuring physiologic parameters.

Aims of the Article

We discuss the use of the Internet and mobile media as a means of delivering CBT, an intervention that helps people with problems to develop and test fresh perspectives, to evaluate underlying beliefs and assumptions, and to question our attributions as to cause and effect. The emergence of the Web, the cloud, mobile and wearable devices, or whatever such immersive systems will be called in the future asks questions of us too, and may challenge and threaten our core beliefs as professionals, for example, "psychological therapy needs to be supervised by a credentialed professional," "it is too risky to have an unmoderated online community," "face-to-face therapy will always be the 'gold standard'" and "this would not work (well or safely) for people with comorbid disorders." Maybe "yes" or maybe "no": we shall see, but it seems wise to be at least open to considering the possibilities that the digital era may bring (we often use the term "digital" instead of "online" to capture native mobile as well as Web-based technologies).

In this article, therefore, we want to consider the opportunity that digital media offer for the delivery of cognitive behavioral insomnia therapies. This opportunity is not confined to a pragmatic alternative for those folks who cannot access traditional care. We have to be open to the possibility that online CBT may be just as effective as face-to-face CBT, and perhaps more effective. We also present our vision for integrated care, whereby clinicians routinely make use of native mobile, wearable, and Web-based technology to support assessment, treatment and real-world implementation. Moreover, this is not just about CBT—it is about any intervention that involves patient participation—nor is it specific to insomnia disorders. The new field of behavioral sleep medicine would do well to grasp what are exciting opportunities spanning treatment, training, and research.

The Rise and Rise of the Internet

In the fifteenth century, the invention of the printing press revolutionized the production of "written" works (previously literally so) and made them much cheaper and more available. Once the press arrived, life would never be the same again. The twenty-first century equivalent is the Internet. We no longer need to rely on the physical printed word but have a choice: e-book or real book. It is largely a matter of preference, because the content is essentially the same. It is only the experience that differs. Where therapy is concerned, the parallel is that we may not need to "see someone" to "get" CBT—perhaps the content can be the same? To help us in our thinking on this point, we shall explore what CBT is at a later point. However, it is worth bearing in mind in the meantime that video can be electronically captured and transmitted, animation can be very engaging, and virtual reality is becoming more and more realistic. The words attributed to Henry Ford, the preeminent automotive entrepreneur, more than 100 years ago, are still worth pondering.

If I had asked my customers what they wanted they would have said faster horses
—Henry Ford.

Web and mobile data access are certainly becoming increasingly ubiquitous. The most recent Oxford Internet Survey (OxIS) report[1] provides methodologically sound UK data. Launched by the Oxford Internet Institute in 2003, OxIS has become an authoritative source of information about Internet access, use and attitudes, and the difference this makes for everyday life, in Britain. Areas covered include digital and social inclusion and exclusion; regulation and governance of the Internet; privacy, trust, and risk concerns; and uses of the Internet, including networking, content creation, entertainment, and learning. The 2011 survey is the fifth in a series, with previous surveys conducted in 2003, 2005, 2007, and 2009. Each used a multistage national probability sample of 2000 people in Britain, enabling estimates to be reliably projected to Britain as a whole.

As can be seen in **Fig. 1**, all age groups, except the oldest, used the Internet in 2011 more than they did in 2009, and considerably more than they did in 2005. As in previous years, younger people continue to use the Internet most; however, usage is stable at about 80% to 85% for people in prime working years (age 25–55 years), before declining in older age groups. Nevertheless, around two-thirds of people aged 56 to 65 years use the Internet, as do one-third of those older than 65 years. Users trust the Internet as much as television and radio media, but they have considerably less trust in newspapers. According to OxIS, use of the internet to search for health information continues to increase. In 2011, it reached 71%, after a sharp increase in 2007 to 68%, when there was a major increase in looking for health information as compared with earlier years (only 37% in 2005). However, people still say that they trust their doctors more than information they find online. As we shall see later, however, perhaps these two should not be seen as competing alternatives. There may be ways that they can be complementary and mutually enhancing. Finally, in the United Kingdom, wireless connectivity has radically transformed the way people connect to the Internet. More than 80% of users now access the Internet at home with WiFi connections and 40% via mobile phones. WiFi access now exceeds telephone line access, which dropped to 73% in 2011. In many places worldwide, mobile technology is already a twenty-first-century norm.

Thinking more globally, the Web site http://www.internetworldstats.com/stats.htm estimated a total of 2.405 billion Internet users as of June 30, 2012, representing a world average penetration rate of 34.3% (global population base, 7.017 billion).[2] The penetration rate in North America was reported as 78.6% and in Europe as 63.2%. Overall growth in accessibility worldwide is estimated at 566% since 2000, with much higher figures for Africa (3606%), the Middle East (2639%), and Latin America/the Caribbean (1310%). By far, the largest absolute number of Internet users of course is in Asia (1.076 billion; **Fig. 2**). The simple fact is that, in a short time,

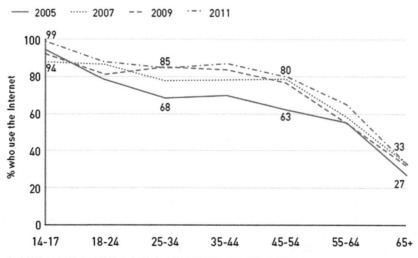

OxIS 2005: N=2,185; OxIS 2007: N=2,350; OxIS 2009: N=2,013; OxIS 2011: N=2,057

Fig. 1. Internet use by age. (*From* Dutton WH, Blank G. Next Generation Users: The Internet in Britain. Oxford Internet Survey 2011. Oxford Internet Institute, University of Oxford.)

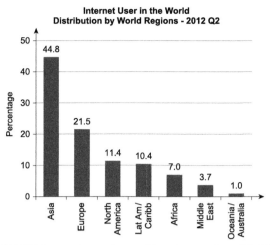

Fig. 2. Distribution of 2,405,518,376 Internet users by world region: on June 30, 2012.

the Internet has become the go to place to get information and to communicate with other people.

Professionals now communicate mainly by e-mail. In addition, however, open access software applications are increasingly used to make voice or video calls over the Internet, rather than the telephone, and online scheduling tools are often used to arrange a date and time to "meet" with multiple people. For the most part, such services are also free. For example, in October 2012, Skype (just one such provider) reached a new peak of 45.5 million concurrent users online at any point in time.[3] Surveys of the 5 busiest search engine providers show that 17.6 billion explicit core searches were conducted in the United States in December 2012 alone, with Google sites ranking first with 11.8 billion.[4] There continues to be an approximate 4% per month growth in such activity. For further information, a readable brief history of the use of social media is available at http://www.uncp.edu/home/acurtis/NewMedia/SocialMedia/SocialMediaHistory.html.[5]

The Internet and Health Care

Formal health care providers have not been slow to embrace eHealth technology. In the NHS in England, £12.8 billion has been invested in a National Programme for Information Technology, and the first Obama administration in the United States similarly committed to a US$38 billion eHealth investment, such investments necessitating continuous systematic investigation.[6] Large-scale expenditure has been justified on the grounds that electronic health records, picture archiving and communication systems, electronic prescribing, and computerized decision support systems help improve quality and safety in health care.[7] Likewise, in the United Kingdom, there are new proposals

from the influential NHS Future Forum that could allow patients to view their medical records online by 2015,[8] and there is a large-scale move that will lead to the telemonitoring of 3 million lives.[9] Although the evidence base for such developments so far is limited, it seems that the die is already cast. Technology is leading reform.

Research, Teaching, and Professional Development Using the Internet

The Internet has made the dissemination and acquisition of new knowledge infinitely easier. Previously labor-intensive "hand-searching" of the literature is largely a thing of the past, and many journals and reference textbooks are now online access only. In the sleep field, *SLEEP* (the official journal of the Associated Professional Sleep Societies in the United States) and the *Journal of Sleep Research* (European Sleep Research Society), for example, are now available only by online subscription or society membership. There has also been an enormous growth in "open access" journals in recent years, now numbering a remarkable 8724 titles (at May 2013: www.doaj.com), and the *Journal Medical Internet Research* (www.jmir.org) launched in 1999 achieved its fifteenth year of publication in 2013 and already has a respectable impact factor (IF) (as of June 2011: IF = 4.7). These serve as examples of how the Internet has revolutionized both the preparation and publication of research.

In terms of research implementation, the Internet provides a means for researchers to amass large datasets, such as the Great British Sleep Survey (www.worldsleepsurvey.com), which applies the Diagnostic and Statistical Manual of Mental Disorders, 5th Edition, criteria to identify insomnia among the sleeping habits and patterns of UK citizens,[10] and the Netherlands Sleep Registry, which uses a range of Web-based assessment, along with high-density (sleep) electroencephalography, transcranial magnetic stimulation, and functional magnetic resonance imaging to explore risk factors, genetic predispositions, and brain mechanisms in sleep disturbances (www.sleepregistry. org). Interests in Web-based methodologies are also becoming more mainstream. For example, the Karolinska Institut and Linkoping University (Sweden) recently launched a Department of Psychiatric Internet Research.

There are new opportunities also to enhance teaching and training, because online courses are more accessible and cost-effective. Again, traditional face-to face lecture, tutorial, workshop, and apprenticeship methods are not necessarily at odds with online learning, but may best be seen as complementary. Professional societies now offer online modules and webinar programs as part of a continuing education approach (eg, American Academy of Sleep Medicine, Australasian Sleep Association), and numerous institutions provide eLearning short courses. There are also degrees available in the sleep field (eg, University of Sydney, Master of Medicine [Sleep Medicine]). We pioneered in Glasgow an eLearning Program in Behavioral Sleep Medicine that was delivered 100% online, and in the first 2 years of operation, health professionals from 12 countries (United Kingdom, Ireland, Netherlands, Germany, Portugal, Spain, Saudi Arabia, South Africa, Hong Kong, Australia, Canada, and the United States) completed the course at Masters or Diploma level. As of 2014, we are proposing a new modular online program at the University of Oxford, Sleep and Circadian Neuroscience Institute (www.ndcn.ox.ac.uk/scni). It should also be noted that many universities worldwide, including Ivy League and Russell Group institutions, are participating in open, free access to online teaching on a wide range of topics. As of May 2013, www.coursera.com listed a total of 337 courses, provided by 62 universities, typically of 5- to 10-week duration. To date, there is no course specifically on sleep, so there could be an opportunity here to raise general awareness of our subject.

THE INTERNET AS A MEANS OF DELIVERING THERAPY

It is clear that Web and mobile technologies are here to stay. Surely this offers a huge opportunity to think creatively about how common problems like insomnia might be managed more effectively and more efficiently. So let us proceed to considering whether or not CBT is a good candidate for Internet delivery. To do so, it may be helpful to take a step back and consider 2 important and related factors. First, what are the generic elements of a psychological intervention and second, how might we understand the concept of a therapeutic dose.

What is Therapy?

Fig. 3 summarizes the core components of a therapeutic intervention and how they may interact. In the upper part of the diagram, the provision of information helps to develop knowledge and understanding, which differs from facts and figures, because knowledge is something personal and meaningful. This is why it lends itself to therapeutic application. There is then mutual feedback between therapy, which promotes existing skills and the acquisition of new ones, and knowledge because the relevance of these skills to the solution of personal problems becomes apparent. In collaborative therapies, such as CBT, this is often referred to as the formulation stage and represents a shared perspective on the problem and its treatment. The third segment in the upper portion of **Fig. 3** refers to real-world implementation. Whatever the therapeutic system or the disorder it is designed to address, shared decision making normally then takes place, and the patient ventures forth encouraged, empowered, and with specific objectives in mind. In CBT, the collaboration and decision making typically take place within session, and the implementation takes place between sessions.

Turning to the lower part of **Fig. 3**, benefit then accrues from interaction among these components. As the individual gains personal understanding, relevant cognitive and behavioral skills, and experience in applying them, alleviation of troublesome symptoms and signs of positive health gain normally emerge. Feedback from real-world experience also yields new information, prompts further support needs, and adaptations of the formulation and treatment plan as required. Progress helps to reinforce successful strategies, and lack of progress may point to gaps in knowledge transfer, understanding, skill acquisition, and or motivational/support needs. The goal of most interventions is to establish some aspect of well-being (eg, good sleep, improved quality of life, and daytime function), the erosion of which, alongside the reemergence of symptoms of the disorder, is often regarded as a relapse. The final component then in this generic therapeutic model is relapse prevention. When viewed as a positive and normalizing element of psychological therapy, a focus on relapse prevention encourages openness to future experiences and provides

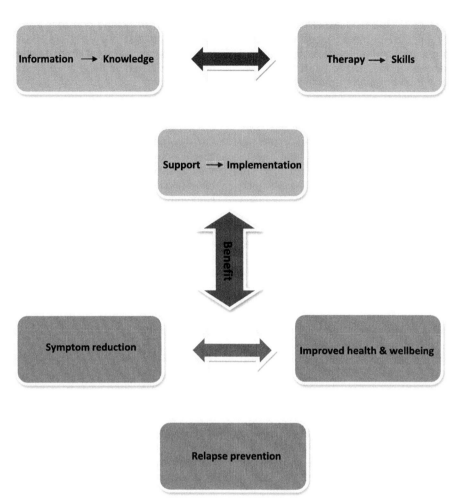

Fig. 3. Generic components of a therapeutic system such as CBT.

assurance that strategies and resources can remain, internalized, or otherwise close at hand, to resolve a future episode.

Why Might the Internet be a Useful Medium to Deliver Therapy?

An important starting point in considering change—and change is always hard—for professionals as much as for patients, is openness to the situation that maintains at present. What are its strengths, and what are its limitations? **Box 1** provides an analysis of at least some of these using the scenario of 8 weekly sessions of CBT with an experienced therapist—what reasonably might be considered the "gold standard" approach.

Suffice to say, there are definite strengths to this approach, but there are also inherent limitations. The strongest endorsement of traditional CBT and the principal reason for it being the gold standard is that it is evidence based. That much is

incontrovertible, although we do not (yet) know that the other listed strengths are prerequisite to its efficacy. Perhaps, the main limitation is that traditional CBT relies heavily on the motivation of the patient to attend, to keep records, and above all to make changes between sessions. The ratio of within:between session time of 1:480 is striking. In any event, we would contend that if you set out to design a therapeutic system to apply the processes and to achieve the outcomes outlined in **Fig. 3**, you would not inevitably end up with traditional CBT.

Box 2 addresses both the strengths and the limitations of traditional CBT, in the context of designing a Web- and mobile-based CBT program. In responding to each of the strengths of traditional CBT, we are not saying that online CBT can (or should) mimic traditional CBT. However, we are suggesting that the technological and scientific challenges associated with achieving that end are feasible. Indeed, such progress is already being made in commercially available

<table>
<tr><td>

Box 1
Strengths and limitations of traditional CBT

Traditional CBT

Eight individual sessions (each 50 minutes) face-to-face and at weekly intervals with an experienced therapist in a clinic setting. Standardized assessment procedures are used at interview, and psychometrically valid scales are administered pretherapy and posttherapy. Diary measures are used on a daily basis. These help to inform treatment progress and implementation. An evidence-based therapeutic model is tailored to the individual's needs.

Strengths

Clinical expertise

Diagnostic evaluation

Eight sessions

Almost 7 hours of therapy

Therapeutic relationship

Tailored intervention

Evaluated for progress

Proved to work

Limitations

Clinic appointments inconvenient, may not attend

People remember relatively little

Hard to keep diaries in practice

Little support during implementation

Seven hours in session to 3360 hours between (1:480)

</td></tr>
</table>

there are challenges that need to be addressed, for any treatment format. For Internet therapy, the challenge may be about tailoring therapy and the management of complex cases; for face-to-face therapy the challenge may be about sustaining behavior change between sessions.

What Constitutes a Therapeutic Dose?

We turn now to some other crucial questions that lie at the heart of this discussion. What is it that makes a difference? What are the active ingredients of CBT, and how much of them do you need to get better?

In pharmacotherapy, a dose response is the relationship between the amount of exposure (dose) to a substance (the active ingredient) and the resulting changes in body function or health (response). It has been suggested that the therapeutic session is the natural quantitative unit of psychotherapy. That is, the number of sessions that a patient attends is stochastically related to exposure to the active ingredients in a psychotherapy.[11] The stepped care model we set out several years ago[12] and more recent variants of the same approach[13,14] likewise envisage the need to allocate more challenging cases to higher intensity treatment at the outset and to increase the dose of intervention for treatment nonresponders. Indeed in the United Kingdom, psychological services provided by the NHS are triaged into low-intensity, high-intensity, and more expert treatment requirements.[15] The logic of this kind of model is that any given patient requires a particular amount of intervention to respond (not less because it does not work, and not more because it does not add anything). Dose, therefore, might be determined by the number of elements in the treatment, the number of sessions, the amount of personal tailoring of treatment, the qualifications and experience of the therapist, and so on. Consequently, it might be assumed that any entry level CBT, at the base of the stepped care pyramid, should be the lowest dose proved to be associated with clinical improvement.

Edinger and colleagues[16] have shown that a brief CBT intervention (4 sessions) is clinically effective in primary insomnia and that an 8-session treatment was not superior in effect. They have also demonstrated that this brief treatment is viable in comorbid insomnia.[17] The Pittsburgh group too have found that brief behavioral therapy for insomnia works well,[18,19] and we have found that 5 sessions of group CBT delivered by a nurse therapist can yield lasting benefit to patients under primary care[20] and patients with cancer[21] and persistent insomnia. Is it then possible then that number of sessions, expertise of therapist, and treatment

products. SHUT-i, for example, uses video-based material from expert therapists to deliver CBT and has interactive components (www.shuti.net), and Sleepio is delivered by an engaging animated therapist, has an active social community of users who support each other during therapy, and uses advanced algorithms to tailor therapy (www.sleepio.com). Moreover, it is worth noting that there are readily accessible technological solutions to many of the problems that beset conventional clinical work, such as missing or incomplete data (eg, text or e-mail prompts and reminders). **Box 3** also highlights potential advantages of online CBT, preeminent among which are 24/7 availability and immersive support, which might enable patients to implement strategies successfully in real life.

Reflecting again on **Fig. 3** then, we would argue that there is no problem in principle with CBT being delivered online, and there may be some practical advantages. We would also argue that

---

Box 2
How Web and mobile-delivered (digital) CBT might emulate the strengths and address the limitations of traditional CBT

Strengths of traditional CBT	Possible solutions using digital CBT
Clinical expertise	Use technology expertise and link to clinical expertise
Diagnostic evaluation	Build algorithmically and validate
Eight sessions	Build dedicated session content and timing
Almost 7 hours of therapy	Titrate amount of therapy to need; theoretically limitless
Therapeutic relationship	Emulate using video, gaming and/or animation technologies, avatars
Tailored intervention	Build algorithmically and adjust contingent on progress
Evaluated for progress	Build web and mobile tools for pre-post and diary
Proven to work	Design and conduct trials
Limitations of traditional CBT	*Advantages of digital CBT*
Clinic appointments inconvenient, may not attend	Can happen anytime, all activity time-stamped
People remember relatively little	Knowledge bank, personal account stores all information
Hard to keep diaries in practice	Prompts, reminders and rewards by SMS and email
Little support during implementation	Immersive; available 24/7. Community/user support
Seven hours in session to 3,360 hours between (1:480)	Immersive; available 24/7

Box 3
Ten research questions relating to digital CBT for insomnia

1. Is digital CBT as clinically and cost-effective as conventional CBT for insomnia?
2. Is digital CBT effective for insomnia in people with other mental health conditions?
3. Is digital CBT effective for insomnia in people with other physical health conditions?
4. Does digital CBT help people reduce and withdraw from sleep medications?
5. Does an active social community enhance outcomes?
6. What are the mediators and moderators of digital CBT treatment outcome?
7. What are the demographic and clinical predictors of improvement with digital CBT?
8. What are the dose-response relationships associated with digital CBT for insomnia?
9. Does digital CBT integrated at various levels with traditional clinical care afford health benefits?
10. Can a fully mobile version of CBT be implemented effectively?

format (individual vs group) may be less critical to outcome than the field has hitherto assumed?

There is, however, a further possible flaw in the argument that the most expert therapy is necessarily a more powerful intervention even than the least (self-help) or that more sessions are inevitably better than few. This is because it may be the cognitive and behavioral work that people actually do, at home and between sessions, which is crucial to treatment effectiveness, not who they see or how often. The dose in CBT could be more associated with the content and execution of CBT than with treatment format. Face-to-face therapy, group therapy, bibliotherapy, and Internet therapy may be simply delivery platforms for the same "substance" (CBT); just as oral pills, oral controlled-release pills, buccal fluid, and intramuscular and intravenous medicines differ administratively, but the compound being administered materially does not.

We suggest that **Fig. 3** may offer a helpful framework for appraising which components of the therapy process need to be prioritized for a patient to get an optimal dose and an optimal response (cf enhanced knowledge, improved skill set, and regular practical implementation). How these components are delivered and enhanced may be a more secondary consideration.

CBT FOR INSOMNIA ON THE INTERNET

The Internet is being used to deliver psychological treatments, CBT in particular, for a wide range of problems. The evidence base for insomnia is in its infancy relative to some other conditions.

Evidence Relating to Online CBT for Other Disorders

In Sweden, Internet-based CBT, standard CBT, and selective serotonin reuptake inhibitor (SSRI) medication are already recommended by the Ministry for Health and Social Affairs as being of equal merit.[22] Likewise, in the United Kingdom, online CBT is a recommended treatment of anxiety and depression, and access to such programs is increasing.[15,23] Such positive results, for both anxiety and depressive disorders, have been reinforced by meta-analytic data,[24] and trials data suggest that Internet-delivered CBT can be equally effective as face-to-face CBT not only in depression[25] but also in panic disorder.[26]

It is for these reasons that Carlbring and colleagues[22] state in their important editorial, "State-of-the-Art Treatment via the Internet: An Optimistic Vision of the Future," "we believe that Internet-based treatment should not be regarded as a third-rate alternative. The general practitioner should not present Internet-based therapy as a fall-back option when standard CBT is costly, or subject to delay, or merely as a means of avoiding the side effects of SSRI medication. On the contrary, Internet-based treatment can be positively promoted as one alternative to choose from among others, because there is clear evidence that this type of treatment does, in fact, produce good results."

Evidence Relating to Online CBT for Insomnia

Early results for online CBT for insomnia are promising. Seven investigations offer encouraging results,[27–33] suggestive of the potential far-reaching benefits of this health technology. In one of the best-designed studies, albeit on a small total sample ($n = 45$), a 16% improvement in sleep efficiency (SE) (proportion of time in bed spent asleep) relative to baseline was observed after CBT (an absolute increase of 12% from pretreatment to posttreatment), compared with 3% (2% in absolute terms) in a wait-listed group.[29] These data were mirrored by significant reductions in insomnia severity. Uncontrolled data also suggested gains were maintained. In 2 larger studies,[30,32] significant effects of CBT over a wait-listed condition were observed, although limited to improvements in sleep quality and reductions in fatigue, rather than sleep parameters per se[30] or showing small-

to-moderate effects.[32] Perhaps the most convincing evidence so far, however, comes from a recent placebo-controlled randomized trial, with a sizable sample ($n = 164$).[33]

In this study, CBT comprised a media-rich Web application with automated support and a community forum (thus making considerable use of the features outlined in **Box 2**). On the primary end point of SE (total time asleep expressed as a percentage of the total time spent in bed), CBT was associated with improvement (+20%; large effect size) relative to both placebo (imagery relief therapy) and treatment as usual (TAU) at posttreatment and at 8 weeks' follow-up. These findings were mirrored across a range of sleep diary measures. The clinical benefits of CBT over IRT and TAU are illustrated in **Fig. 4**.

A Research Agenda

There is some evidence, therefore, that interactive online CBT for insomnia may have beneficial effects that are comparable to face-to-face therapy. Caution, however, is still required because insomnia self-help approaches have historically been associated with less robust effects,[34] perhaps due to variability in methodology. Further work is certainly required to evaluate the objective sleep changes and daytime benefits associated with treatment delivered in this way. In particular, treatment trials of insomnia associated with complex clinical presentations and physical and/or mental health problems are needed to establish any necessary prescreening requirements for access to online therapy, compared with, in-person CBT. A balanced article by Andersson[35] on the promises and pitfalls of Internet therapy offers a helpful research framework, and in **Box 3** we have provided a list of 10 research questions that we believe could be usefully addressed in the insomnia field.

INTEGRATED CBT—USING ONLINE TOOLS IN EVERYDAY PRACTICE

If we as professionals are making increasing use of the Internet, and also as individuals in our private lives, why would we not extend this opportunity to our assessment and treatment of patients, especially when an increasing proportion of the public is becoming proficient in the use of electronic and digital media?

We take it for granted that a whole range of questionnaires, rating scales, and sleep diaries are part of our usual practice. Perhaps we provide these in electronic format or even use a computerized or online data portal to gather such routine information? The advantages of electronic, relative to paper

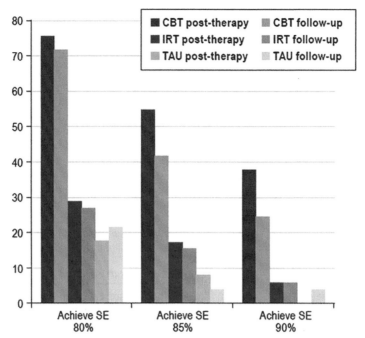

Fig. 4. Percentage of patients within each treatment arm achieving sleep efficiency (SE) clinical end points. CBT, cognitive behavioral therapy; IRT, imagery relief therapy: placebo; TAU, treatment as usual. (*From* Espie CA, Kyle SD, Williams C, et al. A randomized, placebo-controlled trial of online cognitive behavioral therapy for chronic insomnia disorder delivered via an automated media-rich web application. Sleep 2012;35:769–81; with permission.)

and pencil, measures are many, including efficiency, convenience, time-stamping of data, automated scoring, reinforcement of the notion of the patient as his/her own scientist, and so on. Likely, we value the fact that many measures are validated and standardized. Treatment integrity and fidelity might actually be enhanced by this approach.[35] At the very least, having electronic tools available affords flexibility and allows for personal preference. It would not prevent us necessarily from working more traditionally. So it may not be such a large step to consider how digital resources might be harnessed to enhance treatment work.

One reason that might be proffered for not using digital therapy in clinical practice is that in the real world things are complex and that an automated approach might be too simplistic. Indeed, people are complex; they are not like the people who participate in trials. They often have many other problems and may be less motivated. Furthermore, CBT is complex, and so tailoring treatment is a skilled process. In this regard, it is important also to bear in mind that CBT is not a single treatment modality but a family of therapies. Just as pharmacotherapy for insomnia comprises various benzodiazepines, nonbenzodiazepine receptor agonists, antihistamines, hypocretin antagonists, and sedative antidepressants, so CBT comprises

relaxation methodologies (eg, abbreviated progressive muscle relaxation and autogenic training), sleep hygiene (eg, relating to lifestyle and sleep environment), behavioral strategies (eg, sleep stimulus control and sleep restriction), and cognitive therapies (eg, cognitive restructuring and paradoxical intention). Moreover, each of these parts of CBT has subsidiary components (eg, stimulus control—regular sleep timing, avoidance of naps, management of sleep-incompatible behaviors, reinforcement of prosleep behaviors, and prioritizing the bed and bedroom for sleep).

Perhaps it is all too complex—complex problems requiring selectivity from a range of complex solutions? We would argue, however, that it is this complexity that speaks to the need for carefully constructed processes of decision making, that are informed systematically by data. This is how technology can assist, not hinder, and might in fact favor the use of digital resources that are driven by algorithms. One illustration of what is achievable here can be drawn from a section of the Sleepio program where The Prof (an animated character) tutors the user in how to use cognitive restructuring. Associated with one 3-minute piece of interaction, there are more than 2.3 million possible permutations generated by the underlying algorithm, all based on the user's own data.

In our 2009 stepped care article, we proposed that Internet delivery of CBT could be one of several entry-level methods (along with other self-help methods) and that people could be stepped up to more advanced CBT, depending on treatment response and/or treatment preference.[12] The corollary of this was that, further up the stepped care pyramid, face-to-face therapy might be preserved for those in greatest need of dedicated skill and time. We still see merit in this approach. However, in light of the emerging evidence base and the conceptual arguments advanced in this article, we now suggest that the integration of online resources into clinical care may be part of each hierarchical step, as well as forming a self-help base to the care pyramid. This adapted model is presented in **Fig. 5**.

It is proposed that online CBT will form the foundation of future self-help therapy for insomnia. Books and audio resources of course may still play a part at this level. We anticipate that mobile access to therapy will become increasingly popular and convenient for people. We make no assumptions at this point that people accessing help here will necessarily have fewer or lesser problems; research is required to demonstrate whether or not digital therapy (alone) can benefit those with more complex presentations. Either way, however, this is likely to remain for some time the most accessible form of evidence-based CBT, and consistent with the stepped care approach would be expected to manage the highest volume of insomnia cases, at this entry level.

In subsequent tiers, we have represented increased levels of personal therapy, combined with increased expertise. Resource requirements become steadily higher, and the availability of the resource, perhaps, becomes less. We do not intend to be prescriptive about the content of these layers but have illustrated them as best we can. Likewise, there may be fewer, or more, levels to a stepped care system; this is a matter also for local determination. The red 2-way arrows reflect the potential movement/referral pathways within the stepped care model designed to help individuals to find the right approach for them, with stepping up, for example, being associated with an incomplete treatment response at a lower level. We do not regard such movement as a problem, as some people do, who suggest that a poor response from a low-level treatment may reduce acceptance of or hinder response to a higher level CBT. Rather we would see the foundation laid as potentially helpful for more advanced work.

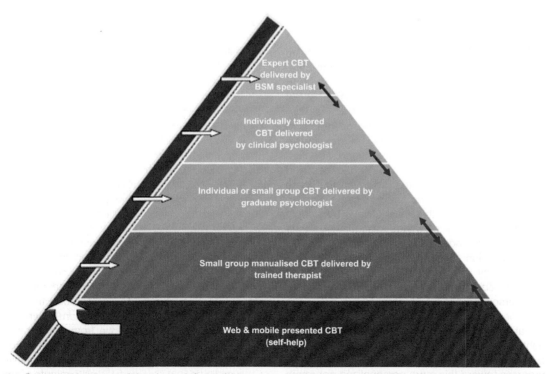

Fig. 5. Stepped care model, adapted for online service integration. Red arrows reflect potential movement/ referral pathways. White arrows illustrate potential integration of digital assessment, treatment, and support components at all levels. (*Adapted from* Espie CA. "Stepped care": a health technology solution for delivering cognitive behavioral therapy as a first line insomnia treatment. Sleep 2009;32:1549–58; with permission.)

Besides, it is worth noting that primary care physicians are able to prescribe the same medicines as are specialists at all levels. Therefore, if we were to compare the stepped care model to pharmacotherapy for most disorders, it is not dissimilar. For example, general practitioners often try their depressed patients on the available pills before referring them to a psychiatrist, and most of the depression is managed (successfully) in primary care.

The white arrows in **Fig. 5** illustrate the potential integration of Web and mobile assessment, treatment, and support components into all levels of the model. We anticipate that this will become the norm within a short time; this again highlights the empirical question of "what is enough" to engender a good clinical outcome.

SUMMARY

CBT has traditionally been delivered by a therapist in a clinic; however, the ubiquitous nature of Web and mobile technology offers new possibilities. We have argued that such change should be seized as an opportunity rather than guarded against as a threat. There is opportunity not only to meet the need and demand for CBT but potentially to improve insomnia care both at the level of the individual patient and at population level. We have proposed that CBT is well suited to online delivery as a stand-alone therapy, and it may have advantages over traditional therapy, but we have also made a strong case for integrated care. High-level expertise in Web and mobile, gaming and animation technologies, and the use of social media may be complementary to clinical skill to enable people to make lasting improvements to their sleep and well-being. There is a provocative and substantial research agenda ahead, attention to which will yield insights on what works best and for whom. It should be noted, however, that there will always be people who prefer to see a clinician or therapist, just as there will always be people who prefer to work on things essentially on their own; so this agenda needs to take account of personal decision making in concert with trials methodology.

Personalized medicine, and here we may substitute personalized therapy, emphasizes giving the right therapy to the right patient for the right problem at the right time and in the right dose to get the right response.[36] We might also add, at the right price. Web and mobile therapy should help us progress toward this more personalized approach because it offers encouraging early data on benefit, introduces practical quantitative tools for tailoring therapy, and provides choice. Moreover,

there is the possibility that self-tracking, using apps, and wearable devices will soon integrate with online therapeutic approaches, thus opening up new opportunities for the dissemination of insomnia treatments (http://www.ucsf.edu/news/2012/10/12913/self-tracking-may-become-key-element-personalized-medicine). Watch this space—remember Henry Ford? We must, however, at all times remain mindful of challenges to our usual ways of ensuring good clinical governance and develop appropriate protocols for managing risk, as well as benefit.

REFERENCES

1. Dutton WH, Black G. Oxford internet survey report - next generation users: the internet in Britain. Oxford (United Kingdom): Oxford Internet Institute; 2011. Available at: http://www.oii.ox.ac.uk/downloads/index.cfm?File=publications/oxis2011_report.pdf. Accessed on May 30, 2013.
2. Miniwatts Marketing Group. Internet World Statistics. 2012. Available at: http://www.internetworldstats.com/stats.htm. Accessed April 2, 2013.
3. Lunden I. Skype reaches a 45M concurrent user peak. 2012. Available at: http://techcrunch.com/tag/p2p/. Accessed May 30, 2013.
4. comScore Inc. December 2012 U.S. Search Engine Rankings. 2013. Available at: http://www.comscore.com/Insights/Press_Releases/2013/1/comScore_Releases_December_2012_U.S._Search_Engine_Rankings. Accessed May 30, 2013.
5. Curtis A. The brief history of social media. Pembroke (United Kingdom): University of North Carolina; 2013. Available at: http://www.uncp.edu/home/acurtis/NewMedia/SocialMedia/SocialMediaHistory.html. Accessed May 30, 2013.
6. Catwell L, Sheikh A. Evaluating eHealth interventions: the need for continuous systemic evaluation. PLoS Med 2009;6(8):e1000126.
7. Black AD, Car G, Pagliari C, et al. The impact of eHealth on the quality and safety of health care: a systematic overview. PLoS Med 2012;8(1):e1000387.
8. NHS Future Forum. Information: A Report from the NHS Future Forum. 2012. Available at: https://www.gov.uk/government/uploads/system/uploads/attachment_data/file/152171/dh_132086.pdf.pdf. Accessed May 30, 2013.
9. Department of Health. A Concordat Between the Department of Health and the Telehealth and Telecare Industry. 2012. Available at: https://www.gov.uk/government/uploads/system/uploads/attachment_data/file/155925/Concordat-3-million-lives.pdf.pdf. Accessed May 30, 2013.
10. Espie CA, Kyle SD, Hames P, et al. The daytime impact of DSM-5 insomnia disorder: comparative

analysis of insomnia subtypes from the Great British Sleep Survey. J Clin Psychiatry 2012;73:e1478–84.

11. Howard KI, Kopta SM, Krause MS, et al. The dose–effect relationship in psychotherapy. Am Psychol 1986;41:159–64.

12. Espie CA. "Stepped care": a health technology solution for delivering cognitive behavioral therapy as a first line insomnia treatment. Sleep 2009;32:1549–58.

13. Vincent N, Walsh K. Stepped care for insomnia: an evaluation of implementation in routine practice. J Clin Sleep Med 2013;9:227–34.

14. Mack LK, Rybarczyk BD. Behavioral treatment of insomnia: a proposal for a stepped-care approach to promote public health. Nat Sci Sleep 2011;26:87–99.

15. Department of Health. Improving access to psychological therapies. IAPT Programme 2012. London: Department of Health; 2012.

16. Edinger JD, Wohlgemuth WK, Radtke RA, et al. Dose-response effects of cognitive-behavioral insomnia therapy: a randomized clinical trial. Sleep 2007;30:203–12.

17. Edinger JD, Olsen MK, Stechuchak KM, et al. Cognitive behavioral therapy for patients with primary insomnia or insomnia associated predominantly with mixed psychiatric disorders: a randomized clinical trial. Sleep 2009;32:499–510.

18. Buysse DJ, Germain A, Moul DE, et al. Efficacy of brief behavioral treatment for chronic insomnia in older adults. Arch Intern Med 2011;171:887–95.

19. Troxel WM, Germain A, Buysse DJ. Clinical management of insomnia with brief behavioral treatment (BBTI). Behav Sleep Med 2012;10:266–79.

20. Espie CA, MacMahon KM, Kelly HL, et al. Randomized clinical effectiveness trial of nurse-administered small-group cognitive behavior therapy for persistent insomnia in general practice. Sleep 2007;30:574–84.

21. Espie CA, Fleming L, Cassidy J. Randomized controlled clinical effectiveness trial of cognitive behavior therapy compared with treatment as usual for persistent insomnia in patients with cancer. J Clin Oncol 2009;26:4651–8.

22. Swedish National Board of Health and Welfare: 2010. Cited in Carlbring P, Andersson G, Kaldo V. Editorial: State-of-the-art treatment via the internet: an optimistic vision of the future. Cogn Behav Ther 2011;40:79–81.

23. National Institute for Health and Clinical Excellence (NICE). Computerised cognitive behaviour therapy for depression and anxiety: guidance. NICE technology appraisal guidance 97. London: Nice; 2006.

24. Andrews G, Cuijpers P, Craske MG, et al. Computer therapy for the anxiety and depressive disorders is effective, acceptable and practical health care: a meta-analysis. PLoS One 2010;5(10):e13196.

25. Spek V, Cuijpers P, Nyklicek I, et al. Internet-based cognitive behaviour therapy for symptoms of depression and anxiety: a meta-analysis. Psychol Med 2007;37:319–28.

26. Bergstrom J, Andersson G, Ljotsson B, et al. Internet- versus group-administered cognitive behaviour therapy for panic disorder in a psychiatric setting: a randomized trial. BMC Psychiatry 2010; 10:54.

27. Strom L, Pettersson R, Andersson G. Internet-based treatment for insomnia: a controlled evaluation. J Consult Clin Psychol 2004;72:113–20.

28. Suzuki E, Tsuchiya M, Hirokawa K, et al. Evaluation of an Internet-based self-help program for better quality of sleep among Japanese workers: a randomized controlled trial. J Occup Health 2008;50: 387–99.

29. Ritterband LM, Thorndike FP, Gonder-Frederick GA, et al. Efficacy of an Internet-based behavioral intervention for adults with insomnia. Arch Gen Psychiatry 2009;66:692–8.

30. Vincent N, Lewycky S. Logging on for better sleep: RCT of the effectiveness of online treatment for insomnia. Sleep 2009;32:807–15.

31. Ritterband LM, Bailey ET, Thorndike FP, et al. Initial evaluation of an internet intervention to improve the sleep of cancer survivors with insomnia. Psychoon-cology 2012;21:695–705.

32. Lancee J, van den Bout J, van Straten A, et al. Internet-delivered or mailed self-help treatment for insomnia? A randomized waiting list controlled trial. Behav Res Ther 2011;50:22–9.

33. Espie CA, Kyle SD, Williams C, et al. A randomized, placebo-controlled trial of online cognitive behavioral therapy for chronic insomnia disorder delivered via an automated media-rich web application. Sleep 2012;35:769–81.

34. van Straten A, Cuijpers P. Self-therapy for insomnia: a meta-analysis. Sleep Med Rev 2009;13:61–71.

35. Andersson G. The promise and pitfalls of the internet for cognitive behavioral therapy. BMC Med 2010;8:82.

36. UCSF Medicine X 2012 Symposium. Available at: http://www.ucsf.edu/news/2012/10/12913/self-tracking-may-become-key-element-personalized-medicine. Accessed May 30, 2013.

Index

Note: Page numbers of article titles are in **boldface** type.

Sleep Med Clin 8 (2013) 421–424
http://dx.doi.org/10.1016/S1556-407X(13)00092-1
1556-407X/13/$ – see front matter © 2013 Elsevier Inc. All rights reserved.

Moving?

Make sure your subscription moves with you!

To notify us of your new address, find your **Clinics Account Number** (located on your mailing label above your name), and contact customer service at:

Email: journalscustomerservice-usa@elsevier.com

800-654-2452 (subscribers in the U.S. & Canada)
314-447-8871 (subscribers outside of the U.S. & Canada)

Fax number: 314-447-8029

Elsevier Health Sciences Division
Subscription Customer Service
3251 Riverport Lane
Maryland Heights, MO 63043

*To ensure uninterrupted delivery of your subscription, please notify us at least 4 weeks in advance of move.

ELSEVIER

Printed and bound by CPI Group (UK) Ltd, Croydon, CR0 4YY

03/10/2024

01040367-0001